Medical histories of Belgium

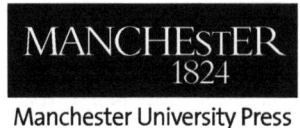

Manchester University Press

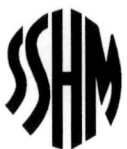

SOCIAL HISTORIES OF MEDICINE

Series editors: David Cantor, Elaine Leong and Keir Waddington

Social Histories of Medicine is concerned with all aspects of health, illness and medicine, from prehistory to the present, in every part of the world. The series covers the circumstances that promote health or illness, the ways in which people experience and explain such conditions and what, practically, they do about them. Practitioners of all approaches to health and healing come within its scope, as do their ideas, beliefs and practices, and the social, economic and cultural contexts in which they operate. Methodologically, the series welcomes relevant studies in social, economic, cultural and intellectual history, as well as approaches derived from other disciplines in the arts, sciences, social sciences and humanities. The series is a collaboration between Manchester University Press and the Society for the Social History of Medicine.

Previously published

Migrant architects of the NHS   *Julian M. Simpson*

Mediterranean quarantines, 1750–1914   *Edited by John Chircop and Francisco Javier Martínez*

Sickness, medical welfare and the English poor, 1750–1834   *Steven King*

Medical societies and scientific culture in nineteenth-century Belgium   *Joris Vandendriessche*

Vaccinating Britain   *Gareth Millward*

Madness on trial   *James E. Moran*

Early modern Ireland and the world of medicine   *Edited by John Cunningham*

Feeling the strain   *Jill Kirby*

Rhinoplasty and the nose in early modern British medicine and culture   *Emily Cock*

Communicating the history of medicine   *Edited by Solveig Jülich and Sven Widmalm*

Progress and pathology   *Edited by Melissa Dickson, Emilie Taylor-Brown and Sally Shuttleworth*

Balancing the self   *Edited by Mark Jackson and Martin D. Moore*

Global health and the new world order   *Edited by Jean-Paul Gaudillière, Claire Beaudevin, Christoph Gradmann, Anne M. Lovell and Laurent Pordié*

Accounting for health: calculation, paperwork and medicine, 1500–2000   *Edited by Axel C. Hüntelmann and Oliver Falk*

Women's medicine   *Caroline Rusterholz*

Germs and governance: the past, present and future of hospital infection, prevention and control   *Edited by Anne Marie Rafferty, Marguerite Dupree and Fay Bound Alberti*

Leprosy and identity in the Middle Ages: from England to the Mediterranean   *Edited by Elma Brenner and François-Olivier Touati*

Patient voices in Britain, 1840–1948   *Edited by Anne Hanley and Jessica Meyer*

Medical histories of Belgium

New narratives on health, care and citizenship in the nineteenth and twentieth centuries

Edited by

Joris Vandendriessche and Benoît Majerus

MANCHESTER UNIVERSITY PRESS

Copyright © Manchester University Press 2021

While copyright in the volume as a whole is vested in Manchester University Press, copyright in individual chapters belongs to their respective authors.

An electronic version of this book is also available under a Creative Commons (CC-BY-NC-ND) licence, thanks to the support of the University of Luxembourg, which permits non-commercial use, distribution and reproduction provided the editor(s), chapter author(s) and Manchester University Press are fully cited and no modifications or adaptations are made. Details of the licence can be viewed at https://creativecommons.org/licenses/by-nc-nd/4.0/

Published by Manchester University Press
Oxford Road, Manchester M13 9PL

www.manchesteruniversitypress.co.uk

British Library Cataloguing-in-Publication Data
A catalogue record for this book is available from the British Library

ISBN 978 1 5261 5108 7 hardback

First published 2021

The publisher has no responsibility for the persistence or accuracy of URLs for any external or third-party internet websites referred to in this book, and does not guarantee that any content on such websites is, or will remain, accurate or appropriate.

Typeset by Newgen Publishing UK

Contents

List of figures — vii
Notes on contributors — x

Introduction – Benoît Majerus and Joris Vandendriessche — 1

Part I: Beyond the nation state

1 Medicine, health and gender – Jolien Gijbels and Kaat Wils — 29
2 Medicine and religion – Joris Vandendriessche and Tine Van Osselaer — 65
3 Medicine and colonialism – Sokhieng Au and Anne Cornet — 99
4 Public health, hygiene and social activism – Thomas D'haeninck, Jan Vandersmissen, Gita Deneckere and Christophe Verbruggen — 134

Part II: Institutions and beyond

5 Ways of knowing medicine – Renaud Bardez and Pieter Dhondt — 171
6 Medicine, money and mutual aid – Dirk Luyten and David Guilardian — 206
7 The material culture of caring and curing – Valérie Leclercq and Veronique Deblon — 244

Part III: Beyond physicians

8 Dis/order and dis/ability – Benoît Majerus
  and Pieter Verstraete   283
9 Medicine, media and the public – Tinne Claes
  and Katrin Pilz   320

Epilogue – Including *all* citizens of Belgium: narratives
beyond the profession and the state – Frank Huisman   358

Timeline of Belgian medical history   372
Index   375

Figures

Unless otherwise stated, all rights are reserved. For permission to reproduce any of these images please contact the rightsholder.

1.1 Painting of Isala van Diest by Pierre-Joseph Steger, ca. 1855 (courtesy of M – Museum Leuven) — 37
1.2 Images of gynaecological objects in the handbook of Rufin Schockaert, *Précis du cours de gynécologie* (Leuven: Feyaerts, 1913), p. 51 (courtesy of KU Leuven Bibliotheken Bijzondere Collecties) — 46
1.3 Poster in favour of the legalisation of abortion, 1979 (courtesy of AVG-Carhif: Archive and Research Centre for Women's History) — 52
2.1 A woman religious operating sterilisation equipment in the Leuven academic hospitals, n.d. (mid twentieth century) (courtesy of Heritage Centre | Sisters of Charity J. M.) — 70
2.2 Postcard of Belgian pilgrims holding mass in a train (collection of Tine Van Osselaer) — 76
2.3 Louise in ecstasy (photograph by Lorleberg, October 1877) (courtesy of Archives Seminary of Tournai) — 79
3.1 Health worker Ruyters visits patient, Beni, 1937 (Province of Costermansville) (AP.0.1.3768, collection RMCA Tervuren) — 110
3.2 Leopoldville. Milk depot and baby clinic, n.d. (AP.0.1.3617, collection RMCA Tervuren) — 115

Figures

3.3 Lomami Recruitment Mission (MOI) for the UMHK, 1930. The doctor carefully examines each native at the preparation camp and thus establishes his robustness index (index of Pignet) (HP.1959.61.264, collection RMCA Tervuren. Photo © UMHK, RMCA Tervuren) — 119

4.1 Portrait of Adolphe Burggraeve (courtesy of Ghent University) — 140

4.2 Portrait of René Sand. From an obituary notice connected with the International Congress of Social Work, 1953 (Wellcome Collection, CC BY 4.0) — 151

5.1 Anatomy lesson at St-Pierre Hospital, 1892 (courtesy of the Université Libre de Bruxelles) — 181

5.2 The Anatomical Institute of Brussels University, 1895 (courtesy of the Université Libre de Bruxelles) — 190

5.3 Pin of G[odelieve] Perneel, one of the nurses who graduated from the Catholic St Elizabeth School in Bruges, 1924 (photo: Pieter Dhondt) — 191

6.1 Poor doctor's certificate, issued for the director of St-Pierre Hospital in Brussels, indispensable for admission, 1837 (ACPASB, Conseil des Hospices, C 339. Courtesy of CPAS Brussels) — 209

6.2 Two possibilities in the 1930s: either the common sick ward, free (as in this picture), or the single room with private bathroom, for paying patients. Ward 14, St-Jean Hospital in Brussels, around 1935 (ACPASB, FI, DONS/1986/6 (Dr Goffart). Courtesy of CPAS Brussels) — 222

6.3 Edmond Leburton (1915–97), the minister who gave his name to a law on financing of the sickness insurance in 1963. Screencap from video 'Conseil des Ministres sur la grève des mineurs du Limbourg', 1970 (Sonuma: Les archives audiovisuelles) — 226

6.4 Construction of a new building for the INAMI inaugurated in 1974, when the economic crisis of the 1970s started (courtesy of Collection Belgian State Archives/CegeSoma) — 228

Figures

7.1 Photograph of a sick ward of the psychiatric facilities of the St-Jean Hospital in Brussels (1930) (courtesy of the Archives du Centre Public d'Action Sociale de Bruxelles, fonds iconographique, H/H.ST-J./67b) — 244

7.2 Vue d'une salle de malade (patient ward of the St-Jean Hospital in Brussels), painting on paper (1863) (courtesy of the Archives du Centre Public d'Action Sociale de Bruxelles, fonds iconographique, H/H.ST-J./8) — 252

7.3 Postcard of a sick ward of a hospital in Oudenaarde (1915) (courtesy of City Archives Oudenaarde) — 261

7.4 Drawing of the children's hospital (academic hospital of Ghent) (© Ghent University Archives) — 265

8.1 Geel – Drève de l'Infirmierie. Postcard (ACPASB – collection Dierckx) — 295

8.2 'Invalide' – drawing by Samuel De Vriendt, dated 1923, Woluwé (collection of Pieter Verstraete) — 299

8.3 Excerpt from the 1971 television programme 'Faits divers' about the Lovenjoel Psychiatric Hospital (© Archives RTBF-Sonuma) — 305

9.1 Newspaper advertisement for a 'breast-enhancing' product, *Le Peuple*, 19 May 1914, p. 6 (Royal Library of Belgium, public domain) — 320

9.2 Félicien Rops, *La Leçon d'hygiène*. Série des Cent légers croquis, 1878–81 (© Musée Félicien Rops) — 325

9.3 Film stills of the public health film on Tuberculosis *Un ennemi public* (1937), 35 mm, b/w, sound, ca. 15 min — 335

Every effort has been made to obtain permission to reproduce copyright material, and the publisher will be pleased to be informed of any errors and omissions for correction in future editions.

Contributors

Sokhieng Au is a lecturer and interim director of the Global Health Studies Program at the University of Iowa, USA. She writes, teaches and researches on global health and the history of medicine, focusing on interchanges between the Global South and the Global North.

Renaud Bardez is a historian of medicine and university teaching at the research centre Mondes Modernes et Contemporains at the Université Libre de Bruxelles (ULB). His main area of expertise is medical education in the nineteenth century, specifically focused on the city of Brussels. He is also in charge of the archives and patrimonial collections of ULB.

Tinne Claes is a postdoctoral fellow of the Research Foundation Flanders at the University of Leuven. Her research concerns the history of medicine, gender and sexuality in the nineteenth and twentieth centuries. Her first book *Corpses in Belgian Anatomy* (Palgrave Macmillan, 2019) reconstructs the stories of the thousands of bodies that ended up in the hands of anatomists in the late nineteenth century. She has published articles on diverse topics, ranging from popular museums to lesbian motherhood.

Anne Cornet is a historian at the Royal Museum of Central Africa (Tervuren, Belgium). Her research concentrates on the history of colonialism in Central Africa (Congo, Rwanda), mainly in the social, missionary and medical domains, with a particular focus on gender issues. She has published, among other works, *Politiques de santé et contrôle social au Rwanda, 1920–1940* (Karthala, 2011).

Thomas D'haeninck is a historian at the Social History since 1750 Research Group of Ghent University. His research focuses on social and moral reformers, cultural mobility and transnational networks in the nineteenth century. Other interests include biographical and network analysis and distant reading techniques. He obtained his PhD in history in 2018, studying transnational networks of social reformers in the nineteenth century.

Veronique Deblon studied history at KU Leuven and the Université de Versailles. She is currently involved in a research project entitled 'Anatomy, Scientific Authority and the Visualised Body in Medicine and Culture (Belgium, 1780–1930)' at the Cultural History since 1750 Research Group of the University of Leuven.

Gita Deneckere is a full professor in the History Department of Ghent University and currently dean of the Faculty of Arts and Philosophy. She is a committed historian who combines scholarly depth with an imaginative, narrative style of writing. Her last book was *From the Ivory Tower: 200 Years of Ghent University* (Ghent, 2018).

Pieter Dhondt is a senior lecturer in general history and head of the Department of Geographical and Historical Studies at the University of Eastern Finland. He has published extensively on the intercultural transfer of university ideas within Europe in the nineteenth century, the history of academic mobility, student revolts and university celebrations. His current research focuses primarily on the history of (dealing with) medical uncertainty in medical training. His recent books include, as editor, *University Jubilees and University History Writing: A Challenging Relationship* (Brill, 2014), and, together with Elizabethanne Boran, *Student Revolt, City, and Society in Europe: From the Middle Ages to the Present* (Routledge, 2017).

Jolien Gijbels is a postdoctoral researcher for the Cultural History Since 1750 research group at the University of Leuven. She recently wrote a doctoral dissertation about religion and obstetrics in nineteenth-century Belgium. Her research interests are in the history of women's health, medical ethics and scientific publishing.

David Guilardian is curator of the Brussels Public Welfare and Hospitals Archives, Libraries and Museum, and is interested in all aspects of local care organisation. He is a member of the SOCIAMM–ULB research group, where he is focusing on the medieval political history of the duchy of Brabant. He is also a member of the board of several scientific journals and societies.

Frank Huisman is a professor in the history of medicine at Utrecht University. He has published on early modern and modern Dutch healthcare. He recently co-edited *Leerboek medische geschiedenis* (Bohn Stafleu van Loghum, 2018), a handbook on medical history for medical students. He is currently working on a book on the transformation of Dutch healthcare between the 1860s and 1940s.

Valérie Leclercq is a post-doctoral researcher in the history of medicine at the Université Libre de Bruxelles. Her areas of interest include nineteenth- and twentieth-century medicine, the history of patients, psychiatry and medical ethics. She is currently attached to the BRAIN research project IMPRESS, dedicated to the study of ideological tensions in nineteenth-century Belgian medicine.

Dirk Luyten is a researcher at the Belgian State Archives/CegeSoma in Brussels. One of his research fields is the history of social policy in Belgium.

Benoît Majerus is a historian of medicine at the Center for Contemporary and Digital History at the University of Luxembourg. He has mainly worked on the history of psychiatry in the twentieth century. He recently co-edited *Material Cultures of Psychiatry* (Transcript Verlag, 2020) with Monika Ankele.

Katrin Pilz is a historian and cultural scientist. After having worked within international projects at the Université libre de Bruxelles (ULB) and the University of Vienna she is currently working as key researcher at the Ludwig Boltzmann Institute for Digital History within the Austrian Science Fund (FWF) project on 'Educational film practice in Austria'. Her lectures, publications and research projects focus on the visual history of medicine and science, as well as urban history, body politics and educational film history in the twentieth century.

Joris Vandendriessche is a research professor at the Cultural History since 1750 Research Group at the University of Leuven. He works on medical history, history of science and health humanities. He is author of *Medical Societies and Scientific Culture in Nineteenth-Century Belgium* (Manchester University Press, 2018) and *Zorg en wetenschap: Een geschiedenis van de Leuvense academische ziekenhuizen in de twintigste eeuw* (Leuven University Press, 2019).

Jan Vandersmissen is a researcher and lecturer at the History Department of Ghent University, for the research group 'Social History Since 1750'. He has published extensively on issues related to the history of science, technology and medicine in imperial contexts from the eighteenth to the twentieth century.

Tine Van Osselaer is a research professor at the Ruusbroec Institute of the University of Antwerp. She works on the history of religion, gender, emotions and pain in the nineteenth and twentieth centuries. She recently co-published *The Devotion and Promotion of Stigmatics in Europe, c.1800–1950: Between Saints and Celebrities* (Brill, 2020).

Christophe Verbruggen is director of the Ghent Centre for Digital humanities and associate professor at the research unit 'Social History Since 1750'. He is currently working on the history of social and cultural reform movements and the development of virtual research environments for the study of transnational and entangled history.

Pieter Verstraete is a historian of education at the Research Unit for Education, Culture and Society (KU Leuven). His research interests are the history of special education in the nineteenth and twentieth century. Currently he is working on a book project about the history of silence from an educational perspective. He is also curator of the annual Leuven disABILITY Film Festival.

Kaat Wils is professor of contemporary European cultural history at KU Leuven. She works on medical history, gender history and the history of education. She co-edited *Bodies Beyond Borders: Moving Anatomies, 1750–1950* (Leuven University Press, 2017) and *Sign or Symptom? Exceptional Corporeal Phenomena in Religion and Medicine in the 19th and 20th Centuries* (Leuven University Press, 2017).

Introduction

Benoît Majerus and Joris Vandendriessche

In 1837, the Antwerp physician Jean-Corneille Broeckx published his *Essay on the History of Belgian Medicine Before the 19th Century*. Broeckx left no doubt as to his motives. He wanted to prove that 'in medicine, as in the other sciences, Belgium is capable of bringing forth its share of famous men.'[1] Published only seven years after the Belgian Revolution of 1830 – during which the southern parts of the United Kingdom of the Netherlands broke away to form a new nation state – Broeckx's *Essay* is the earliest example of 'Belgian' medical history. It is a work pervaded by patriotism and professional pride, one of the products of an expanding historical culture comprising also paintings, statues, parades, public lectures, plays and history books, which was to affirm the new country's *raison d'être* alongside its European neighbours. The history of medicine was 'nationalised' in the writings of Broeckx and his colleagues. From the mediaeval surgeon Jan Yperman to the sixteenth-century anatomist Andreas Vesalius and the seventeenth-century physician and chemist Jan Baptist van Helmont, these writings have presented us with a series of 'Belgian' medical heroes, representatives of the Belgian nation in the (internationally competitive) field of the medical sciences.[2]

This book does not intend to offer – like Broeckx's work – a glorifying and legitimising narrative of 'Belgian medicine'. Yet, it does take the national level as its starting point and point of synthesis by offering a set of medical histories that treat the Belgian medical field in the nineteenth and twentieth centuries. The book presents a broad view of medical history both *of* Belgium and *in* Belgium, and does not reduce the country to a matter of socio-political context for medical developments or to state infrastructure in public health. Its aim is rather to assemble narratives that go beyond such traditional 'national' overviews, which tend to focus on state–profession interactions, and explore the relation between medicine and sociopolitical views and realities, treating a variety of themes such as gender, religion, disability, media and colonialism. It goes without saying that a 'national' medical history of this kind bears a resemblance to Broeckx's *Essay* in name only. The narratives in this book are intended as critical and accessible historical overviews of medicine and health in modern Belgium.

A focus on national frameworks does not exclude contributing to a wider historiography. On the contrary, by developing the Belgian case study more deeply and broadly, we seek to offer insight into a European historiography of medicine for the twenty-first century. We do this, first, by engaging thoroughly with the second half of the twentieth century. Medical history often remains stuck within the perspective of the long nineteenth century, from the 1830s until the 1940s. The second half of the twentieth century too often only appears as an appendix. Yet, the post-1945 period was marked by a crucial rethinking of medicine and of the social role of medical institutions and their boundaries. What was the meaning of 'cure', 'care' and 'therapy'? Who determined what was to be considered medical knowledge?[3] This brings us to a second, related point on which this book innovates: the attention to a multiplicity of actors, places and media. This heterogeneity seems evident for the last thirty years but constitutes an equally valuable perspective to apply to the past two centuries: which role does the carpenter play in psychiatry by constructing a bed, the accountant in the hospital when introducing new management methods, the designer in public hygiene when developing a television programme on human immunodeficiency virus (HIV)? One could multiply the examples of professions that until now have rarely been taken into account when historians write about medicine.

Finally, this book aims to enrich and 'decentre' the European historiography of medicine by adding the perspective of a particular region, of a particular country, to the mix. The narratives of medical historiography as found in most syntheses are organised around the European triad of Great Britain, France and Germany, to which comparisons with the case of the United States are added. This book does not want to replace Germany by Belgium in a new history full of 'facts and firsts'. Rather, it makes a plea to include other localities – be it Belgium, Finland, Albania or Portugal – to introduce new chronologies, heterodox practices, unknown places. The benefit of such a regional perspective to the history of medicine, this book shows, is precisely that it allows us to study how different (foreign) medical traditions have intersected, for example in medical and hygiene education. It also enables scrutiny of how issues such as the gender balance in the medical field or the organisation of medical services developed in ways specific to that region's sociocultural and political traditions.

Physicians and the state

In Belgium, as in other European countries, a historiography of medicine developed in the 1980s that challenged older notions of medical progress. Medical sociologists and social historians denounced the 'triumphalist' discourses that underpinned the growing social power of the medical profession (see also the Epilogue). This social history of medicine, written by professional historians, developed against a backdrop of an uneasy relationship to medical power (in particular with regard to psychiatric institutions). Since the 1960s, a growing criticism on the latter institutions, and the organisation of healthcare more generally, had been linked to calls for more extensive patient rights and to worries about the sustainability of the welfare state. Karel Velle, among others, developed a critical historiography of medicine, scrutinising the processes of 'professionalisation' of medicine and the 'medicalisation' of Belgian society.[4]

These social histories of medicine produced a new, strong metanarrative about Western medicine in which the national level was very present. In these histories, the central evolution of the nineteenth and twentieth centuries was the joint development of the medical profession and the state. In other words, the rising social status of physicians developed in parallel with the expansion of government intervention in healthcare. Their relationship was one of mutual legitimising. Medical expertise underpinned state expansion into new social realms. State legislation, in turn, strengthened physicians' position in the medical marketplace. Belgium appeared as a case study that confirmed broader, Western, narratives already well proven for Great Britain, Germany or France. This main narrative of the social history of medicine has resulted in a series of representations that have also found their way into more general (political) histories of Belgium. Given the attention historians paid to the government regulation of public health, the image of the physician as a social expert, as embodied by public health specialists, became the dominant representation of the medical profession as a whole.[5] As a by-product of the theory of the medicalisation of society, which was said to reinforce an ongoing process of secularisation, the physician has also been represented as a substitute for the priest, suggesting a competitive relationship between the medical and religious fields. A third and related imagery concerns the progressive 'medicalisation' of the hospital. This narrative stressed a rather one-sided evolution of the hospital from a space of religious and social 'care' (by women religious) to one of 'cure' (by doctors and lay nurses).

Research into the social history of Belgian medicine has resulted in a thorough understanding of the creation of medical legislation, public healthcare institutions and professional organisations of physicians. Medical reforms introduced in the mid nineteenth century have received particular attention, such as the foundation of the Royal Academy of Medicine of Belgium in 1841 and the Belgian Medical Federation in 1863, the introduction of the unified academic degree of Doctor of Medicine, Surgery and Obstetrics in 1849 (see Chapter 5) and the Medical Treatment Act in 1850 (see Chapter 8).[6] More recently, a second series of legislative reforms that reshaped the medical field almost a century later have been scrutinised. In 1936, the Belgian Ministry of Public Health was founded; in 1938, the Order of Physicians was established; in 1944, mandatory health insurance was introduced for all employees, effectively creating a form of Belgian social security; in 1957, after long debates dating back to the interwar years, medical specialists were legally recognised; and in 1963, the Leburton Law (named after secretary Edmond Leburton) further expanded health insurance, leading to a nationwide physicians' strike (see Chapter 6).[7]

Over the last two to three decades, historians' interests have expanded beyond legal shifts, state developments and professional struggles in the Belgian medical field. This work clearly built on the groundwork of the social history of medicine, but also challenged its established categories and narratives. Without going into too much historiographical detail, for which we refer to the discussion of the literature in the chapters, we will here point to some main trends. A first observation is that medicalisation has continued to act as an important analytical framework, but now with much more attention to the social role of medical discourse and the construction of medical knowledge. By studying the intellectual origins of medical metaphors and their different uses in society, Belgian historians of medicine have addressed new topics such as science, art and gender in relation to an expanding medical field.[8] More recently, a rich historiography of the body has emerged at the crossroads of gender history, the history of sexuality, the history of religion and the history of science.[9] In these studies, historians not only look at intellectual medical discourse, but also pay attention to medical practice and caregivers' performance as professionals. While the term 'performance' may refer to different types of medical conduct in this book – such as the performance of a professional identity or of scientific expertise, and the performance of healing – it is clear that in moving beyond the history of a profession, the history of medicine does not return to a narrow view of medical knowledge, but has embraced a more complex understanding of the interplay between medicine as science and practice in different settings. This includes looking at how knowledge about the body circulates between different academic and public contexts, for example in medical subfields such as anatomy (see Chapter 9).[10]

A second general observation about medical historiography in recent years concerns the actors that historians have put on the stage. A growing diversity of themes has gone hand in hand with a greater variety of players; hydropaths and naturalists operating at the medical fringe, novelists and artists engaging with the body within the performing arts, social scientists, legal experts and academics from different backgrounds, missionaries and politicians from diverse ideological strands have entered medical history. More recently, this diversity has expanded even further together with new methodological approaches to the history of medical institutions. Roy Porter's call to make the patients' voices heard has been integrated into histories of Belgian medicine. By paying attention to the materiality of medical practice and to the agency of the different actors involved in clinical encounters, patients' perspectives and their asymmetrical power relation to caregivers in the past have been brought to light. To this end, the rich archives of the public welfare institutions in Brussels offered many opportunities. In writing a new type of institutional history, historians also moved beyond the classic duo of the sick person and the physician, and brought new actors to the fore such as women religious and lay nurses, medical students and hospital attendants, architects, accountants and psychologists.[11] The result of this attention to a greater variety of actors has been that historians have 'decentred' medical history, placing the pivotal position of doctors, their professional organisations and the state into perspective.

This book builds on these efforts. In presenting a series of medical histories, it adopts a much broader view of the medical field than previous accounts. From the missionaries who travelled to the Belgian Congo and combined the provision of medical care with efforts for conversion, to the popular anatomists who simultaneously entertained and educated the public with their fairground shows, each account shows the (sometimes surprising) ways in which issues of health and illness were tied up with sociopolitical shifts and cultural developments in Belgium. It goes without saying that physicians continue to appear in these histories. They remain central players, but their roles and identities become more complex once we consider them as more than only experts in public health or advocates of the medical profession.[12] In this book, they take on roles as educators, scientists, designers, ethicists, caregivers and politicians, and interact with people far beyond the strictly professional medical milieu.

The broadening of actors and themes, however, has inevitably also led to more fragmentation. This is illustrated by the fact that, compared to the social historiography of the 1980s and 1990s, the national level has become far less central to medical historians. Recent hospital histories, histories of medical faculties and histories of medical subfields such as gynaecology and anatomy tend to focus on the local (often the urban) level for the exploration of medical practices and interactions, using these sites as illustrations of international trends.[13] When writing a history of a psychiatric institution from below, for example, one tries to capture a clinical reality that seems quite distant from political debates on health on the national level.[14] In such histories, the level of the nation state has tended to be rather absent. To a lesser extent, the same is true for the transnational histories that have emerged on topics such as colonial medicine or social reform. Historians highlighted the development of expert communities across national boundaries (e.g. at international conferences). Here again, the local and the international are interconnected in more direct ways.[15]

The absence of attention to the national level is not a problem in itself. For some topics, the impact of government policies was simply limited or offered no added value because Belgian trends followed international trends closely, without national particularities. But the fact that the broadening of our understanding of the medical field has not yet resulted in a new overview, which takes the national level as its point of reference, does have its disadvantages. It hampers a strong profiling of Belgian medical historical research – a small field – both within the general historiography of Belgium and within the international historiography of medicine. Even more important is the danger that when historians present Belgian medicine to an international audience (e.g. in scholarly articles), the older narratives of state–profession interactions and their related representations of physicians, medical institutions, reforms and laws, reappear as the (sole) contextual 'frames'. This means that the sociopolitical particularities of Belgian medicine are reduced to questions of legislation, state intervention and professional union – a representation that is contrary to the gains in historians' understanding of medicine's diverse roles in Belgian society. In other words, while Belgian historians have succeeded in opening up the medical world in their case studies, they have yet to summarise their findings and reassess the stories they tell about the Belgian medical field as a whole.

This volume aims to fill this void and establish new narratives about the Belgian medical field in the nineteenth and twentieth centuries. As Belgian medical historiography matures as a scholarly subfield, we need more effective and nuanced ways of situating our case studies and discussing general trends without reducing them to matters of legislation or state expansion. Here the national level, situated in between local dynamics and international shifts, offers new opportunities as a shared point of reference for Belgian scholars and as a means of mid-level analysis.[16] The challenge this book takes up is therefore also an exercise in connecting medical developments to the sociopolitical realities that shaped Belgium's history as a modern nation, an exercise in broadening our understanding of the political embeddedness of Belgian medicine beyond the well-known story of physicians and the state. In the next two sections, we discuss some of the ways in which the authors took up this challenge: first, by including a broad perspective on the 'politics' of Belgian medicine and by paying particular attention to the care provided by different actors; second, by looking more closely at the scales and levels on which health and healing took place in – and indeed beyond – Belgium.

The politics of (health)care

The weakness of the Belgian nation state is a recurring theme in Belgian history, which emerged well before the many government reforms that transformed the country into a federal state from the 1960s onwards.[17] Two reasons may be identified for this weakness: first, private initiative – whether in the form of Catholic initiatives or by different players in the economic realm – played a powerful role in the country. Second, the Belgian state often functioned at a lower level than the level of the national government; many responsibilities were left to local authorities.[18] The social history of medicine that emerged in the 1980s can be said to have challenged this image. It was characterised by a firm national perspective and depicted the nation state as a powerful player. Medical history therefore casts critical doubt on the notion of a weak Belgian state. The new medical histories in this book again paint a more nuanced picture. They emphasise, above all, the diversity of players involved – especially the strong Catholic influence – and the interplay between different levels, with a particular focus on local players and transnational currents.

When the Belgian state was created in 1830, the political elites devised a twofold system for medicine and health, spearheaded by the two dominant ideological trends of the time: liberalism and Catholicism. Private initiative was not stifled; on the contrary, it was encouraged. Mental asylums in nineteenth-century Belgium, for example, were not state-run institutions like in France; they were generally run by religious congregations. In 1876, these congregations managed three-quarters of all the country's psychiatric patients.[19] The psychiatric infrastructure shows that in Belgium, more than elsewhere in Europe, Catholicism had a massive impact on the provision of healthcare (see Chapter 8). Historians of nineteenth-century Belgian Catholicism Vincent Viaene and Peter Heyrman have shown how a shared resistance to state intervention among liberals and Catholics – a key feature of the Belgian nation state – allowed the Catholic Church to develop extensive charitable initiatives (including hospitals, schools, homes for elderly people, etc.), many of which were subsidised by the state. They rightly speak of a Catholic 'empire by invitation'.[20] Catholic influence was at least as decisive in the colonies, via the missions set up in the Congo. Since the colonial governance structures were not well developed, these missions served several purposes, including the provision of healthcare.[21] In the first half of the twentieth century, when secularisation began to take hold in Belgium, there was a significant rise in religious vocations for the colonial missions: the number of Belgian missionaries increased from 2,686 in 1922 to 10,070 in 1961 (see Chapter 3).[22] Parallel yet in contrast with these rising colonial vocations, the impact of secularisation became visible in Belgium itself. First, the number of people entering religious life, in both congregations and healthcare institutions, began to drop. Second, a movement led by urban, liberal middle classes called for the secularisation of hospital staff. In Brussels, from 1887 onwards, classes were offered to nurses with the specific aim of breaking the monopoly of religious congregations.

Given the importance of Catholicism, one of the challenges this book takes up is to bring the history of care into the narratives about the Belgian medical field.[23] Several chapters illustrate how attention to care allows historians to complicate the narrative of the medicalisation of society, as a linear evolution 'from care to cure', and pay more attention to the religious motives that underpinned medical practice. Taking care of someone's body was closely linked to spiritual care. The figure of the nun-nurse, who has been somewhat marginalised in a medical history focusing on doctors – a neglected position that Barbra Mann Wall counters in her work in on American religious congregations and their involvement in (colonial) healthcare – represents this connection most clearly (see Chapter 2).[24] In a colonial setting, moreover, medical care went hand in hand with conversion. But traditions of care were not solely inspired by religion. The link between care and femininity was made in a variety of debates over women's access to the medical profession, and more generally to different areas of social life (see Chapter 1). Furthermore, reassessing the relationship between 'care' and 'cure' from a religious or gender perspective guides our attention to lesser-known aspects of Belgian medical history with considerable research potential, such as the history of home care, medical ethics and the history of pain.[25] The perspective of care also has the potential of writing intertwined histories of psychiatry and disability by transcending a too narrow view of medicalisation and by pointing to the shared trajectories of the institutionalisation and deinstitutionalisation of care, and to the role of a variety of caregivers (see Chapter 8).

The Belgian government gave considerable autonomy to the local authorities, some of which played a major role in the organisation of the medical field. Charitable organisations, especially the committees of civil hospitals, were important local players. In Belgium's major cities, these committees managed huge hospital complexes, the most significant example being Brussels, where the General Council of Hospices and Assistance was responsible for a vast hospital empire. Although local authorities took the lead in the development of public hospital infrastructure, they did so in close collaboration with (wealthy) private players, who acted as philanthropists (see Chapter 6). This also held true for medical education and research. The medical sciences initially developed within an engaged urban civil society, through the activities of 'private' learned societies that cooperated with state-subsidised institutions such as the Royal Academy of Medicine of Belgium (set up in 1841), a space where Catholic and liberal doctors could meet. The model of the research university was only introduced in the late nineteenth century in Belgium, and in the case of the ideologically opposed Catholic University of Leuven and Free University Brussels, its infrastructural development largely depended on private capital. As an intellectual field, Belgian medicine had its particular dynamics of compromise and competition, infused by competing ideologies and the room given to private initiative (see Chapter 5).

Turning to the twentieth century, the century of the welfare state, the Belgian national government did more actively intervene in the field of healthcare. The development of health insurance companies involved a considerable degree of state intervention, through the establishment of a regulatory legal framework and the allocation of state subsidies. Yet the organisation of these companies remained firmly in the hands of Catholic, socialist and, to a lesser extent, liberal communities – the so-called ideological pillars of Belgian society (see Chapter 6). With regard to hospital infrastructure, religious congregations managed to reinvent themselves and maintain a grip on the sector. Unlike in Quebec, another region where these congregations played a key role in the nineteenth and early twentieth century, Belgian congregations retained their hold over healthcare institutions despite the upheavals of 1968 and the rapidly falling numbers entering religious orders.[26] This nineteenth-century Belgian model – involving both public and private players, with a key role played by local authorities – therefore went on to characterise the medical field until the end of the twentieth century. Of course, the development of the welfare state gave greater influence to the national government. But a strong centralised system was never set up in Belgium. While the 1944 Mandatory Health Insurance Act was undoubtedly a key moment in the creation of a social security system in Belgium, this system never exerted the same degree of control as in the United Kingdom or France. Considerable responsibility was left to private players, in particular the socialist and Catholic mutual health insurance funds. Since the late 1960s, the national set-up has also begun to splinter as a result of successive government reforms that have created federal entities. The latter have been given increasing responsibilities in the fields of medicine (university education) and health (mental health and elderly people).[27]

So, while this book challenges the tendency of Belgian medical historiography to focus on the state, it also emphasises that over the past two centuries, healthcare has been one of the areas in which different forms of citizenship and access to medical service have been under constant discussion. Do women and colonised people have the right to be integrated into the nation state? To what extent does the state have the right to intervene on and in the bodies of individuals to guarantee the health of the nation? The moments of exclusion and inclusion that define the nation state in the nineteenth and twentieth centuries can often be seen in terms of Belgian biopolitics. These specific Belgian characteristics run through most chapters of the book as subtext, while developments in the field of medicine are also considered as part of a broader European history.

From the local to the international level

It is clear, therefore, that while those writing the history of medicine in Belgium cannot ignore the role of the nation state, other perspectives must also be considered. Indeed, the specific national characteristics of Belgium can be attributed precisely – in part – to the absence of a strong state and the delegation of responsibilities to local players such as municipal authorities or to transnational players such as religious congregations. The interplay between different levels – which for at least thirty years has been posited as one of the best ways for historical narratives to incorporate the experiences of key players and for historians to take account of influences beyond the national framework – is particularly pertinent in the case of Belgium.[28]

The levels that came into play varied hugely in the nineteenth and twentieth centuries, and their relationship was often complex. In scientific publishing, for example, the first 'national' medical journal, the *Bulletin médical belge* (1834), appeared as an annex to a Brussels-based journal with international ambitions, the *Encyclographie des sciences médicales* (1833). It was designed to compensate for the lack of publishing space for Belgian scholars as the *Encyclographie* reprinted articles from across the Western medical world by making use of the absence of international copyright. The journals of 'local' Belgian medical societies, while mostly comprised of regional authorship, attracted a readership that was surprisingly national and even international (see Chapter 5).[29] After a century marked by a certain degree of nationalisation, scientific exchange in the period after the First World War was equally complex. On the one hand, international political tensions hampered relations within the medical field. On the other hand, internationalisation and specialisation increased, in particular in terms of research. Within this changing context, no Belgian medical journal gained scientific recognition in the competitive world of international academic publishing, yet many continued to exist (such as the *Bulletin of the Belgian Academy of Medicine*) as a means of debate among local academic and professional audiences.

When incorporating these different levels in medical historiography, the challenge is to move past a narrative of a gradual increase in scale. The development of the medical field, in fact, continued to be characterised by a significant degree of localism. In the nineteenth century, several professional associations, whether for pharmacists or physicians, initially emerged at the local level before meeting at the national level. New national professional associations for medical specialisations – such as the Society for Mental Illness (1869) or the Belgian Society of Gynaecology and Obstetrics (1889) – initially served as spaces of sociability for fledgling communities, which were spread geographically unevenly across the country and at the same set up international contacts (see Chapters 1 and 8).[30] Until the mid twentieth century, some of the country's more influential professional medical journals were developed in a highly local setting, such as the Liège-based *Le Scalpel* (1848). And in the second half of the twentieth century, the reform of the psychiatric field was essentially centred on Brussels, where favourable local circumstances (the existence of a university, social players open to experiences in psychiatry and political majorities interested in developments in public health) can explain the establishment of non-hospital-based structures, which remained extremely rare in the rest of the country.[31]

Beyond the local and national levels, the transnational level has proven to be particularly stimulating in recent years for Belgian historiography. Belgium has often been seen as a 'mini Europe' that is transnational by definition, and there is no doubt that the Belgian medical community has at times been particularly open to its neighbouring countries.[32] In the nineteenth century, as the medical sector was in the throes of nationalisation, several first editions of international medical and hygiene conferences were held in Brussels.[33] In addition to highlighting Belgium's role as 'a key site for international conferences, world's fairs and the headquarters of international associations', as social and political historians have argued, the attention to transnational movements has also put the nation state into perspective regarding its colonial project in the Congo (and for two decades in Ruanda-Urundi) (see Chapter 4).[34] The history of medicine in the colonies is a field in which the transnational approach has proved to be particularly effective for telling the story of Belgium. In the colonies, local Belgian initiatives coincided with projects spearheaded by the British and French, but that were also conducted within the imperial space (see Chapter 3).[35]

While at times Belgium has been at the crossroads of new developments, at other times it has found itself on the sidelines. The topos of the 'Belgian latecomer' is a recurrent narrative pattern in medical and political debates: whether with the 1850 Mental Treatment Act or the development of public health films in the early twentieth century, Belgium has regularly been presented as a country that is lagging behind. While the use of such imagery was often politically inspired, the impact of foreign influences is an important aspect of medical historians' work, especially when a strong 'national' production is lacking as in the case of health exhibits or medical cinematography (see Chapter 9). As a country that belongs to two linguistic areas and is surrounded by larger neighbours such as France, the United Kingdom and Germany, Belgium can be seen in medical history as a 'seismograph' that enables historians to identify, examine and reconstruct transnational developments as well as local adaptations.

Finally, moving beyond the realm of medical history, paying attention to the different levels at which healing and healthcare took place may be of great value for investigating the history of Belgium in general, and especially the Belgian state. When Belgian historiography first emerged in the nineteenth century, the strength of local entities was immediately emphasised.[36] While this book to some extent reflects that view, an examination of medicine and health also enables us to emphasise moments when the nation state assumed a stronger role, especially after the two world wars and also during the rise of the welfare state: at these points, the state appears as a strong player rather than a weak entity (see Chapter 6).

Medical histories of Belgium

This book reflects a renewed interest in Belgian medical history over the past twenty years. At different levels, ranging from master's and PhD theses to published articles and monographs, historians have engaged with questions of health and healing, science and the body.

For this book, we brought together twenty-one authors from both the French-speaking and Dutch-speaking academic communities of Belgium, and asked them to compare their approaches and sketch the state of the art for various topics. Our intention was not to create a single standard account of Belgian medical history, but to bring more synthesis to the existing scholarship in the form of accessible *histories* of the medical field. Each chapter, moreover, ends with a selected bibliography of key works, providing easy access to further reading.

As expected, clear gaps in the historiography emerged during the process of making this book. At the very start, as we conceptualised its structure, it became clear that while for some topics considerable research existed, other topics had only scarcely been looked at. It is a telling fact of itself that we could find no authors to write an overview chapter on the history of pharmacy and illegal drugs in Belgium – topics that we would have liked to see combined in a single chapter. For other possible subjects as well, such as rural medicine or medicine and age, we hit upon a similar lack of research.[37] Moreover, as we organised two workshops to discuss texts, we were surprised to find that the history of disease has in fact been relatively little developed within Belgian historiography. In line with historians' attention to state interference, some diseases that have been framed as public health threats such as acquired immune deficiency syndrome (AIDS), tuberculosis or sleeping sickness in the Belgian Congo have been well studied. In addition, there exists an established tradition of demographic historical research into health, disease and mortality in Belgium.[38] Yet, few studies have appeared on the experience of and changing medical views on diseases such as cancer, polio, diabetes or migraine, in a way comparable to the rich Anglo-Saxon historiography of disease.[39] Similarly, the history of everyday medical practice and 'alternative medicine' is relatively little explored.[40] Finally, traditional subjects that are recurrent in Belgian historiography, such as the linguistic conflict between the Francophone and Dutch-speaking (Flemish) communities make only a brief appearance in Belgian medical history.[41]

Taking these gaps into account, each chapter attempts to fulfil three criteria: to review the current state of the historiography, to offer an overview that includes recent research findings and to highlight any persistent blind spots. This threefold approach provides readers with a critical snapshot of current research and indicates areas that could benefit from further investigation. Other than that, the authors made their own choices in line with their topics, for example in the way they composed the narrative of their chapter and structured the period treated. To bring more unity to the volume as a whole, and as an additional tool to the navigate the history of the Belgian medical field, we also drew up a timeline together with the authors. This timeline includes not only the major events, typical of the social history of medicine (e.g. acts of legislation, foundations of professional bodies), but also events specific to the topics of the chapters (e.g. the graduation of the first female Belgian physician). In addition, cross-references between the chapters indicate that many evolutions were closely related and that the authors treated the same wide themes (e.g. the relation between medicine and sexuality) from different angles.

The book is organised in three thematic parts. This thematic approach focuses on the three traditional players in medical historiography – namely the nation state, the hospital and the physician – but viewed from a decentralised perspective, with the aim of proposing innovative narratives. The titles of the three parts – 'Beyond the Nation State', 'Institutions and Beyond', and 'Beyond Physicians' – serve as idealistic exhortations to produce new histories. But in all three sections, the difficulties in moving beyond these 'pillars' of medical history, which continue to dominate the narrative, became clear. The fact that not all parts of the book have an equal number of chapters is in itself symptomatic of the current state of the field. It reflects the fact that Belgian historians have been more successful in employing wide frameworks to write medical history (instead of looking only at state–profession interactions) than in broadening the range of players beyond institutionalised settings or adopting an approach that looks at the field 'from below' (e.g. through patients' eyes). While historians' analyses increasingly reveal the cultural anxieties, religious beliefs and gendered stereotypes that have underpinned much medical discourse, they are still strongly centred on physicians. Here lies an agenda for further research.

Part I, 'Beyond the Nation State', highlights those dynamics in the medical field that transcended Belgian borders, yet impacted Belgium in a particular way. The four chapters show how medical knowledge was intimately connected to colonial conquest, notions of gender, religious views and expanding state power in public health. Specialisms such as tropical medicine, gynaecology and 'hygienism' may be considered as products of these social views and transformations, but at the same time played an important role in legitimising them. While histories revealing this complex entanglement between medicine and modern society may be written for many countries, Belgian particularities also appear. These include the clear impact of Catholicism on the ways in which views about the healthy body were constructed, resulting in sexual codes that were framed in moral and religious terms, and the dominance of religious congregations in healthcare both in Belgium and the Belgian colonies of Congo and Ruanda-Urundi. Focusing on gender, reproductive medicine and sexuality, in Chapter 1 Jolien Gijbels and Kaat Wils present a history in which medicine becomes both a tool of power and inequality (e.g. of men constructing the female body and medical insights underpinning labour divisions), but also a means of gaining more control for women and men over their bodies (e.g. the attention paid by the feminist movement to abortion). In Chapter 2, Joris Vandendriessche and Tine Van Osselaer write a history of Catholicism in Belgian healthcare in more than only political terms. By looking at the evolution of Catholic institutions, at the medical meanings that were ascribed to religious practices and rituals, and at Catholic medical ethics and professional identity, they present a varied overview of the many interactions between medicine and religion.

In addition, the chapters in Part I of the book engage with the notion of the relatively weak Belgian state. In Chapter 3 on medicine and colonialism, Sokhieng Au and Anne Cornet make clear how a lack of political will to invest in healthcare in the colonial territories, which was tied to a relative 'indifference' towards the colony, left all the room to private players such as religious missions, industrial companies and universities to develop health programmes and infrastructure. One of the implications of this indifference was that for a long time Belgian state citizenship remained inaccessible for colonial subjects – who Au and Cornet suggest were rather treated as 'objects'. As for the weak state in Belgium itself, in Chapter 4 Thomas D'haeninck, Jan Vandersmissen, Gita Deneckere and Christophe Verbruggen move beyond a narrative of slow or speedy developments in public health, or of strong or hesitant state interventions. Instead, they structure their chapter according to changing networks and modes of exchanging knowledge of 'reformers', many of which (but certainly not all) were physicians. In this way, the history of public health shifts between local medical societies, international conferences and transnational health programmes – in which the nation state forms only one level or actor.

In Part II, 'Institutions and Beyond', the authors highlight most clearly those aspects of the Belgian landscape of medicine and healthcare that make it unique. In seeking ways to turn the history of respectively medical faculties, mutual societies and hospitals into a broad analysis with different actors and covering two centuries, they come to a defining characteristic of Belgian medicine: the strong influence of ideology. In Chapter 5, on medical education in Belgium, Renaud Bardez and Pieter Dhondt argue that the ideologies of liberalism and Catholicism, and the struggle between them, are key to understand the changes and particularities in the medical curriculum of the state universities and of the private and ideologically opposed Free University of Brussels and the Catholic University of Leuven. Catholic viewpoints, for example, underpinned the latter university's hesitance in the nineteenth century towards far-reaching scientific training at the expense of broad and practical clinical courses designed to educate 'conscious' practitioners. In Chapter 6, Dirk Luyten and David Guilardian equally refer to competing ideologies and their translation into particular systems of financing healthcare, to explain historically how mutual societies have come to occupy such a strong position in Belgian healthcare. In a long-term perspective, they show how the Belgian state supported private initiatives (mostly Catholic and socialist) through a system of 'subsidised liberty' since the late nineteenth century and extended this system in 1944 when Belgian social security was introduced. While 1944 is often seen as a foundational moment of the Belgian welfare state, in terms of the political and financial logic there was no clear 'break' with the past. In Chapter 7, Valérie Leclercq and Veronique Deblon show expressions of ideology in healthcare in unexpected places, as they write the history of Belgian hospitals – institutions that have socially and medically completely been transformed over the past two centuries – by focusing on their material outlook. Strikingly, the influence of Catholicism becomes clear even in the public hospitals of the liberal stronghold of Brussels in the form of religious symbols (e.g. crosses) and practices (e.g. communion) that were introduced on request of patients. Somewhat contradictory, the modernist hospital architecture of these same institutions propagated an image of (anti-religious) progress.

While the chapters in Part II politically ground Belgian medicine within competing ideologies, they also pay attention to medicine as a profession. By also including this more traditional perspective, they show that Belgian physicians were above all trained to be practising professionals – an ambition that had to be balanced with their scientific schooling. Physicians furthermore organised themselves as actors in an economic market, where they sometimes clashed with other players (mutual societies, political parties) on the modalities of democratising the access to healthcare. New perspectives, such as attention to the financing of healthcare and the material culture of healthcare institutions, allow historians to renew this history of professional struggles. This innovative potential becomes most clear in the image of the hospital presented in these chapters. As more diverse patients' groups found their way to the hospital to receive specialised care, the involvement of physicians increased as well, along with the development of different functions of these institutions as spaces of instruction, healing and science.

The chapters in Part III, 'Beyond Physicians', put into practice most clearly the ambition to give agency to non-professional actors, patients in particular, in the history of medicine.[42] In Chapter 8, Benoît Majerus and Pieter Verstraete boldly bring together the histories of disability and mental illness, and in doing so include the voices of disabled people and people with mental illnesses. They pay attention to the very different experiences of these people (e.g. in their relation to their own bodies and to social prejudice and governmental structures in Belgium), but also to their shared historical trajectories of segregation and classification as 'subgroups', and the growing unease in the course of the twentieth century with such institutionalised segregation. In Chapter 9, Tinne Claes and Katrin Pilz draw attention to curators, to patients in their role as consumers of information about health and the body and to journalists and film-makers. They call for a history of the 'popularisation' of medical knowledge in Belgium that avoids a top-down relationship between professionals and laypersons, and between science and the public. Their analysis of health exhibitions (such as the Spitzner Museum in Brussels) and medical films (such as the first Belgian public health film *Un ennemi public* from 1937) reveals how different audiences were not passive consumers, but instead chose and adapted the available views on health, responding to them in unexpected ways.

Given the focus in both chapters in this final part on experiences 'from below', they also question – more clearly than elsewhere in the book – the narrative of medicalisation and point to its limitations. To understand the experiences of disabled people, for example, a medical gaze excludes too many social aspects related to being categorised as 'disabled' in Belgian society. A narrative of boundaries and people's agency in coping with these structures and reacting against them offers an alternative. To understand the function of medical knowledge within Belgian society, a gaze through the eyes of experts and scientists is similarly insufficient. Instead, narratives of travelling knowledge, and of the adaptation and consumption of medical information by users, seem more suited to bring to light that medicine and health had a 'demand side' as well – besides the better-studied 'supply side' as offered by physicians.

To place Belgian medical historiography in a wider European perspective and wrap up this book, we asked the Dutch historian of medicine Frank Huisman to write an epilogue. Huisman does so eloquently by identifying how the chapters reflect the different 'turns' that medical historiography has taken since the social history of the 1970s and 1980s. Huisman comments how new understandings of the body as an object of biomedical knowledge, as a gendered construct, as something fragile and prone to care, have impacted medical historiography and resulted in much more varied and dynamic histories. He concludes by discussing the book's ambition to look beyond the profession and the state and refers to Roy Porter's work, stating that such an effort also means – in Porter's words – reflecting and redefining the goals and limits of medicine. By presenting a new set of narratives about 'Belgian medicine', this book hopes to contribute to such reflection.

Introduction

Notes

1 J.-C. Broeckx, *Essai sur l'histoire de la médecine belge avant le XIXe siècle* (Ghent: Hebbelynck, 1837), iii.
2 J. Vandendriessche, *Medical Societies and Scientific Culture in Nineteenth-Century Belgium* (Manchester: Manchester University Press, 2018), 206–17.
3 Overviews of twentieth-century medicine include R. Cooter and J. Pickstone (eds), *Companion to Medicine in the Twentieth Century* (London: Routledge, 2003); and L. Monnais, *Médecine(s) et santé: Une petite histoire globale – 19e et 20e siècles* (Montréal: Les Presses de l'Université de Montréal, 2016). On the particularities of the twentieth-century history of medicine in the Low Countries, see F. Huisman, J. Vandendriessche and K. Wils, 'Blurring boundaries: towards a medical history of the twentieth century', *BMGN-LCHR (Bijdragen En Mededelingen van de Geschiedenis Der Nederlanden: Low Countries Historical Review)*, 132:1 (2017), 3–15. Specifically on the field of psychiatry in the twentieth century, see V. Hess and B. Majerus, 'Writing the history of psychiatry in the 20th century', *History of Psychiatry*, 22:2 (2011), 139–45.
4 K. Velle, *De nieuwe biechtvaders: de sociale geschiedenis van de arts in België* (Leuven: Kritak, 1991); C. Havelange, *Les figures de la guérison (XVIIIe–XIXe siècles): une histoire sociale et culturelle des professions médicales au pays de Liège* (Paris: Lettres Liège, 1990); R. Schepers, *De opkomst van het medisch beroep in België. De evolutie van de wetgeving en de beroepsorganisaties in de 19de eeuw* (Amsterdam: Rodopi, 1989).
5 See, for example, J. Craeybeckx, A. Meynen and E. Witte, *Political History of Belgium from 1830 Onwards* (Brussels: ASP, 2009).
6 R. Schepers, 'Towards unity and autonomy: the Belgian medical profession in the nineteenth century', *Medical History*, 38 (1994), 237–54; J. Demolder and B. Pattyn, 'Het ontstaan van de psychiatrie in België', in *Psychiatrie, godsdienst en gezag*, ed. P. Vandermeersch (Leuven: Acco, 1984), 153–69. Another Belgian medical institution founded in the mid nineteenth century was the Superior Health Council (1849), see E. Bruyneel and L. Dhaene, *Le Conseil Supérieur de la Santé (1849–2009): trait d'union entre la science et la santé publique* (Leuven: Peeters, 2009).
7 I. Meul and R. Schepers, 'De opkomst en consolidering van medische specialisten in België (1857–1957)', *Belgisch Tijdschrift Voor Nieuwste Geschiedenis*, 43:2 (2013), 10–45; G. Marchildon and K. Schrijvers, 'Physician resistance and the forging of public healthcare: a comparative

analysis of the doctors' strikes in Canada and Belgium in the 1960s', *Medical History*, 55 (2011), 203–22.
8 L. Nys, H. de Smaele, J. Tollebeek and K. Wils (eds), *De zieke natie: over de medicalisering van de samenleving 1860–1914* (Groningen: Historische Uitgeverij, 2002); J. Tollebeek, G. Vanpaemel and K. Wils (eds), *Degeneratie in België 1860–1940: een geschiedenis van ideeën en praktijken* (Leuven: Leuven University Press, 2003).
9 K. Wils (ed.), *Het lichaam (m/v)* (Leuven: Leuven University Press, 2001); E. Peeters, *De beloften van het lichaam: een geschiedenis van de natuurlijke levenswijze in België 1890–1940* (Amsterdam: Bert Bakker, 2008); E. Peeters, L. van Molle and K. Wils (eds), *Beyond Pleasure: Cultures of Modern Asceticism* (New York: Berghahn, 2011); De Ganck, *Le sexe, une invention moderne? Histoire des réactions face aux anomalies sexuelles et à l'hermaphrodisme en Belgique contemporaine (1830–1914)* (Brussels: Université des femmes, 2012).
10 T. Claes, *Corpses in Belgian Anatomy, 1860–1914: Nobody's Dead* (Basingstoke: Palgrave Macmillan, 2019); K. Wils, R. De Bont and S. Au, *Bodies Beyond Borders: Moving Anatomies, 1750–1950* (Leuven: University Press, 2017).
11 See, for example, S. Richelle, *Hospices. Une histoire sensible de la vieillesse: Bruxelles, 1830–1914* (Rennes: Presses Universitaires de Rennes, 2019); and J. Vandendriessche, *Zorg en wetenschap. Een geschiedenis van de Leuvense academische ziekenhuizen in de twintigste eeuw* (Leuven: Leuven University Press, 2019).
12 J. Vandendriessche and K. Wils, 'Een traject van onderhandeling. Hygiënisme als wetenschap, Antwerpen 1880–1900', *BMGN: Low Countries Historical Review*, 128:3 (2013), 3–28.
13 Some recent studies include: J. De Ganck, 'Cultiver la différence. Histoire du développement de la gynécologie à Bruxelles (1870–1935)' (PhD diss., Université libre de Bruxelles, 2016); L. Nys, *Van mensen en muizen: Vijftig jaar Nederlandstalige Faculteit Geneeskunde aan de Leuvense universiteit* (Leuven: UPL, 2016); and R. Bardez, 'La Faculté de Médecine de l'Université Libre de Bruxelles: Entre Création, Circulation et Enseignement ses Savoirs (1795–1914)' (PhD diss., Université libre de Bruxelles, 2015). We refer to Chapter 5 in this volume for a discussion of the literature on the history of medical education, to Chapters 6 and 7 for an overview of Belgian hospital history and to Chapter 1 for a discussion of historical studies on gynaecology in Belgium.
14 B. Majerus, *Parmi les fous. Une histoire sociale de la psychiatrie au 20e siècle* (Rennes: PUR, 2013).

15 On public health reformers and their networks, see, for example, N. Randeraad, 'Triggers of mobility: international congresses (1840–1914) and their visitors', *Jahrbuch für Europäische Geschichte/European History Yearbook*, 16 (2015), 63–82. On international networks of colonial doctors and missionaries, see, for example, S. Au, 'Medical orders: Catholic and Protestant missionary medicine in the Belgian Congo', *BMGN: Low Countries Historical Review*, 132:1 (2017), 62–82.

16 When it comes to synthesising historical knowledge and moving beyond the level of the case study, Robert Kohler and Kathryn Olesko make a plea for such mid-level analysis instead of composing a new 'big picture'. See R. E. Kohler and K. M. Olesko, 'Introduction: Clio meets science', *Osiris*, 27:1 (1 January 2012), 1–16.

17 M. Beyen and B. Majerus, 'Weak and strong nations in the Low Countries: national historiography and its "others" in Belgium, Luxembourg, and the Netherlands in the nineteenth and twentieth centuries', in *The Contested Nation: Ethnicity, Class, Religion and Gender in National Histories*, ed. S. Berger and C. Lorenz (Basingstoke: Palgrave Macmillan, 2008), 283–310.

18 For a nuanced discussion of municipalism in Belgium, see M. van Ginderachter, 'An urban civilization: the case of municipal autonomy in Belgian history 1830–1914', in *Nationalism and the Reshaping of Urban Communities in Europe, 1848–1914*, ed. W. Whyte and O. Zimmer (London: Palgrave, 2011), 110–30.

19 *Onzième rapport sur la situation des asiles d'aliénés du Royaume (1874–1876)* (Brussels: Fr. Gobbaerts, 1878), 8.

20 P. Heyrman, 'Catholic private poor relief and the state in 19th-century Belgium: reconquest, competition and complementarity' (forthcoming); V. Viaene, *Belgium and the Holy See from Gregory XVI to Pius IX (1831–1859): Catholic Revival, Society and Politics in 19th-Century Europe* (Leuven: Leuven University Press, 2001), 177.

21 Au, 'Medical orders'.

22 G. Vanthemsche, *Belgium and the Congo, 1885–1980* (New York: Cambridge University Press, 2012), 67.

23 For a recent historiographical overview, see A. Jusseaume, P. Marquis and M. Rossigneux-Meheust, 'Le soin comme relation sociale: bilan historiographique et nouvelles perspectives', *Histoire, médecine et santé*, 7 (15 November 2015), 9–15; and R. L. Numbers and D. W. Amundsen, *Caring and Curing: Health and Medicine in the Western Religious Traditions* (Baltimore, MD: Johns Hopkins University Press, 1998).

24 B. M. Wall, *Into Africa: A Transnational History of Catholic Medical Missions and Social Change* (New Brunswick, NJ: Rutgers University

Press, 2015); B. Mann Wall, *Unlikely Entrepreneurs: Catholic Sisters and the Hospital Marketplace, 1865–1925* (Columbus: Ohio State University Press, 2005), 5.

25 In the international historiography, much more attention has been paid to such subjects. See, for example, M. Stolberg, *A History of Palliative Care, 1500–1970: Concepts, Practices, and Ethical Challenges* (Cham: Springer International, 2017).

26 On religious congregations in Québec, see A. Charles and F. Guérard, 'Les religieuses hospitalières du Québec au XXe siècle: une main d'œuvre active à l'échelle international', in *L'incontournable caste des femmes: Histoire des services de santé au Québec et au Canada*, ed. M.-C. Thifault (Ottawa: Presses de l'Université d'Ottawa, 2012), 79–102.

27 M. Mormont, 'Régionalisation, bonne pour la santé', *Alter Échos*, 377 (2014), 29–32.

28 Historians have, for example, written the political history of Belgium 'from below'. See M. van Ginderachter, *The Everyday Nationalism of Workers: A Social History of Modern Belgium* (Palo Alto, CA: Stanford University Press, 2019); M. van Ginderachter and M. Beyen, *Nationhood from Below: Europe in the Long Nineteenth Century* (Basingstoke: Palgrave Macmillan, 2012).

29 J. Vandendriessche, 'Turning journals into encyclopaedias: medical editorship and reprinting in the Low Countries (1815–1860)', *Centaurus*, 62:1 (2020), 82–97; J. Vandendriessche, 'Setting scientific standards: publishing in medical societies in nineteenth-century Belgium', *Bulletin of the History of Medicine*, 88:4 (2014), 626–53.

30 E. Andersen, 'De Société de Médecine Mentale de Belgique in transnationaal perspectief (1869–1900)', *BTNG-RBHC: Journal of Belgian History*, 47:4 (2017), 50–84; Vandendriessche, *Medical Societies and Scientific Culture*, 250–78.

31 B. Majerus, 'La désinstitutionnalisation psychiatrique: un phénomène introuvable en Belgique dans les années 1960 et 1970?', in *La fin de l'asile? Histoire de la déshospitalisation psychiatrique dans le monde francophone*, ed. A. Klein, H. Guillemain and M.-C. Thifault (Rennes: Presses Universitaires de Rennes, 2017), 143–55.

32 P.-Y. Saunier, 'The next big thing … historians, let us all be Belgians! A few comments about Belgium's heuristic power', *Journal of Belgian History*, 4 (2014), 150–4.

33 For example Brussels (1899), the first International Congress on Radiology and Ionization, Liège (1905), the first International

Congress of Pedology, Brussels (1911), the first International Congress of Catholic Physicians, Brussels (1935), etc.
34 C. Verbruggen, D. Laqua and G. Deneckere, 'Belgium on the move: transnational history and the belle époque', *Revue Belge de Philologie et d'Histoire*, 90 (2012), 1219; D. Laqua, *The Age of Internationalism and Belgium, 1880–1930: Peace, Progress and Prestige* (Manchester: Manchester University Press, 2013); N. Randeraad, *States and Statistics in the Nineteenth Century: Europe by Numbers* (Manchester: Manchester University Press, 2010).
35 M. Mertens and G. Lachenal, 'The history of "Belgian" tropical medicine from a cross-border perspective', *Revue Belge de Philologie et d'Histoire*, 90:4 (2012), 1249–71.
36 Beyen and Majerus, 'Weak and strong nations'.
37 Sophie Richelle's work on care for elderly people in public institutions in Brussels forms an exception, see Richelle, *Hospices*. A historiography as reflected in the chapters 'Childhood and Adolescence' and 'Medicine and Old Age' in the *Oxford Handbook of the History of Medicine*, ed. M. Jackson (Oxford: Oxford University Press, 2011) is lacking for Belgium.
38 See, for example, I. Devos and A. Janssens (eds), 'Reconsidering the Burden of Disease in the Low Countries in Past Centuries', special issue of *Low Countries Journal of Social and Economic History* 14:4 (2017); and I. Devos, *Allemaal beestjes: mortaliteit en morbiditeit in Vlaanderen, 18de-20ste Eeuw* (Ghent: Academia Press, 2006).
39 We refer here, for example, to the historiography of cancer developed by Ilana Löwy, Carsten Timmermann, David Cantor and Elizabeth Toon, among others. Belgian scholars, however, have not engaged in writing disease histories or 'biographies' of disease as have been published in the series of Johns Hopkins University Press or Oxford University Press over the past decades.
40 Scarce examples of such research are the work by Anne-Hilde van Baal on homeopathy and Evert Peeters on Catholics' openness to more holistic approaches to medicine such as hydropathy. See A.-H. van Baal, *In Search of a Cure: The Patients of the Ghent Homoeopathic Physician Gustave A. van den Berghe (1837–1902)* (Rotterdam: Erasmus, 2008); and E. Peeters, *De beloften van het lichaam: een geschiedenis van de natuurlijke levenswijze in België, 1890–1940* (Amsterdam: Bakker, 2008). For a more elaborate discussion of the relation between orthodox medicine, alternative healers and the public, see Chapter 9 in this volume.

41 A counterexample to this observation is the role played by physicians in the splitting up of the University of Leuven in the 1960s, an event with nationwide political consequences. See J. Vandendriessche and L. Nys, 'Expansion through separation: the linguistic conflicts at the University of Leuven in the 1960s from a medical history perspective', *BMGN: Low Countries Historical Review*, 132:1 (2017), 38–61.
42 A. Bacopoulos-Viau and A. Fauvel, 'The patient's turn: Roy Porter and psychiatry's tales, thirty years on', *Medical History*, 60:1 (January 2016), 1–18.

Part I

Beyond the nation state

1

Medicine, health and gender

Jolien Gijbels and Kaat Wils *

In 1875, the entrance of women to the medical profession was discussed in the Belgian parliament. Along with discussions within medical societies, this public debate is an important source to study gendered views about women's involvement in medicine. About three-quarters of a century before women's suffrage was fully granted in Belgium, it was evident that women were not allowed at the negotiating table. Such public discussions thus pose a methodological challenge for historians who study the intersections of gender and medicine and aim to give women a voice. Due to a scarcity of personal documents and publications by female healthcare professionals and feminists, it remains a challenge to work with a corpus of sources in which men's voices dominate.

The parliamentary debate of 1875 took place in the aftermath of international developments in favour of women's access to medical studies; the American Elizabeth Blackwell being the first woman who, in 1849, obtained a medical degree. In the margin of a debate on a bill that was to regulate the awarding of academic degrees, the liberal deputy Eudore Pirmez suggested to offer women access to at least some branches of the medical profession. Pirmez's plea consisted of different types of arguments. He started by referring to the natural capacities of women to fully devote themselves to the care for others, a degree of dedication that men rarely attained. The availability of women physicians would also lower the barriers for women to consult a doctor when confronted with intimate medical issues, as concerns with indecency would no longer be at play, Pirmez argued. At the end of his plea he referred to the American situation, where more than three hundred women doctors proved to be talented and successful practitioners. 'Physicians will agree with me,' he continued, 'that there are no anatomical or physiological differences between American and

Belgian men and women, and hence no reasons to continue to organise the medical field in a different way.'[1]

Parliamentary opinions on Pirmez's proposal were divided and it was decided to ask the four Belgian universities and the Royal Academy of Medicine for advice. Responses were mainly negative.[2] The most elaborate arguments against women's entrance in the profession came from the Academy. In a lengthy discussion in which in fact all participants agreed, Pirmez's three main arguments were reversed. Women's nature was indeed inclined to care for others, but it was precisely her nature that made her physically, intellectually and emotionally unfit for both the studies and the hard profession of medicine. Women's bodies and minds were mainly, and naturally so, determined and preoccupied by the heavy demands of menstruation, reproduction and lactation. Their nervous system was much more delicate than that of men, as the exclusive occurrence of hysteria among women made clear. In order to become a physician, masculine qualities were needed. The rare woman who by accident succeeded in becoming a doctor, could no longer be considered a woman – she would be 'a virago', a 'monstrous being'.

Academy members also countered Pirmez's argument that women doctors would lower the barrier for female patients to consult a physician. Wasn't it telling, they stated, that while lower-class women relied on female midwives to deliver their babies, more distinguished women, who could not be suspected of having less modesty, all preferred male doctors? Problems of indecency would arise when female students were being exposed to male bodies in the anatomical theatre. And who wanted female students to have to study sperm and syphilis together with male students? Pirmez's reference to the situation abroad was equally turned down. The so-called emancipation of women had indeed advocates in Germany, England, France, Russia and the United States, but should not be seen as a model, on the contrary. Belgium had so far been spared of such aberrations. It was no coincidence that the few women who had applied for an authorisation to exercise the medical profession in Belgium were 'fanatics' from abroad.[3]

The debate of 1875 not only offers an excellent insight in prevailing male opinions on the issue, but it also constitutes a good introduction in the many ways in which gender, health and medicine have been intertwined over the past two centuries. In a first, very explicit way, the discussion dealt with the social division of medical labour. Power relations within the medical field have indeed been structured along class and gender lines, and the definition of both the internal and the external boundaries of the medical profession has often been informed by cultural representations of men's and women's roles and their so-called nature. In the case of the 1875 debate, physicians' elaborate argumentations on the physical and mental inferiority of women point to a second pattern: medical knowledge, medical practices and medically informed discourses have always been gendered. Specific cultural representations of men and women have indeed informed medical knowledge. While nineteenth-century physicians constructed hysteria as a typically female disease associated with women's supposedly natural emotionality, men's mental problems were related to 'manly behaviour' such as violent experiences or sexual excessive activity. Inversely, an apparent gender neutrality could result in inequalities when research, for instance, tended to concentrate on diseases that occur more in men than in women, or when medication was tested exclusively on men. These often invisible but structural historical inequalities have been laid bare by feminist scholars such as Londa Schiebinger and Ilana Löwy; they remain a topical issue within contemporary health research and theory.[4] The explicitly feminist engagement of many scholars points to a third issue, which was also apparent in the 1875 debate, where fear of female emancipation was so obvious. Since the nineteenth century, feminists indeed have included questions of reproduction and health in their social activism. While medicine has often functioned as an instrument of male power over women's bodies, it has also functioned as a space where both women and men could gain more control over their bodies, and the ways in which biological sex and gender relate to each other.

These three interrelated themes – the social division of medical labour, the gendered character of medical knowledge and practice, and feminist activism to claim and redefine the body – will structure this chapter. On each of these themes, an extensive body of literature has appeared since at least the 1970s – and in fact earlier. Substantive studies on, for instance, the history of female physicians did appear as early as 1900.[5] Globally, this historiography has moved from a focus on the underestimated role of women in the field of healthcare to more structural analyses of the gendered nature of knowledge, scientific cultures and medical practices. While path-breaking studies such as Ludmilla Jordanova's *Sexual Visions* (1989) and Alison Bashford's *Purity and Pollution* (1998) demonstrated the interrelatedness of these questions, new and exciting research on more 'classical' topics such as women surgeons in the nineteenth century continues to be done.[6] Here as elsewhere in the field of medical history, scholars based in the United Kingdom and the United States have played an important role in the development of the field.[7] Their studies, which often privilege English-speaking regions, depict historical evolutions which also occurred in Belgium, albeit at a different pace and with different accents, given the long-standing dominance of Catholicism, the slow pace of women's political emancipation and the major role of ideological pillars in the organisation and financing of healthcare. On the contrary, within Belgian historiography there hardly exists a tradition of historical research on intersections of gender and medicine in which these recent historiographical insights and perspectives are incorporated. Whereas female medical practitioners mainly figure in histories of medical professionalisation and medicalisation, the doctoral dissertation of Tommy De Ganck on nineteenth-century gynaecology in Brussels is one of the sole examples of historical scholarship on medicine's role in the production of gendered cultural representations.[8] Feminists' activism to legalise birth control and abortion in Belgium – the third and last theme of this chapter – has received most historical attention, yet their medically informed views remain largely unexplored.

The division of medical labour

In the Southern Netherlands – the region that would become Belgium in 1830 – childbirth was women's work. Officially recognised midwives mainly operated in cities, while unlicensed birth attendants assisted at deliveries in villages. In Belgium, as elsewhere, the medicalisation and professionalisation of midwifery coincided. International historiography has traced how physicians in Europe and the United States increasingly gained control of traditional female birthing practices in the nineteenth century.[9] Early-modern attempts of doctors and surgeons to control (il)legal birth deliveries having been unsuccessful, it was under Dutch rule (1815–30) that medical supervision on the medical practice of childbirth was installed in the Southern Netherlands (see Chapter 5, pp. 177–9). The legal framework of 1818 established the education and practice of midwifery for the nineteenth century. The royal decree of 1823 further determined the organisation of two years of training. Female students mainly had to follow practical courses at an important maternity ward in their province.[10] Similarly to French laws but unlike in the United States and Britain, Dutch legislation recognised midwifery as a distinct field of medical practice.[11] The second part of the nineteenth century witnessed further calls for the improvement of midwifery training. In 1884 these attempts resulted in a royal decree that established stricter admission requirements and a broadening of the curriculum. At a time when the number of official midwives had increased in such a way as to – at least theoretically – replace non-official birth attendants, the sterner requirements for student midwives now slowed down a further growth in an age in which the number of doctors continued to rise.[12]

The professionalisation of midwifery was intertwined with the development of gendered hierarchies limiting the competences of female birth attendants vis-à-vis their male counterparts. The Dutch law of 1818 differentiated between three groups of obstetric practitioners: the doctor of obstetrics, the male midwife and the midwife. Unlike male practitioners, midwives had to confine their practice to 'normal births' that did not require specialised instruments. When confronted with difficult deliveries, they had to call a doctor or a male midwife.[13] Taking such restrictions for midwives into account, historian Karel Velle has argued that the declining social role of midwives almost points at a process of 'deprofessionalisation'.[14] Throughout the nineteenth century the majority of doctors in the Academy of Medicine and in the provincial medical commissions, which supervised medical practice and advised the government on matters of public health, continued to defend such a gendered division of labour. The medical debate in the Belgian Academy in the 1870s on a proposition introduced by the physicians Hyacinthe Kuborn and Louis Mascart is exemplary in this respect. The proposition put forward the authorisation for midwives to use forceps when confronted with an emergency situation and an absence of doctors. Both physicians mainly argued that such an extension of midwives' competences was necessary since midwives often stood alone in the countryside. It would, moreover, be an effective means to combat illegal birthing practices that mainly took place outside the cities. Most doctors disagreed, among other things arguing that midwives were ignorant and disposed of weak intellectual capabilities. Finally, in 1879, the proposition was rejected by the majority of academy members and midwives' access to the forceps was formally prohibited.[15] In 1908, a law that replaced the law of 1818 confirmed the supposedly limited competences of midwives.[16] Recurring arguments about women's 'ignorance' and medical debates about midwives' insecure financial position make clear that social inequality was constructed on the intersection of gender and class hierarchies. Recently, however, historians have argued that studies privileging these medical sources have exaggerated the precarious social status of midwifery. Research into the social background of female birth attendants in Belgium has shown that while midwives operated within local communities of poor people, they themselves often originated from and married within the social environment of skilled laborers.[17] Moreover, the fees midwives charged for a delivery were not necessarily different from what a doctor received for a delivery and were equivalent to what a day labourer earned in two to four working days.[18]

While male doctors solidified their dominance over the nineteenth-century domain of childbirth, nursing was an almost exclusively female domain consisting mainly of women religious (see Chapter 2, pp. 69–71). The first training programmes emerged in the context of tense ideological debate in the 1880s on the nursing competences of women religious. Early initiatives for lay nurses in the liberal settings of Liège and Brussels were followed by Catholic training programmes after 1900. Historians and feminists have often explained this gendered division of labour by underlining the hierarchy between caring and curing. Caring tasks of nursing were traditionally associated with 'female' maternal qualities, while the responsibility of curing patients belonged to the male-dominated field of medicine.[19] In Belgium, as elsewhere, representations of the profession of nursing were indeed peppered with gendered notions of maternal care, altruistic dedication and female compassion.[20] Recently, however, historians also challenged these gendered notions of care by paying more attention to the practices and discourses of male nurses who were most clearly visible in psychiatric hospitals.[21] The Belgian mental institutions of the Brothers of Charity, for instance, were almost all-male spaces, both in terms of patients and nurses. A first exploration of the Brothers of Charity's journal for nurses has shown that existing gender ideals informed the construction of a professional identity. 'Male' characteristics such as discipline and physical strength were associated with the care for mentally ill patients. At the same time, however, male nurses were also described as 'mothers' who cared for their children: the – equally male – patients.[22] Outside psychiatric settings, male nurses were present as well. About 30 per cent of the first generations of qualified nurses were men.[23] The gendered discourse on these nurses awaits research.

In the twentieth century, the position of Belgian independent midwives who assisted at home deliveries was increasingly threatened by the rapid professionalisation of nursing, on the one hand, and the medicalisation of giving birth in hospitals, on the other. The first process was accelerated by the development of midwifery as a specialisation within the nursing training programme as of 1951.[24] The medicalisation of birth comprised the isolation of birthing women in hospital delivery rooms, the introduction of new medical technologies and the increasing use of anaesthesia during deliveries.[25] In most countries – the Netherlands being a notable exception – the medicalisation of childbirth implied an increasing employment of midwives in hospital settings, where they were put in a subordinate position to physicians.[26] A Belgian law of 1944 promoted deliveries in maternity clinics by offering mothers a compensation for all costs within the first ten days of a hospitalised stay, while home deliveries by midwives were not covered. Shortly afterwards, independent midwives were allowed to assist at deliveries in maternity departments. As a result, midwives preferred a paid employment in hospitals above poorly paid self-employment. From 2,513 independent midwives in 1900, there remained around 80 in 2000.[27] The profession of midwifery remains a remarkably stable 'feminine' domain. In contrast to the domains of medicine and nursing, very few men practise midwifery at present. In France, for instance, there has been an increase of male students since the profession was opened to men in 1982, yet the actual number of male practitioners remains limited. In Belgium, male midwives also form a minority. In 2017, about 1 per cent of the qualified Belgian midwives were men.[28]

Testimonies of midwives themselves complicate the dominant narrative of medicalisation. In contrast to France, where historians have been able to integrate the professional experiences of midwives into their work,[29] Belgium disposes of only a couple of oral and written testimonies of female birth attendants and their family members in the nineteenth and twentieth century.[30] The few available testimonies display a more balanced view of being an independent midwife in the countryside before, during and after the Second World War. Their socially vulnerable position – low wages, hard work and stressful situations – was definitely an important facet of their lives. Yet, the testimonies also show expressions of commitment and a high internal motivation. Midwives took pride in the many roles they fulfilled and for which they were recognised and appreciated in their community. Those who worked among large poor families, for instance, did additional tasks as social workers by providing them with material help and advice. Midwives in rural territories hardly ever called upon doctors, except when medical intervention was necessary.[31] Moreover, recent research based on witness statements of unqualified midwives in the context of court cases on infanticide and the illegal practice of medicine suggests that in urban contexts collaborations between doctors and (unqualified) midwives sometimes occurred until the beginning of the twentieth century.[32]

Since the 1990s, the existing power hierarchies between physicians and midwives have been challenged. In 1994, a European law determined that midwives were qualified to assist deliveries autonomously and decide whether it was necessary to call a doctor. At the same time Belgian midwives adopted new roles in counselling future parents. They opened the first birth centres, providing for prenatal consultations, workshops, specific courses and information sessions. There, they offered their services by giving parents information and care before, during and after home deliveries.[33] For the setting up of these birth centres midwives looked for inspiration abroad – the Netherlands, Scandinavia, Britain and the United States – where home deliveries were more common.[34]

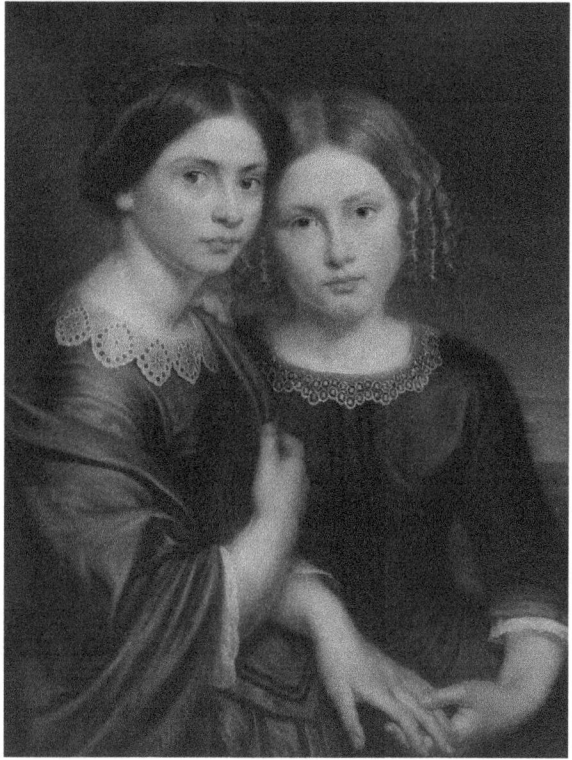

Figure 1.1 Painting of Isala van Diest by Pierre-Joseph Steger, ca. 1855.

In contrast with the professions of midwifery and nursing, the field of medicine was for a long time closed to women. From an international perspective, Belgian medical education opened up quite late. Medical schools in Switzerland and France admitted women early on in the 1860s. The first woman to receive a French medical degree was the British Elizabeth Garrett, who had been unsuccessful in her attempts to enter a British medical school.[35] In Belgium too, Isala van Diest had been denied access in Leuven in 1873. She went to Bern, where she took her degree in 1877 (Figure 1.1). Garrett and Van Diest fit in a broader pattern of the first generations of female students who studied abroad.

Around the same time, an initiative offering a minimal medical education to women was launched by the Brussels doctor Constant

Crommelinck. In 1875 he opened a 'free school of medicine' that offered female students a two-year elementary training in 'natural medicine' consisting of weekly conferences.[36] This initiative was, however, short-lived and remained marginal vis-à-vis mainstream medicine. In 1880, the right of women to enter academic studies would be recognised, although Van Diest had to wait until 1884 to be allowed to exercise her profession in Belgium and it would take another six years, until 1890, before the access of women to the medical profession was regulated. In 1887 the first female student, Clémence Everart, started at the Free University of Brussels. Soon other students followed in Brussels, Liège and Ghent, while the Catholic University of Leuven would only welcome female students from 1920 onwards.

Yet, it was too early for a real influx of women into medical studies, as there were hardly any secondary schools that provided girls the required qualifications to enter university. On the eve of the First World War, 27 Belgian women physicians had received medical qualifications out of a total of more than 4,400 Belgian physicians.[37] This was a small number, also in comparison with the number of foreign female students who studied in Belgium. In the twentieth century, the number of female students enrolled in medicine increased gradually, with an acceleration in the 1960s. After 1970 male enrolment started to decline, which resulted in a majority of female medical students as of 1990.[38]

Little is known about the experiences of the first women physicians in Belgium. The few interviews that historian Denise Keymolen conducted with physicians in the 1970s indicate that the first female students were approached as equals by fellow male students.[39] It took longer for women to become accepted as medical practitioners. Prejudices about women's 'limited capabilities' among doctors and patients hindered the efforts of the very first female doctors to run an independent medical practice. In an interview published in the Brussels liberal newspaper *La Réforme*, Isala van Diest testified to her difficulties with setting up her own practice. She started working in a refuge for prostitutes, which probably damaged her reputation among bourgeois families. Her later private practice mainly attracted British and American female patients who were more used to women doctors.[40] A sociological study of the professional life of graduates of the Catholic University of Leuven in the first half of the twentieth century confirms that most of the sick in a hospital or sanatorium preferred a man above a woman when first encountering their doctor.[41] There were, however, exceptions. At the end of the nineteenth century, doctor Marie Derscheid not only attracted numerous patients, but she also participated in (male) scientific sociability and was a member of the editorial board of the *Journal Médical de Bruxelles*.[42] Yet, her success was probably partly made possible thanks to her marriage with the notable physician and Brussels professor in medicine, Albert Delcour. More generally, family networks have been important for many 'first' women doctors. It was probably no coincidence that Belgium's first female doctor, Isala van Diest, was the daughter of a doctor.[43]

In 1921, Derscheid would become the first president of the Belgian Federation of University Women (Fédération Belge Des Femmes Universitaires).[44] The Belgian Federation was one of the many women's organisations in Europe that arose following the birth in 1919 of the International Federation of University Women (IFUW), a British–American initiative aimed at the formation of a female educated elite and the promotion of ideals of peace and progress. In those early years, doctors formed the largest professional group within the Belgian Federation. As of 1922 they participated in conferences of the Medical Women's International Association (1919), where critical reflections were made on the need for international cooperation and female empowerment within each country. Members combined their efforts to achieve equality of women physicians within the medical profession with broader claims for women's professional rights.[45]

Despite these efforts, women doctors continued to struggle with career opportunities throughout the twentieth century. The difficult entrance of female researchers to medical faculties is a case in point. At Ghent University, as of 1900, women were allowed to specialise after their general medical training, yet their efforts to continue an academic career remained fruitless. Unspoken gendered divisions in academia discouraged women to aspire to a position in high academic ranks.[46] Yvonne Desirant, for instance, who in the interwar period succeeded in becoming first assistant ('chef de travaux') at Ghent University, later testified that she had never hoped for a career as a professor. There were, however, differences between universities: while in Ghent the medical faculty appointed a female professor, Irène van der Bracht, in 1925, this would take another forty years in Leuven. Yet Van der Bracht had no medical training and she was appointed to teach educational gymnastics to female students. Early academic recognition of women doctors occurred at the margins of the medical profession.[47]

By contrast, the Belgian colony of Congo seems to have offered new employment opportunities for both men and women (see Chapter 3, pp. 106–20). The demand of medical care rose as the establishment of a series of colonial hospitals in Congo was envisioned. Organisations such as the Union of Belgian Colonial Women (L'Union Des Femmes Coloniales) (1923–40) and later on the Union of Women of the Belgian Congo and Ruanda-Urundi (L'Union des Femmes du Congo Belge et du Ruanda-Urundi) promoted colonial employment for women.[48] However, as articles in the journal of this latter organisation indicate, women were expected to practise 'essentially feminine' medical professions such as midwifery and nursing.[49] The case of sister Marie Guido – known by the local population as 'the mother doctor' – is a counterexample showing that religious congregations could empower female religious doctors. Marie Guido obtained her medical degree in the 1940s and worked in the Congolese locality of Musienene, where she performed medical operations such as caesarean sections and amputations.[50]

Women's entrance into the medical profession was not only a slow process, it was also marked by disciplinary hierarchies. Women gained access most easily to disciplines such as paediatrics and gynaecology, which were considered to be 'natural' fields of specialisation for women in and beyond Belgium, while 'masculine disciplines' such as surgery, urology and orthopaedics remained highly closed to them. In a recent interview, Ilse Kerremans recalled the patronising words of fellow male colleagues when she started a specialisation in surgery in the 1970s.[51] Up until today the medical profession is marked by gendered divisions of labour and prestige. Telling in this respect is the underrepresentation of women in the numbers of professors at Belgian medical faculties.[52]

The gendering of medical knowledge and medical practices

From the 1990s onwards scholars have shown the role of modern biomedicine in the production of ideas about men's and women's 'nature'. Thomas Laqueur's famous (and heavily debated) study *Making Sex* (1990), for instance, has highlighted the naturalisation of sexual difference since the end of the eighteenth century.[53] Enlightenment brought about the dominant view of the so-called two-sex model, which accentuated fundamental sexual difference. Corporeal and physiological observations of female genitals increasingly served as evidence of the 'natural' roles of women as housewives and mothers. As Ornella Moscucci and others have shown, the nineteenth-century discipline of gynaecology provided a scientific basis for these cultural ideas about maternity and femininity.[54] Contrary to existing medical disciplines that took the male body as a model for men and women, gynaecology was designed to study woman's distinctive physical and mental characteristics through a focus on her reproductive functions. It became the 'science of woman'. A similar discipline devoted to men's sexual organs – andrology – arose only during the second half of the twentieth century.

Contrary to international trends, the Belgian gynaecological profession developed rather late. From the 1860s on, gynaecology acquired a status in most large cities as an autonomous specialty based on the first successes of modern surgery. In this context practitioners favoured an interventionist surgical approach to alleviate disorders in women.[55] In Belgium, gynaecology emerged twenty years later with the establishment of a scientific gynaecological society (1889) and the organisation of the first clinical courses at the state universities of Liège and Ghent.[56] In the 1890s, private hospitals were set up, and in collaboration with the universities specialised services in public hospitals were established. At this time the study of women's diseases was not necessarily identified with the older branch of obstetrics. Belgian universities provided students with a general medical training in medicine, surgery and obstetrics, after which doctors could specialise in women's pathologies through professional and scientific activities. In line with the international trend, gynaecological services in the public hospitals existed separately from the older obstetric services. While midwives and obstetricians in maternity wards took care of women's deliveries, gynaecologists concentrated on diseases centred in the sexual system of women and problems following childbirth or medical abortion. To treat 'women's diseases' they employed both methods preserving women's fertility, such as the use of pessaries and curettage, and radical surgical therapies such as ovariotomy and hysterectomy, the surgical removal of the ovaries and the uterus. In Brussels, the focus of these early gynaecologists on abdominal surgery is exemplified by the placement of the first gynaecological service in an operating room.[57]

At the time of the institutionalisation of gynaecology, biological sex differences increasingly marked discourses in medicine and society. Belgian physicians started to accentuate women's social mission as mothers by relating this mission to their 'nature'. In this way doctors also came up with an answer to existing medical and political anxieties regarding the so-called degeneration of the Belgian nation. In the second half of the nineteenth century, degeneration was considered to be a process of degradation from a physical, psychological and moral point of view. According to degeneration theories, degenerated persons could contaminate healthy citizens through social interaction and sexual intercourse. Belgian and other physicians became fascinated by heredity and accentuated women's reproductive 'essence' as a vital instrument to safeguard the survival and health of future generations.[58] Unlike in France, population decline was not yet at stake before 1900, but it soon afterwards became an element of medical concern. Within the same context, Belgian physicians and politicians would start to actively intervene in the domain of infant care after the First World War.[59] Gendered medicalised discourses equally marked reformatory politics. In response to the growing social protest of workers in the 1880s, ideals of home-centred maternity as a weapon against social disorder and immorality were promoted by political elites. Belgium's first social legislation bore traces of this medicalised and gendered perspective. As of 1889, girls younger than twenty-one were forbidden to work in the mines and female workers who had given birth were obliged to stay at home for four weeks, without any financial compensation.[60]

Medically informed ideals of women's important social roles as mothers were often countered by reality. The clientele of Brussels gynaecologists in public hospitals mainly consisted of poor women suffering from the physical effects of numerous successive pregnancies. These labouring women had neither the time nor the money to undergo a long gynaecological treatment. The research of Tommy De Ganck on gynaecology in the Brussels hospitals, where prostitutes and other working women were provided with free care, has shown that social inequalities determined doctor's choice for radical treatments. To cure women who were incapable of working because of pelvic pain, physicians easily turned to the surgical removal of their ovaries and uterus, rather than investing in time-consuming and costly treatments that were offered to bourgeois women in private clinics. As this example shows, class differences often intersected with gender hierarchies, reinforcing each other.[61]

The case of ovariotomy is interesting from a different perspective as well, as it testifies to the role of medicine in producing 'female' pathologies and mental disorders.[62] For the first time successfully performed in 1809 in the United States, the operation initially aimed at extirpating ovarian tumours. Starting in the 1870s, however, Anglo-Saxon surgeons also executed ovariotomies to amputate healthy ovaries of women who experienced mental problems.[63] In Belgium and elsewhere in Europe it was also common to explain the causes of mental illness by referring to a woman's defective reproductive physiology – among other things menstruation problems or specific injuries to the genitals. 'Hysteria', an umbrella term that was continuously redefined throughout history, was sexualised as a 'female' disease. It was linked with all sorts of deviant behaviour.[64] Doctors therefore believed women could be cured by using localised genital therapies, of which ovariotomy was a radical example. Contrary to physicians in the United States and Britain, however, most Belgian gynaecologists were sceptical about ovariotomy as a treatment for non-gynaecological complaints. The research of Tommy De Ganck has shown that there is little evidence of actual operations for the purpose of curing hysteria in Belgium. By the time that ovariotomy became a regular operation in Belgium – the first known successful surgical removal of a cyst took place in 1870 – gynaecological explanations for hysteria had lost ground in international medical circles.[65]

Belgian and other doctors had instead adopted the neurological explanation of hysteria by the French doctor Jean-Martin Charcot in the 1880s. Years of clinical observations had convinced Charcot that both men and women could experience hysteria. His first descriptions of hysteria in adult men were highly controversial in the medical world. Notwithstanding this inclusion of men, Charcot's published case studies do reveal the gendered nature of his diagnoses. Women were not only diagnosed much more frequently with hysteria than men, but his etiological theory differed for men and women. The neurologist mostly applied the hysteria diagnosis to males who had undergone traumatic physical accidents at work. Hysteria among women, on the other hand, was the result of an overpowering emotional experience in domestic settings. Moreover, erotic antics of several female hysterics clearly reveal a sexual component.[66] Like French physicians, Belgian doctors diagnosed hysteria with men who had undergone physical trauma such as soldiers, a topic that appeared in the medical press in 1888. While Belgian military neurologists did not often refer to the traumatic effects of war in their own work, they did refer to foreign studies on the devastating psychological effect of traumatic war experiences. During the First World War, this type of psychological disorder would become known as 'shell shock' (see Chapter 8, pp. 298–300).[67] In contrast, hysteria, depression and melancholy in women was related to their 'emotional' nature.[68] Sexualised representations of female hysterics would remain visible in popular museum exhibitions, such as the travelling Spitzner Museum, where wax figures represented hysterical women.[69]

For both men and women, a healthy sex life within marriage was seen as the main solution to cope with mental problems. It follows that physicians were concerned about sexual behaviour that departed from this ideal, such as sexual abstinence, promiscuity and masturbation. While abstinence was associated with frigid upper-class women, physicians pathologised excessive sexual activity and masturbation among men. In Great Britain those men were regularly diagnosed with spermatorrhea.[70] The disease, with an excessive loss of sperm as the main symptom, was understood to elicit, among other things, anxiety, nervousness and impotence. It is unclear to what extent spermatorrhea determined medical practice in Belgium, yet research has shown that masturbation and sexual excess were seen as causes for mental illness in men.[71]

Excessive sexual behaviour was also seen as a major cause of the spread of venereal diseases. Prostitutes in particular were held accountable for this, even though they were increasingly perceived not only as seductresses, but also as victims. In Belgian debates on the problems of prostitution in the army – an all-male space – inebriety was seen as part of the problem.[72] Physicians argued that alcohol made soldiers more susceptible to both careless sexual behaviour and infections.⁷³ As elsewhere, Belgian regulations on alcohol and prostitution were supposed to prevent the outbreak of diseases. In Brussels, the first Belgian city to regulate prostitution in 1844, registered prostitutes were subjected to medical examination twice a week. In case of sickness, they were isolated in hospitals until they recovered. In other Belgian cities similar medical procedures were introduced. In 1948 – after more than fifty years of political protest – the system of forced medical supervision was abolished.⁷⁴

The gynaecological examinations also point at an issue that was at the heart of the discipline of gynaecology in Belgium and abroad. Physicians were concerned about the chastity of 'respectable' women. While prostitutes were not considered to be modest, visual examinations of the private parts of middle-class women were seen as offensive to women's sexual pudency. Especially the reintroduction of the speculum in medical practice from 1820 onwards aroused international moral concerns over the exposure of respectable women's bodies to visual inspection (Figure 1.2). Until the end of the century, gynaecologists preferred other tactile procedures above ocular examinations.⁷⁵ Concerns about modesty also influenced the management of hospital spaces, where sexual segregation was to protect female dignity. In the 1900s in the public hospitals of Brussels, for instance, gynaecological consultations were held at specific times as to prevent the presence of male patients. Private rooms for surgery and curtains were installed for the same purpose.⁷⁶

In the interwar years, the medical protection of maternity took on a new dimension. In this period, stagnating infant and maternal mortality rates were seen as a problem for the survival of the nation by physicians and politicians alike. Belgian physicians for the first time linked the survival of children with the health of women during the whole process of pregnancy. Prenatal consultations for future mothers were therefore installed in hospitals and maternity departments.⁷⁷ As in Great Britain, this political climate of scrutinising and pathologising pregnancy seems to have facilitated the unification of gynaecology and obstetrics in hospitals and universities. The law of 1957 officially reunited and recognised gynaecology and obstetrics as one specialty along with other specialties in Belgium. Little is known, however, about the specific reasons for the rapprochement between the two disciplines.⁷⁸

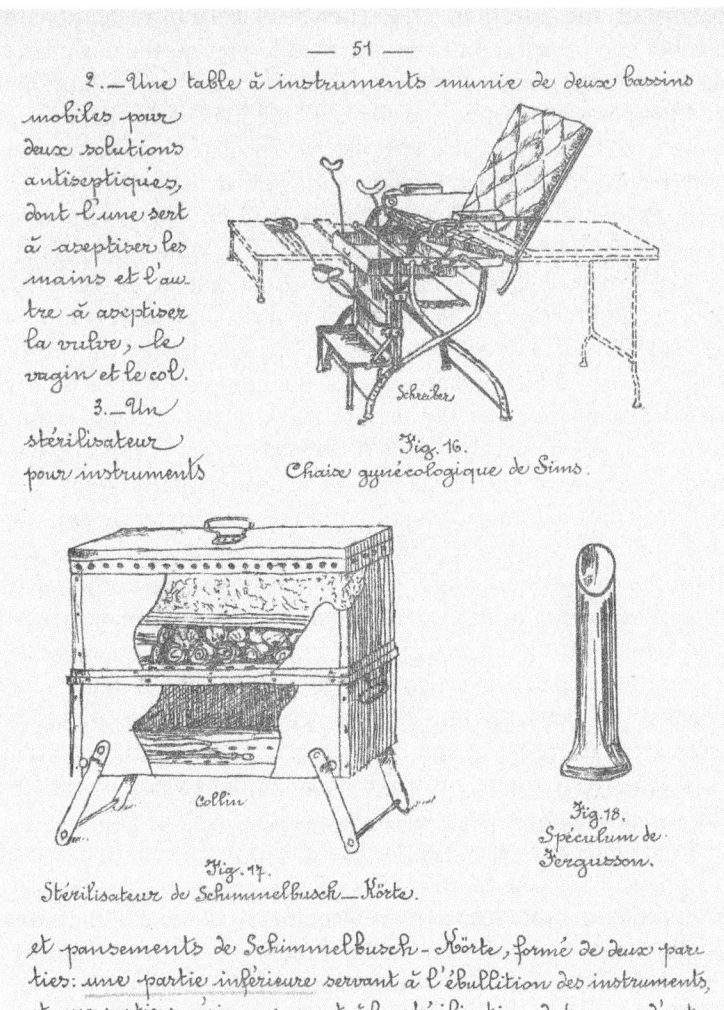

Figure 1.2 Images of gynaecological objects in the handbook of Rufin Schockaert, *Précis du cours de gynécologie* (Leuven: Feyaerts, 1913), p. 51.

The twentieth-century history of Belgian medical specialisation is a promising avenue of future research. With the exception of a recent study of the Leuven academic hospitals, it has mainly been researched from a legal perspective.[79]

In the same context of pro-natalist policies, Belgian gynaecologists made an important contribution to a moralising sexualised discourse regarding birth planning. Different from other countries, Belgian gynaecologists, such as the Leuven professor Rufin Schockaert, undertook a leading role in promoting a Catholic vision on sexuality. According to this vision, reproduction was the sole purpose of marriage, implying the condemnation of birth control and contraception (see Chapter 2, pp. 82–4). The scant Belgian literature on this subject has revealed the dominance of Catholic approaches in twentieth-century medicine,[80] and medico-ethical debates on infertility.[81] Neo-Malthusianism – the movement that originated in Great Britain in the 1870s and aimed at expanding knowledge on and the dissemination of contraceptives – had limited success in Belgium. Historians have explained this by referring to the condemnation of the movement by Belgian church representatives, legal opposition by Catholics and socialists and the mobilisation of Catholic doctors and midwives against abortion and birth control.[82] Small organised neo-Malthusian movements emerged after 1900. These organisations consisted of a limited number of liberals and a stronger representation of socialist members, including some prominent socialist doctors such as Fernand Mascaux.[83]

Feminism and bodily self-determination

Birth control and related questions were also explicit concerns of the first and in particular the second wave of organised feminism in Belgium, and of women's activism throughout the twentieth century. Actors involved in political debates about women's rights had to fight against stereotypical, often medically legitimised views about women's moral and physical weaknesses and their incapacity to assume various social roles. An exemplary legal dispute in this respect is the so-called Popelin Affair of 1888. In that year Marie Popelin claimed the right to practise as a lawyer in court. Having obtained a doctoral degree in law she was refused to take the oath as an attorney. She decided to challenge this decision legally. In its refusal of Popelin's request, the court of appeal used a language that was interspersed with sexualised visions of women. The battles and hard work of the bar were considered incompatible with women's nature and their social mission in the household. Several historians have argued that this decision was partly motivated by the then dominant association between masculinity and the public sphere. To open up the public profession of a lawyer to women was inconceivable. The medical profession by contrast could be linked with 'feminine qualities' of care and with advantages for the modesty of female patients.[84] Notwithstanding this difference, at the time of the Popelin Affair the legal position of women physicians was still uncertain and a matter of dispute in medical and political circles.

The Popelin Affair was the starting point for feminists to organise themselves politically in order to press for legal reforms. Starting from 1892 with the Belgian League for the Rights of Women (Ligue Belge du Droit des Femmes), this and other politically 'neutral' associations were founded, alongside socialist and Catholic women's organisations. Neo-Malthusianism was marginal within first-wave feminism in and beyond Belgium. The socialist feminist Emilie Claeys was one of the only Belgian pioneers who defended the use of contraceptives in the early 1890s. She associated voluntary motherhood with women's emancipation. In the socialist journal *De Vrouw* she published under a pseudonym, whereas the same journal featured some publications on family planning by the Dutch female doctor Aletta Jacobs. These feminist ideas on reproductive self-determination were very contentious, as they radically separated sexuality from reproduction. Many Western European feminists chose to remain silent on the matter and focused instead on themes such as equal political rights, women's education and work.[85]

That does not mean that contraception and abortion were non-existent at that time. Contraceptive methods such as coitus interruptus, sexual abstinence and – since the 1860s – condoms were often used. Abortion, however, remained the most accessible method of birth control. Social and liberal newspapers featured weekly advertisements for self-made abortionists and abortive products. At first, many practitioners were unqualified midwives. At the end of the century, abortion also became the working terrain of doctors. To compete with these physicians, unqualified midwives started to present themselves as experts by adding medically related titles to their names such as 'former intern of hospitals'. Abortionists were rarely convicted for their practices. Despite the penal law of 1867 that criminalised abortion, illegal abortionists were not actively pursued.[86] Convictions were also rare in countries such as Britain where criminal law on abortion was among the severest in Europe.[87]

Until the interwar period, Belgian feminists wrote little on the subject of birth control. In their pleas in favour of women's rights, they often reappropriated traditional and biologically based images of gendered differences. For instance, Isabelle Gatti de Gamond, one of the leading Belgian feminists, provided argumentation in favour of specific public roles – teaching, nursing and curing – that were harmonious with women's 'natural' domestic capacities.[88] In line with the political and moral discourse of the time, the aforementioned working-class feminist Claeys promoted birth control by pointing at the well-being of the children and the benefits for a harmonious relationship between wife and husband. Nevertheless, her plea for birth control in the socialist journal *De Vrouw* was so controversial in the 1890s that she risked a legal sentence. After having been accused of maintaining an extramarital relationship, her marginalisation within the socialist and feminist movement came as no surprise.[89] Although more research needs to be done on the topic, it seems that the first generations of female doctors – including those united in the Belgian Federation of University Women – did not publicly engage in favour of women's reproductive rights. The achievement of professional recognition in the male-dominated medical field was probably felt as a more pressing issue.

During the interwar years, it was lone voices who discussed women's reproductive and sexual rights. Referring to contemporary and older sexologists such as Mary Stopes and Henry Havelock Ellis, a handful of self-made sexologists, among whom Marc Lanval and Geert Grub, pleaded for the legalisation of abortion and the female right to sexual pleasure. They advocated female sexual liberation by opposing a bourgeois anti-physical masculinity. According to them, the sexual taboo had caused men to hide their sexuality in the nineteenth century. By contrast, the 'new man' was responsible for the sexual satisfaction of his wife. For women this implied that they had equal rights to sexual pleasure. At the same time, however, the discourse of Lanval and Grub was marked by nineteenth-century biological and social hierarchies between men and women.[90]

Nevertheless, the ideas of the sexologists on abortion and sexuality were very controversial in the 1920s and 1930s. Fear of population decline led the post-war Belgian governments to pursue pro-natalist policies. In 1923, a law banned the selling, disseminating and advertising of contraceptives and abortion. Maternity-oriented policies connected with the long-standing efforts of the Catholic Church and Catholic doctors to counter the use of contraceptives. For instance, in 1931, the Society of Saint-Luc, an association of Catholic doctors, organised a conference where Catholic doctors along with jurists, philosophers and religious leaders discussed the causes and solutions of the falling birth rate. At the conference, doctors underlined women's role in procreation by pointing at the manifold harmful effects of birth planning. The Leuven physician Schockaert argued that birth control made women sick, which eventually prevented their sexual organs from functioning normally.[91]

Women's movements between 1918 and 1960 were partly encapsulated within maternity-oriented discourses. Especially Catholic feminists but also feminists within socialist women's organisations advocated socio-economic measures that complied with women's role as housewives.[92] From the 1930s onwards, some socialist women such as Vogelina Dille-Lobe and Isabelle Blum took up the theme of 'conscious maternity' and tentatively argued in favour of birth planning. Twenty years later, Dille-Lobe developed into a more ardent advocate of the liberalisation of contraceptives. Gradually, feminist publications placed women's reproductive rights at the heart of the issue of birth control.[93] Socialist women and especially the Socialist's Women Federation (SVV) would also play an important role in sex education. In the 1960s the Belgian Society for Sex Education (Belgische Vereniging voor Seksuele Vorming) (BSSE, 1955) and its French-speaking counterpart La Famille Heureuse (1962) founded consultation bureaus in diverse Belgian cities that provided information on birth control and distributed contraceptives.[94]

Yet, in the 1950s and 1960s the influence of the Catholic Church on sexual morality remained extensive (see Chapter 2, pp. 84–5). The most read literature on sex education was Catholic and progressive voices remained exceptional, as the limited numbers of members of the BSSE show.[95] According to Catholic doctrine, calendar-based methods (which had been improved in the 1930s) were the only accepted form of contraception. Not surprisingly, the contraceptive pill had little success when it was introduced to the Belgian market in 1961. In the beginning, mainly doctors linked to the BSSE and La Famille Heureuse prescribed the pill.[96] Yet, recent research on the Leuven hospitals shows that the contraceptive pill also became an accepted reality among Catholic doctors. In the Leuven hospitals gynaecologists were quite open to women's concern of unwanted pregnancies.[97] Moreover, the devout Catholic gynaecologist Ferdinand Peeters made an important contribution to the development of Anovlar – the successful pill produced by the company Schering AG – out of concern for health problems in women and social strains related to family growth.[98] These shifts have to be understood in relation to more lenient Catholic positions regarding contraception during the papacy of the progressive pope John XXIII (1958–63) and the second Vatican Council (1962–65). In that climate of openness, progressive efforts, such as the medically informed sexology under impulse of the Belgian archbishop Leo Jozef Suenens, were welcomed. Suenens pleaded in favour of a revision of the Catholic doctrine regarding birth control. Pope Paul VI, however, made an end to hopes of reform with *Humanae Vitae* (1968) which reaffirmed the earlier ban on contraception of *Casti Connubii* (1930).[99]

In the 1970s the theme of abortion was taken up by a coalition of new mediagenic feminist movements such as Dolle Mina and Marie Mineur, older movements of socialist women and freethinking doctors linked to centres of family planning. Their pleas for the legalisation of abortion resulted in a first bill for law reform in 1971, which went largely unnoticed in parliament. The arrest of 'abortion doctor' Willy Peers in 1973 served as a catalyst for mobilising both supporters and opponents of abortion (Figure 1.3). Women indeed looked for 'underground' solutions, such as a secret abortion by doctors like Peers in Belgium or 'abortion tourism' in Great Britain and later also the Netherlands.[100] Abortion practices at the academic hospital of Brussels are well documented. At the Catholic academic Leuven hospitals, doctors also performed abortions, for example in the case of severe genetic defects. An institutional policy of secrecy, however, made sure that no publicity was given to such practices.[101]

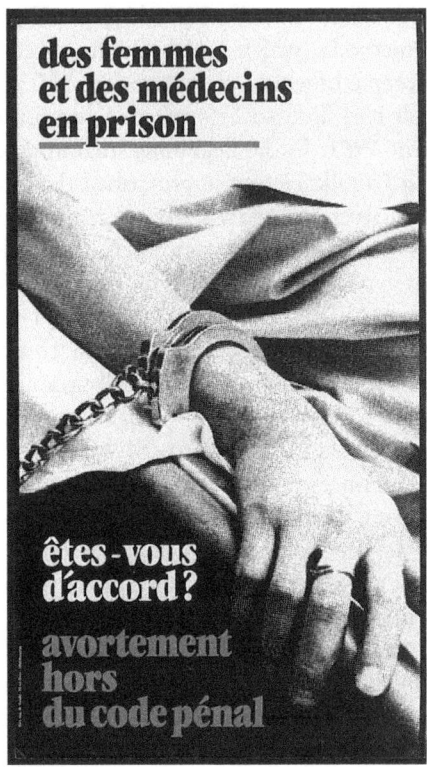

Figure 1.3 Poster in favour of the legalisation of abortion, 1979.

In the first parliamentary discussions on abortion in 1971 and 1973, the traditional parties were completely polarised on the issue. The socialist party was clearly in favour of the liberalisation of abortion, while the Catholic party took the opposite side. As a sort of compromise, in 1973 the government lifted the legal ban on selling and advertising contraceptives. In the following years, the political debate was repeatedly revitalised. Continuing protest of pressure groups, qualitative improvements to the practice of abortion and the rise of actual abortions reinforced the position of proponents of abortion. In the 1980s times had clearly changed. Abortion was more openly discussed in newspapers, on the radio and on television. In medicine there was increasing attention for the patient's right to make informed decisions, an argument that was also present in the political debate on abortion. In politics the advocates of abortion grew in numbers, while the Catholic party became ever more isolated. In 1990 abortion was partially depenalised (until twelve weeks of pregnancy), a measure that was taken quite late compared with several other European countries. In 2018 a further step was undertaken to decriminalise abortion. Previously considered as a criminal offence outside of the legal restrictions of 1990, the clauses on abortion were taken out of the penal code and converted into a specific law on abortion. Up till now the legalisation of abortion remains contested by 'pro-life' groups.[102]

Conclusions

In the last decades a shift in gender identities has occurred. The increasing visibility and achievements of transgender activism and the important role of medicine in answering health concerns of transsexual, transgender and gender non-conforming people invite us to think beyond the persistent gender binary. The historical analysis presented in this chapter shows that notions of femininity and masculinity have in fact never been stable categories. On the intersection of medicine and gender, medical practitioners and feminists have renegotiated gender hierarchies, while medicine as a body of expert knowledge has often participated in the historical construction of gender difference. And it continues to do so, for instance by developing medical aesthetic treatments that reinforce the normativity of Western feminine beauty ideals.

Within Belgian historiography, the field of gender and medicine awaits further research. In traditional sources such as meeting reports of parliament or medical societies the voice of women is mostly absent. Historians' dependence on these sources has for a long time hindered more complex stories of interaction and competition between male and female medical practitioners. In the domain of childbirth, recent research has for instance shown that largely unexplored sources such as witness statements can lead to cases where physicians and (illegal) birth attendants collaborated during deliveries. Together with the few available testimonies on professional experiences, these sources provide us with tools to look at actual practices and bypass top-down narratives of medicalisation and professionalisation. In the same vein, legal sources can illuminate the role of medical knowledge by laywomen. In cases of rape and sexual assault of minors, for instance, recent research has shown that the physical examination by mothers of their children's body was considered as reliable evidence by coroners.[103]

The history of sexuality might also be a promising avenue to broaden such histories of medicine and gender by adding a health perspective. Patient registers, in which physicians took regular notes on the health of patients with mental or other problems, can for instance inform historical knowledge about medical ideas on a healthy sex life. Although patient registers first and foremost reflect the doctor's voice, they also reveal much about patients' sexual experiences and expectations. The promising results of histories from below, however, do not alter the fact that female voices remain difficult to trace for the nineteenth and the early twentieth century. When it comes to medically informed ideas about gender, feminists and historians have started to uncover the constructions of gender difference in relation to other social hierarchies such as class and ethnicity. In Belgium, as elsewhere, medicine played an important role in the production of gendered diseases and in the promotion of 'natural' social roles of women of different classes and ethnicities. In particular, the role of ethnicity in the gendered history of medicine awaits research, not only in relation to Belgium's colonial past, but also with regard to the more recent multi-ethnic composition of the population.

Notes

* We would like to thank Tommy De Ganck, who played an important role in the conceptualisation of this chapter. Thanks also to Marjoleine Delva and Dorien Jaenen for their research assistance.
1 'Séance du 19 février 1875', *Annales Parlementaires* (1875), 429–31.
2 D. Keymolen, 'Feminisme in België. De eerste vrouwelijke artsen (1873–1914)', *Bijdragen en Mededelingen betreffende de Geschiedenis der Nederlanden*, 90:1 (1975), 38–58; H. de Smaele, 'Het Belgische politieke discours en de "eigenheid" van de vrouw aan het einde van de negentiende eeuw', *Tijdschrift voor Genderstudies*, 1:4 (1998), 27–38.

3 'Rapport de la commission nommée par l'Académie', *Bulletin de l'Académie Royale de Médecine de Belgique*, 9 (1875), 351–412.
4 L. Schiebinger, *Has Feminism Changed Science?* (Boston: Harvard University Press, 1999); I. Löwy, 'Le féminisme a-t-il changé la recherche biomédicale? Le Women Health Movement et les transformations de la médecine aux Etats-Unis', *Travail, Genre et Sociétés*, 14:2 (2005), 89–108. See, for instance, the structural attention to feminism and gender in F. Collyer (ed.), *The Palgrave Handbook of Social Theory in Health, Illness and Medicine* (Basingstoke: Palgrave Macmillan, 2015).
5 See, for instance, M. Lipinska, *Histoire des femmes médecins depuis l'antiquité jusqu'à nos jours* (Paris: Librairie G. Jacques, 1900).
6 L. Jordanova, *Sexual Visions: Images of Gender in Science and Medicine Between the Eighteenth and Twentieth Centuries* (Hemel Hempstead: Harvester Wheatsheaf, 1989); A. Bashford, *Purity and Pollution: Gender, Embodiment and Victorian Medicine* (Basingstoke: Macmillan, 1998); C. Brock, *British Women Surgeons and Their Patients, 1860–1918* (Cambridge, UK: Cambridge University Press, 2017).
7 On the danger of extrapolating English research findings on the history of women's healthcare to other European countries, and on the problematic character of straightforward narratives of the gradual marginalisation of women from healthcare since the eighteenth century, see e.g. M. H. Green, 'Gendering the history of women's healthcare', *Gender and History*, 20:3 (2008), 487–518.
8 J. De Ganck, 'Cultiver la différence. Histoire du développement de la gynécologie à Bruxelles (1870–1935)' (PhD diss., Université Libre de Bruxelles, 2016).
9 J. Donnison, *Midwives and Medical Men: A History of Inter-Professional Rivalries and Women's Rights* (London: Heinemann, 1977); J. W. Leavitt, *Brought to Bed: Childbearing in America, 1750 to 1950* (New York: Oxford University Press, 1986).
10 G. Pluvinage, 'La profession de sage-femme en Belgique au XIXe siècle. De l'accoucheuse traditionnelle à l'auxiliaire médicale', *Sextant*, 23–4 (2007), 177–81.
11 M. J. van Lieburg and H. Marland, 'Midwife regulation, education, and practice in the Netherlands during the nineteenth century', *Medical History*, 33:3 (1989), 298–300.
12 Pluvinage, 'La profession de sage-femme', 182–5; K. Velle, *De nieuwe biechtvaders. De sociale geschiedenis van de arts in België* (Leuven: Kritak, 1991), 343
13 Van Lieburg and Marland, 'Midwife regulation', 298–9.
14 K. Velle, 'De vroedvrouw in de 19e eeuw. Een beroep in de verdrukking?', *Oostvlaamse Zanten*, 5:2 (1990), 75, 84–5.

15 Pluvinage, 'La profession de sage-femme', 189–92.
16 Ibid., 192–5.
17 C. Matthys and S. Gryson, 'Het spanningsveld van de reproductieve gezondheidszorg. Vroedvrouwen, artsen en achterwaarsters in Vlaanderen tijdens de 19de eeuw', *Journal of Belgian History*, 48 (2018), 77–81.
18 C. Matthys, 'Pay the midwife! The cost of delivery in nineteenth-century rural West Flanders: the case of midwife Joanna Mestdagh', *TSEG/Low Countries Journal of Social and Economic History*, 15:2–3 (2018), 16–17.
19 M. C. Versluysen, 'Old wives' tales? Women healers in English history', in *Rewriting Nursing History*, ed. C. Davies (London: Croom Helm, 1980), 188–9; C. Gilligan, *In a Different Voice: Psychological Theory and Women's Development* (Cambridge, MA: Harvard University Press, 1982).
20 S. De Graeve, 'Professionele zorgverstrekking en gender. Dienende liefde bij verpleegsters en vroedvrouwen 1907–1946' (master's thesis, KU Leuven, 1998), 30–9, 61–74; L. De Munck, *Altijd troosten. Belgische verpleegsters tijdens de Eerste Wereldoorlog* (Amsterdam: Amsterdam University Press, 2018), 109–16.
21 B. Mann Wall, *American Catholic Hospitals: A Century of Changing Markets and Missions* (New Brunswick, NJ: Rutgers University Press, 2011), 55–72.
22 De Graeve, 'Professionele zorgverstrekking', 151–6; B. Majerus, *Parmi Les fous. Une histoire sociale de la psychiatrie au 20e siècle* (Rennes: PUR, 2013), 98–108; J. van Gucht, 'Van zielenverpleger tot ziekenverpleger. De psychiatrische verpleger van de Broeders van Liefde (1924–1972)' (master's thesis, KU Leuven, 2018), 39–40.
23 L. De Munck, ' "Soms genezen, dikwijls verlichten, altijd troosten." Belgische verpleegsters tijdens de Eerste Wereldoorlog' (master's thesis, KU Leuven, 2017), 29.
24 S. De Graeve, 'Gefnuikte zelfstandigheid. Vroedvrouwen en verpleegsters in de marge van de vrije beroepen (1908 1974)', in *Vrouwenzaken-zakenvrouwen. Facetten van vrouwelijk zelfstandig ondernemerschap in Vlaanderen, 1800–2000*, ed. L. van Molle and P. Heyrman (Ghent: Provinciebestuur Oost-Vlaanderen, 2001), 148–50.
25 A. Labisch, 'From traditional individualism to collective professionalism: state, patient, compulsory health insurance and the panel doctor question in Germany 1883–1931', in *Medicine and Modernity: Public Health and Medical Care in Nineteenth- and Twentieth-Century Germany*, ed. M. Berg and G. Cocks (Cambridge, UK: Cambridge University Press, 1997), 18–34.

26 R. De Vries, *A Pleasing Birth: Midwives and Maternity Care in the Netherlands* (Amsterdam: Amsterdam University Press, 2005), 59–64.
27 De Graeve, 'Professionele zorgverstrekking', 147–8; Pluvinage, 'La profession de sage-femme', 196.
28 P. Charrier, 'Comment envisage-t-on d'être sage-femme quand on est un homme? L'intégration professionnelle des étudiants hommes sage-femmes', *Travail, Genre et Société*, 12:2 (2004), 105–24; P. Charrier, '103 hommes sage-femmes en Belgique', *La Capitale* (21 June 2017).
29 Y. Knibiehler, *Accoucher. Femmes, sages-femmes et médecins depuis le milieu du XXe siècle* (Rennes: Presses de l'Ecole des hautes études en santé publique, 2007).
30 A. Neuberg, *Naître autrefois. Rites et folklore de la naissance en Ardenne et Luxembourg* (Bastogne: Musée en Piconrue, 1993); P. van Eyck, *Clara* (Turnhout: Heibrand, 1995); E. Reusens, 'Een profiel van Oost-Vlaamse vroedvrouwen. Levensloopanalyse van 31 vroedvrouwen uit Oost-Vlaanderen' (master's thesis, Ghent University, 2008), 91–113; see also the theme issue on midwives in *Chronique Féministe* (2008), which includes different Belgian testimonies such as the story of Marie-Louise Blatter: F. Huart, 'Vécu et pénibilité du métier de sage-femme dans l'après-guerre en Ardenne', *Chronique Féministe*, 100 (2008), 45–9.
31 Reusens, 'Een profiel van Oost-Vlaamse vroedvrouwen', 95; Huart, 'Vécu et pénibilité du métier', 48.
32 Matthys and Gryson, 'Het spanningsveld van de reproductieve gezondheidszorg', 85–6.
33 A. Vanthienen, 'Vroedvrouwen, het oudste beroep ter wereld?', *Rosa Factsheet*, 45 (2006), 8–9, www.yumpu.com/nl/document/read/19740582/vroedvrouwen-het-oudste-beroep-ter-wereld-rosa (accessed 9 June 2021).
34 L. E. Ettinger, *Nurse-Midwifery: The Birth of a New American Profession* (Columbus: Ohio State University Press, 2006), 189; De Vries, *Pleasing Birth*, 243.
35 T. N. Bonner, *To the Ends of the Earth: Women's Search for Education in Medicine* (Cambridge, MA: Harvard University Press, 1992); L. L. Clark, *Women and Achievement in Nineteenth-Century Europe* (Cambridge, UK: Cambridge University Press, 2008), 210–22.
36 Keymolen, 'Feminisme in België', 45.
37 Velle, *De nieuwe biechtvaders*, 343.
38 *Bureau de statistiques universitaires. Rapport annuel* (Brussels: Fondation Universitaire, 1937–90); L. Goovaerts, 'Het glazen plafond doorbroken? De eerste generatie vrouwelijke hoogleraren aan de UGent, een oral history project' (master's thesis, Ghent University, 2016), 41.

39 Keymolen, 'Feminisme in België', 51–2.
40 *La Réforme* (19 September 1894), 2.
41 C. Leplae, *Les femmes universitaires. Étude sociologique des diplômées de l'Université de Louvain* (Leuven: Nauwelaerts, 1950), 37.
42 Keymolen, 'Feminisme in België', 55–6.
43 Ibid., 41; E. Gubin, V. Piette, J. Puissant, S. Dupont-Bouchat and J.-P. Nandrin (eds), *Dictionnaire des femmes belges. XIXe et XXe siècles* (Brussels: Racine, 2006), 188.
44 V. Di Tillio, 'La Fédération Belge des Femmes Universitaires. Naissance et essor (1921–1940)', *Sextant*, 9 (1998), 83–4, 91.
45 K. Jensen, 'War, transnationalism and medical women's activism: the Medical Women's International Association and the Women's Foundation for Health in the aftermath of the First World War', *Women's History Review*, 26:2 (2017), 224.
46 A. S. van der Meersch, 'La carrière universitaire des femmes à l'Université de Gand. Un plafond de verre?', in Gubin et al., *Femmes de culture et de pouvoir*, 283.
47 P. Delheye and H. Vangrunderbeek, 'Struggling with science and status: physiotherapy – including radiology and cancer treatment – and physical education at the State University in Ghent, Belgium, 1906–1936', *International Journal of the History of Sport*, 32:6 (2015), 818; M. Bruneel, 'Witte raven in zwarte toga's. De eerste vrouwelijke professoren van de Leuvense universiteit (1960–1985)' (master's thesis, KU Leuven, 2018), 95.
48 C. Jacques and V. Piette, 'L'Union des Femmes Coloniales (1923–1940). Une association au service de la colonisation', in *Histoire des femmes en situation coloniale: Afrique et Asie, XXe Siècle*, ed. A. Hugon (Paris: Karthala, 2004), 95–117; S. Heyvaert, 'Belgisch feminisme, 1892–1960. Imperialisme als referentiekader? Over de houding van feministen ten opzichte van kolonialisme' (master's thesis, Ghent University, 2011), 145.
49 M. H. Delva, 'Le travail professionnel de la femme blanche au Congo', *L'Union des Femmes du Congo Belge et du Ruanda-Urundi*, 132 (1951), 6.
50 R. Darolle, 'Dans cet hôpital du Congo... Le chirugien est ... une religieuse', *L'Union des Femmes du Congo Belge et du Ruanda-Urundi*, 156 (1957), 23–4.
51 D. Noltinckx, 'Les femmes médecins à Bruxelles (1890 à nos jours)', *Sextant*, 3 (1995), 168; L. Nys, *Van mensen en muizen. Vijftig jaar Nederlandstalige Faculteit Geneeskunde aan de Leuvense universiteit* (Leuven: Leuven University Press, 2016), 116.
52 Nys, *Van mensen en muizen*, 40, 116, 295–6; R. van Damme-Lombaerts, J. Eggermont, I. Haesendonck and R. Veugelers, 'Arts-Specialisten in

Opleiding. Verschillen M/V', *Delta: Tijdschrift Voor Hoger Onderwijs*, 19 (2008), 39–42.
53 T. W. Laqueur, *Making Sex: Body and Gender from the Greeks to Freud* (Cambridge, MA: Harvard University Press, 1990); Jordanova, *Sexual Visions*.
54 W. Mitchinson, *The Nature of Their Bodies: Women and Their Doctors in Victorian Canada* (Toronto: University of Toronto Press, 1991); O. Moscucci, *The Science of Woman: Gynaecology and Gender in England, 1800–1929* (Cambridge, UK: Cambridge University Press, 1993).
55 G. Weisz, *Divide and Conquer: A Comparative History of Medical Specialization* (Oxford: Oxford University Press, 2006), 203–5.
56 De Ganck, 'Cultiver la différence', 142–61.
57 Ibid., 157, 374.
58 L. Nys, 'De Ruiters van de Apocalyps? Alcoholisme, tuberculose, syfilis en degeneratie in medische kringen, 1870–1940', in *Degeneratie in België 1860–1940: een geschiedenis van ideeën en praktijken*, ed. J. Tollebeek, G. Vanpaemel and K. Wils (Leuven: Leuven University Press, 2003), 24–6, 35.
59 C. Marissal, *Protéger le jeune enfant. Enjeux sociaux, politiques et sexués (Belgique, 1890–1940)* (Brussels: Editions de l'Université de Bruxelles, 2014), 129–48.
60 E. Gubin, 'Home, sweet home. L'image de la femme au foyer en Belgique et au Canada avant 1914', *Journal of Belgian History*, 22:3–4 (1991), 521–68; N. Bracke, 'Koningin van het huisgezin of volwaardige arbeidskracht? De visies van de Belgische Werkliedenpartij op de fabrieksarbeid van vrouwen: 1885–1914', *Brood en Rozen : Tijdschrift voor de Geschiedenis van Sociale Bewegingen*, 1:3 (1996), 8–25; H. Moors, 'Drempels van de droom. Vrouwen, vrouwelijkheid en socialisme 1830–1870', in *Begeerte heeft ons aangeraakt: socialisten, sekse en seksualiteit*, ed. D. De Weerdt (Ghent: Provinciebestuur van Oost-Vlaanderen, 1999), 17–58; L. Peiren, 'Socialisme en vrouwen(beweging) in de tweede helft van de 19de eeuw', in Marissal, *Protéger le jeune enfant*, 17–58; T. Van Osselaer, *The Pious Sex: Catholic Constructions of Masculinity and Femininity in Belgium, C. 1800–1940* (Leuven: Leuven University Press, 2013), 40–2, 79.
61 T. De Ganck, 'Souffrir de folie ou souffrir à la folie? La chirurgie gynécologique à Bruxelles au tournant du XXe siècle', *Histoire, Médecine et Santé*, 12 (2018), 39–56.
62 There are other examples such as the gendering of cancer that was reinforced by a nineteenth-century model of cancer underlining its reproductive origins: I. Löwy, 'Le genre du cancer', *Clio. Femmes, Genre, Histoire*, 37 (2013), 65–83; O. Moscucci, *Gender and*

Cancer in England, 1860–1948 (London: Palgrave Macmillan, 2016), 1–13.
63 S. Frampton, 'Defining difference: competing forms of ovarian surgery in the nineteenth century', in *Technological Change in Modern Surgery: Historical Perspectives on Innovation*, ed. T. Schlich and C. Crenner (Rochester: Boydell & Brewer, 2017), 51–70; S. Frampton, *Belly-Rippers, Surgical Innovation and the Ovariotomy Controversy* (Cham: Palgrave Macmillan, 2018).
64 J. Guislain, *Leçons orales sur les phrénopathies ou traité théorique et pratique des maladies mentales: cours donné à la clinique des établissements d'aliénés à Gand* (Ghent: Hebbelynck, 1852), 74–9.
65 J. Falleyn, 'Hysterie en de medische wereld in België 1855–1914' (master's thesis, KU Leuven, 1999), 27–33; De Ganck, 'Souffrir de folie?', 50–1.
66 M. S. Micale, *Hysterical Men: The Hidden History of Male Nervous Illness* (Cambridge, MA: Harvard University Press, 2008), 143–45, 156–61, 179–80.
67 R. Debusschere, 'De militaire psychiatrie in België voor de Eerste Wereldoorlog. Verkenning van een discipline in wording' (master's thesis, KU Leuven, 2013), 46–7; C. van Everbroeck and P. Verstraete, *Verminkte stilte. De Belgische invalide soldaten van de Groote Oorlog* (Namur: Presses universitaires de Namur, 2014), 82–5.
68 Falleyn, 'Hysterie en de medische wereld', 91–2, 101; J. Stappaerts, 'Het evenbeeld van Ophelia: de medische beeldvorming over geesteszieke vrouwen in de instellingen van de Zusters van Liefde in Gent en Melle,1900–1920' (master's thesis, KU Leuven, 2018), 16–20.
69 E. Jonckheere,'Van narrenschip tot waanzinnige coureur: het (schouw) spel van waanzin en arbeid', in *Het spel voorbij de waanzin. Een theatrale praktijk?*, ed. E. Jonckheere, C. Stalpaert and K. Vuylsteke Vanfleteren (Ghent: Academia Press, 2010), 88–90.
70 E. B. Rosenman, 'Body doubles: the spermatorrhea panic', *Journal of the History of Sexuality*, 12:3 (2003), 365–99; E. Stephens, 'Pathologizing leaky male bodies: spermatorrhea in nineteenth-century British medicine and popular anatomical museums', *Journal of the History of Sexuality*, 17:3 (2008), 421–38.
71 C. Verbruggen, 'De volstrekt normale mensch bestaat niet: een analyse van de medische registers uit de psychiatrische instelling van de Broeders Alexianen te Boechout (1875–1899) en van het Stuivenbergziekenhuis in Antwerpen (1907–1914)' (master's thesis, KU Leuven, 2005), 47–9.
72 J. Hoegaerts, *Masculinity and Nationhood, 1830–1910: Constructions of Identity and Citizenship in Belgium* (Basingstoke: Palgrave Macmillan, 2014), 43–56.

73 Nys, 'De Ruiters van de Apocalyps?', 20–2; L. Nys, 'De grote school van de natie. Legerartsen over drankmisbruik en geslachtsziekten in het leger, 1850–1950', in Tollebeek et al., *Degeneratie in België 1860–1940*, 82–4.
74 K. Pittomvils, 'Tussen repressie en permissiviteit: socialisme, socialisten, prostitutie en geslachtsziekten (eind 19de eeuw – 1997)', in De Weerdt, *Begeerte heeft ons aangeraakt*, 216–22; C. Machiels, *Les féminismes et la prostitution 1860–1960* (Rennes: Presses universitaires de Rennes, 2016); M. Rodriguez Garcia and K. Gillis, 'Morality politics and prostitution policy in Brussels: a diachronic comparison', *Sexuality Research and Social Policy*, 15:3 (2017), 259–70.
75 A. Carol, 'L'examen gynécologique XVIIIe–XIXe siècle: techniques et usages', in *Les nouvelles pratiques de santé: acteurs, objets, logiques sociales, XVIIIe–XXe Siècles*, ed. P. Bourdelais and O. Faure (Paris: Belin, 2005), 60–6; K. Yeniyurt, 'When it hurts to look: interpreting the interior of the Victorian woman', *Social History of Medicine*, 27:1 (2014), 22–40.
76 De Ganck, 'Cultiver la différence', 219–24.
77 Marissal, *Protéger le jeune enfant*, 67–76, 194–203.
78 Moscucci, *The Science of Woman*, 184–5; De Ganck, 'Cultiver la différence', 445–6.
79 I. Meul, 'De professionalisering van het medisch-specialistisch beroep in het kader van de verplichte ziekte- en invaliditeitsverzekering in België (1944–2014)' (PhD diss., University of Antwerp, 2016); J. Vandendriessche, *Zorg en wetenschap. Een geschiedenis van de Leuvense academische ziekenhuizen in de twintigste eeuw* (Leuven: Leuven University Press, 2019).
80 J. Stengers, 'Les pratiques anticonceptionnelles dans le mariage au XIXe et au XXe siècles. Problèmes humains et attitudes religieuses', *Revue Belge de Philologie et d'Histoire*, 49 (1971), 403–81, 1119–74; R. Christens, 'De orthodoxie van het zaad. Seksualiteit en sekse-identiteit in de rooms-katholieke traditie', in *Het lichaam m/v*, ed. K. Wils (Leuven: Leuven University Press, 2001), 231–49.
81 I. Brosens, *The Challenge of Reproductive Medicine at Catholic Universities: Time to Leave the Catacombs* (Leuven: Peeters, 2006), 71–142; Nys, *Van mensen en muizen*, 143–50; Vandendriessche, *Een geschiedenis van de Leuvense academische ziekenhuizen*. Current postdoctoral research at KU Leuven by Tinne Claes focuses on infertility.
82 Stengers, 'Les pratiques anticonceptionnelles', 1161–6; K. Celis, 'Socialisme en seksuele fraude: de houding van de Belgische socialisten tegenover abortus en anticonceptie (1880–1990)', in De Weerdt,

Begeerte heeft ons aangeraakt, 191–5; C. Vanderpelen-Diagre and C. Sägesser (eds), *La Sainte Famille: sexualité, filiation et parentalité dans l'Église catholique* (Brussels: Editions de l'Université, 2017).

83 P. van Praag, 'The development of Neo-Malthusianism in Flanders', *Population Studies*, 32:3 (1978), 467–80.

84 E. Gubin, 'Signification, modernité et limites du féminisme belge avant 1914', *Sextant*, 1 (1993), 49–50; J. Carlier, 'Moving beyond boundaries: an entangled history of feminism in Belgium, 1890–1914' (PhD diss., Ghent University, 2010), 45–51.

85 H. Peemans-Poullet, 'Féminisme et contrôle des naissances', in *Corps de femmes: sexualité et contrôle social*, ed. M. Coenen (Brussels: De Boeck, 2002), 131–57; Celis, 'Socialisme en seksuele fraude'; Carlier, 'Moving beyond boundaries', 151–7.

86 K. Celis, 'Abortus in België, 1880–1940', *Journal of Belgian History*, 26:3 (1996), 209; Celis, 'Socialisme en seksuele fraude', 192–5.

87 R. Sauer, 'Infanticide and abortion in nineteenth-century Britain', *Population Studies*, 32:1 (1978), 84.

88 K. Wils, 'Science, an ally of feminism? Isabelle Gatti de Gamond on Women and Science', *Revue Belge de Philologie et d'Histoire*, 77:2 (1999), 435.

89 Carlier, 'Moving beyond boundaries', 156.

90 E. Peeters, 'Een dubbelzinnige erfenis. Belgische seksuologen over vrouwenemancipatie en nieuwe mannelijkheid in het interbellum', *Journal of Belgian History*, 38:3 (2008), 437–59.

91 C. de Borchgrave, *God of Genot: Vlaanderen 1918–1940: een kerk in strijd met de moderne zinnelijkheid* (Leuven: Van Halewijck, 1998), 100–1; V. Piette and E. Gubin, 'La politique nataliste de l'entre-deux-guerres', in M. Coenen, *Corps de femmes*, 115–29.

92 Peemans-Poullet, 'Féminisme et contrôle des naissances', 148–50.

93 Celis, 'Socialisme en seksuele fraude', 196.

94 Ibid., 197; L. Blancquaert, R. Goris and W. Trommelmans, *Vlaanderen vrijt! 50 jaar seks in Vlaanderen* (Leuven: Van Halewyck, 2006), 12, 48.

95 Blancquaert et al., *Vlaanderen vrijt!*, 50; C. Matthys and I. Devos, ' "Gij doet u plichten niet, man?" De houding van mannen ten opzichte van seksualiteit en geboortebeperking in Vlaanderen, 1900–1940', *EED Working Papers Series* (2012), 1–15.

96 Blancquaert et al., *Vlaanderen vrijt!*, 48.

97 Vandendriessche, *Een geschiedenis van de Leuvense academische ziekenhuizen*.

98 K. van den Broeck, D. Janssens and P. Defoort, 'A forgotten founding father of the pill: Ferdinand Peeters, MD', *European Journal of Contraception and Reproductive Health Care*, 17:5 (2012), 321–8.

99 W. Dupont, 'Catholics and sexual change in Flanders', in *Sexual Revolutions*, ed. G. Hekma and A. Giami (Basingstoke: Palgrave Macmillan, 2014), 81–98.
100 E. Witte, 'De liberalisering van de Abortus-wetgeving in België (1970–1990)', in *Abortus. Rapporten en perspectieven omtrent vrouwenstudies*, ed. M. Scheys, vol. 4 (Brussels: VUB press, 1993), 23–38.
101 M. Temmerman, J. J. Amy and P. De Quint, 'Profiel van de aanvragen voor vrijwillige zwangerschapsafbreking in een Brussels ziekenhuis in 1984', in *Rapporten en perspectieven omtrent vrouwenstudies*, ed. M. Scheys, vol. 1 (Brussels: VUB press, 1988), 93–8; Vandendriessche, *Een geschiedenis van de Leuvense academische ziekenhuizen*.
102 K. Celis, 'The abortion debates in Belgium (1974–1990)', in *Abortion Politics, Women's Movements and the Democratic State: A comparative Study of State Feminism*, ed. D. Stetson (New York: Oxford University Press, 2001), 39–61; J. Vandendriessche, 'Genetic counselling in Belgium: the Centre for Human Genetics at the University of Leuven, 1960–1990', in *History of Human Genetics: Aspects of its Development and Global Perspectives*, ed. H. Petermann, P. Harper and S. Doetz (Heidelberg: Springer, 2017), 455.
103 L. Tuybens, 'Verloren intimiteit. Medische expertise bij aanrandings- en verkrachtingszaken in België (1850–1900)' (master's thesis, KU Leuven, 2017).

Selected bibliography

Celis, K., 'The abortion debates in Belgium (1974–1990)', in D. Stetson (ed.), *Abortion Politics, Women's Movements and the Democratic State: A Comparative Study of State Feminism* (New York: Oxford University Press, 2001), 39–61.

De Ganck, T., 'Souffrir de folie ou souffrir à la folie? La chirurgie gynécologique à Bruxelles au tournant du XXe siècle', *Histoire, Médecine et Santé*, 12 (2018), 39–56.

Dupont, W., 'Catholics and sexual change in Flanders', in G. Hekma and A. Giami (eds), *Sexual Revolutions* (Basingstoke: Palgrave Macmillan, 2014), 81–98.

Gijbels, J., 'Medical compromise and its limits: religious concerns and the post-mortem caesarean section in nineteenth-century Belgium', *Bulletin of the History of Medicine*, 93:3 (2019), 305–34.

Keymolen, D., 'Feminisme in België. De eerste vrouwelijke artsen (1873–1914)', *Bijdragen en Mededelingen betreffende de Geschiedenis der Nederlanden*, 90:1 (1975), 38–58.

Marissal, C., *Protéger le jeune enfant. Enjeux sociaux, politiques et sexués (Belgique, 1890–1940)* (Brussels: Editions de l'Université de Bruxelles, 2014).

Matthys, C., 'Pay the midwife! The cost of delivery in nineteenth-century rural West Flanders. The case of midwife Joanna Mestdagh', *Tijdschrift voor Sociale en Economische Geschiedenis*, 15:2–3 (2018), 5–32.

Peeters, E., 'Een dubbelzinnige erfenis. Belgische seksuologen over vrouwenemancipatie en nieuwe mannelijkheid in het interbellum', *Journal of Belgian History*, 38:3 (2008), 437–459.

Pluvinage, G., 'La profession de sage-femme en Belgique au XIXe siècle. De l'accoucheuse traditionnelle à l'auxiliaire médicale', *Sextant*, 23–4 (2007), 177–96.

Stengers, J., 'Les pratiques anticonceptionnelles dans le mariage au XIXe et au XXe siècles. Problèmes humains et attitudes religieuses', *Revue Belge de Philologie et d'Histoire*, 49:2 (1971), 403–81 and 49:4, 1119–74.

2

Medicine and religion

Joris Vandendriessche and Tine Van Osselaer

On 1 October 1928, a community of women religious arrived in Leuven to run the newly built Institute of Cancer, the first of a series of institutes that made up the St Raphael Hospital of the Catholic University of Leuven. Like all monastic communities of the Sisters of Charity of Jesus and Mary, it kept a memorial book to chronicle exceptional events: the consecration of a baptismal font in the maternity ward, the thousandth patient of the Institute of Cancer, the visits from royalty and bishops to inaugurate new hospital buildings, the anniversaries of sisters' vows, etc. The book evokes a community drawing strength from faith to offer medical care as a form of missionary work. 'The shrine [in the chapel]', Mother Superior wrote in 1934, 'infuses life and generates energy for divine Charity to rule and spread'. The book is a telling record of the interwoven histories of Belgian medicine and Catholicism. Entries from the 1930s adopt a militant and expansionist rhetoric at a time of Catholic Action, the movement to re-Christianise society in the face of secularisation: 'Charity is victorious and St Raphael dreams of an ever-growing place under the blue sky.' Later entries point to public practices of devotion in healthcare. In 1955, a statue of Mary with child was placed on the monastery's facade, 'which one can see from a long way and seems to reassure the ill who are on their way to the clinic.' In 1958, a procession of doctors, patients, nurses and sisters – together more than 450 people – made its way across the hospital buildings and inner courts, praying and carrying candles to celebrate the beginning of May, the month of Mary.[1]

The women religious' memorial book hints at the importance of religious beliefs and practices in Belgian medicine and healthcare.[2] Such importance should hardly come as a surprise: up until the 1960s, when the speed of secularisation increased, Belgium was a profoundly Catholic country. For most Belgians, the experience of illness and medical care was closely connected to their (Catholic) faith. For many doctors and caregivers as well, religion occupied an important position in the way they conducted their professional lives. Recent historical analyses have gradually come to acknowledge this relation between medicine and religion. These histories follow an international trend in moving from a representation of both domains as 'opposites' to narratives of interaction and collaboration. In that sense, they break with older representations of the physician as a modern substitute for the priest, or of the lay nurse as a replacement for sisters and friars – representations that imply an understanding of medicalisation and secularisation as mutually reinforcing processes.[3] Historians have also started to paint a broad picture of the place of ideology in medicine that goes beyond the political conflicts between liberals, socialists and Catholics over the provision of medical care.[4] Within an older historiography, attention to the imagery that was used in political strife (i.e. of the rise of modern medicine going hand in hand with the secularisation of medical institutions, e.g. of lay nurses replacing nuns), had precisely underpinned an oppositional reading of the relation between medicine and religion.

Recent historical scholarship has started exploring the variety of interactions between the medical and religious fields. These could lead to conflict, but also to productive exchange.[5] Entries from the memorial book of the Sisters of Love reveal women religious' pride in working within 'modern' equipment and in 'up-to-date' hospitals. In 1932, the order took over the St Elizabeth School for Nursing, founded in 1922 in Leuven. In 1939, it opened a college for 'nursing instructors'. Both were spaces where a Christian tradition of care, morality and responsibility was integrated into the professional training of (lay) nurses. While the order faced the effects of secularisation, with diminishing callings and with the resulting decision in 1966 to leave the Leuven hospitals, the development of Catholic nursing education gained traction. At the college's twenty-fifth anniversary in 1964, 'the formation of a Christian senior staff of nursing, who devote themselves to mankind and the Holy Church' was seen as its major achievement. A narrative of lay nurses merely replacing women religious as care providers does not fully do justice to this trajectory. As Barbra Mann Wall has shown for American religious congregations, women religious acted as 'entrepreneurs' over the past two centuries in developing modern healthcare.[6]

In taking stock of this historiography, this chapter attempts a varied overview of the historical relation between medicine and religion in Belgium. To an extent, this is an exercise in balancing out a too strong political reading of the history of healthcare, which has focused on strive or compromise between oppositional forces, with more attention to 'productive' intellectual encounters. To develop the latter perspective, the chapter draws on recent scholarship from the history of science and medicine, sexuality and religion that has turned to venues of debate and identity formation such as scientific academies (e.g. the Belgian Academy of Medicine) and professional societies (e.g. the Belgian Society of Saint-Luc, a society of Catholic doctors). In these spaces, the encounter between medicine and religion took on a less polemical style and inspired new approaches on both sides. Only limited attention within Belgian historiography has gone to studying archival (patient) records, looking for the space of rituals or devotion in medical practice (see Chapter 7, pp. 261–3). As such, the chapter brings a particular set of Catholic historical actors into the limelight: Catholic doctors, missionaries, women religious, theologians, etc. Their integration into medical history, however, does not mean that moments of conflict are left out. It is key to acknowledge that ideological tensions had a clear impact on the Belgian medical field, shaping its institutional outlook since the second half of the nineteenth century and still resurfacing in debates on medical ethics in the late twentieth and twenty-first centuries.

The chapter distinguishes three levels of interaction between the medical and religious spheres, each treated in a separate section. First, we sketch the evolution of Catholic organisations and institutions in Belgian healthcare, most notably the changing role of religious orders, which in Belgium have held a firm grip on the medical field. We describe evolving Catholic views on 'care' along with political conflicts over an expanding welfare state and changing views on the growing role of lay medical personnel. Second, we turn to religious practices, rituals and exceptional phenomena such as miracles, and the medical debates these inspired. From a medical perspective, and in some cases depending on one's personal religious convictions, religion could be a source of health (e.g. 'moral therapy' to treat mental illness) or disease (e.g. 'Christomanie', a nervous disease said to result from excessive religious behavior). Third, we discuss how Catholic doctors and caregivers gave their religious views a place in their professional work and identities. Here we turn to medical ethics and professional codes of conduct, and the ways in which these have been inspired by Catholic thinking. We pay particular attention to questions related to reproductive medicine and the end of life. The presence of the Catholic University of Leuven, the largest Catholic university in the world, ensured that these debates were followed closely far beyond Belgium, most notably in the Vatican.

Traditions of *Caritas*

Caritas, the care for the sick and the poor, has been central to Catholic teachings for centuries and has stimulated Catholic involvement in this field.[7] Since the *Ancien Régime* (and even long before that) religious orders have been actively engaged in social and healthcare provision in the Southern Netherlands.[8] The French regime incited a structural change as public health became the responsibility of the public authorities (localities and departments). As a result, many of the independent institutions became public institutions, ruled by a municipal commission (see Chapter 6, pp. 208–9). In a second phase, the religious orders that had hitherto been involved in caretaking (like the hospital sisters) were expelled and replaced by lay personnel.[9] There was, however, never a complete expulsion as the hospital sisters could count on the sympathy of the population and their replacements soon proved costly and inexperienced.[10] Older orders like the hospital sisters resumed their activities after their initial (yet only partial) suppression under French rule. Most of them were active again by 1810. In nineteenth-century Belgium, as in France, most public medical institutions were thus run by religious congregations at the request of the authorities.[11] Many of these were new congregations: the Sisters of Charity of Jesus and Mary were founded in 1803; the Hospital Brothers of St Vincent in 1807, who were later called the Brothers of Charity; and the Sisters of St Vincent de Paul in 1818.[12] In 1846, approximately 5,298 of the 11,968 religious orders (45 per cent) were involved in the provision of medical care.[13]

The growth of these new religious orders occurred against the background of a young nation state with a profoundly liberal constitution. These liberal freedoms allowed congregations to expand without being opposed by the state, laying the basis of the Catholic dominance in the provision of medical care. In the field of psychiatry, the activities of the mentioned Sisters and Brothers of Charity, founded by Canon Petrus-Joseph Triest, form a telling example. Both orders started their work in Ghent, taking care of the city's mentally ill, but soon developed activities across the country and abroad. The Sisters of Charity were asked to run an asylum in Tournai in 1818 as well as the state-owned psychiatric institution of Mons in 1866. They also founded private institutions in Sint-Truiden in 1838, in Melle in 1911, in Beau-Vallon in 1914 and in Lovenjoel in 1926.[14] The Brothers of Charity followed a similar trajectory. By 1924, they ran ten institutions in Belgium and were responsible for the medical care of nearly five thousand patients.[15] The governance of such networks of hospitals required considerable financial and administrative expertise. Religious orders developed an almost 'entrepreneurial' spirit.[16] Both orders merged the ideal of *caritas* with the values of social engagement and of leading a moral life that were central to a developing civil society. *Caritas*, embodied by the zealous work of the religious, became in this way a means by which the Catholic Church expanded its influence on Belgian society.[17]

The strong rise of female religious orders in the nineteenth century, the 'century of the nun',[18] has been well documented. Already in 1976, André Tihon made an in-depth study of the Belgian 'feminisation' of the religious profession. He concluded that the largest number of these religious women were working in the field of education, but the orders involved in hospitals came in second place (Figure 2.1). Tihon's extensive study includes convincing statistics: in 1846 these nuns formed 28.19 per cent of the female religious; in 1900 this dropped to 18.30 per cent, in 1947 their number rose again to 20.46 per cent of the total of female religious. Still, even though their relative importance diminished, their numbers rose in those years: in 1846 they counted 2,359 members, in 1900 there were 5,738 and in 1947 10,155.[19] In comparison with lay staff of the hospitals, in 1910, 1,644 laywomen were active as caretakers, nurses and helpers in all medical establishments,

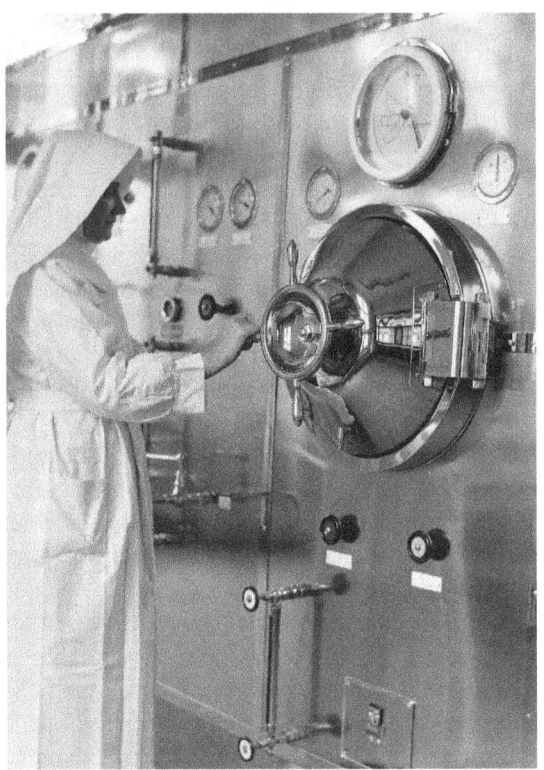

Figure 2.1 A woman religious operating sterilisation equipment in the Leuven academic hospitals, n.d. (mid twentieth century).

hospices and poor relief services. Apart from these institutions, 3,328 women worked as birth helpers, masseuses, pedicurists and carers. In total their number rose to 4,972, whereas there were 8,121 members of female orders that were exclusively focused on hospitals.[20] Just like in other European countries such as Germany and France, ecclesiastical *caritas* carried a 'female face'.[21] A similar trend might be detected in the lay charity movements that developed in the second half of the nineteenth century. These were a means for Catholic men and women from the bourgeoisie and upper classes, conducting home visits, to alleviate the needs of the poor and by doing so diminish social tensions.[22] Nursing and caring seem to have been central to women's movements.

Described as a continuation of their 'feminine' task of caring for others (see Chapter 1, pp. 34–5), an extension of their motherly duties, these movements provided women with a space of action beyond their homes. Tellingly, of the 144 charity works that were initiated by *dames d'œuvres* (charitable ladies from the aristocracy and bourgeoisie), 111 focused on healthcare at home, one took care of pilgrims, 23 worked in the colonies of sick children and 9 were part of Work of the Calvary (who helped cancer patients in the homes that they had created).[23]

While the competence of these voluntary laywomen as care providers was rarely questioned, the capabilities of women religious as nurses were subject to considerable debate, certainly from the late nineteenth century onwards. Such debates paralleled the introduction of new technologies into the hospital (e.g. for radiotherapy) and, more generally, the rise of the 'general hospital' as a space for medical treatment (in particular surgery) rather than of social care. The medical training of women religious is one of those topics for which ideological conflict has formed the dominant framework in historiography. Even if not to the same degree as in France, where the image of the unqualified nun featured prominently in the politicised debates over healthcare in the late nineteenth century,[24] Belgian politicians and physicians – mostly liberals – did criticise the competence of the religious as care providers. The most telling example is perhaps the attacks by the socialist doctor-politician Modeste Terwagne, which earned him the nickname of *nonnenvreter* ('nun-eater').[25] It is also clear that the setting up of training programmes for (lay) nurses started in the liberal settings of Liège and Brussels in the 1880s. The first Catholic initiatives for the schooling of nurses date from the early twentieth century; these included the St Camille School in Brussels in 1907 and the aforementioned St Elizabeth Institute in Leuven in 1922.[26] But within congregations as well, formal training courses were organised for new brothers and sisters in addition to the informal ways in which hands-on knowledge was passed on. Luc De Munck's ongoing research engages with these Catholic educational initiatives to improve patient care. The many journals that were developed to this end since the early twentieth century, such as *Catholic Nursing* (*De katholieke ziekenverpleging*), *Caritas* and *Caring for the Ill* (*Ziekenverpleging*), offer a wealth of source materials.

After the First World War, the Catholic Church strongly emphasised the religious nature of healthcare institutions operated by religious orders. At a moment when coalition governments with socialists and liberals replaced the hegemony of the Catholic party, which had held the majority in the Belgian parliament between 1884 and 1914, the dominance of religious orders in the provision of medical care seemed threatened. New medical institutions of a different nature appeared, such as socialist outpatients' clinics and the institutes of the ideologically neutral Red Cross. As the Catholic world felt forced on to the defensive, stronger organisational structures were developed. In 1922, the Belgian Society of Saint-Luc, a professional organisation for Catholic physicians, was founded. In 1932, the Catholic Service for Hygiene and Aid, soon renamed Caritas Catholica following international trends, was established to group all Catholic initiatives in healthcare. In 1938, the League of Health Care Institutions was created as a subdivision of Caritas Catholica to assist Christian hospitals and defend their interests.[27] The organisation seems comparable to the Catholic Hospital Association, established in 1915 in the United States to help institutions keep up with the pace of hospital modernisation and nursing education.[28] At a time when state initiatives were regarded as too 'materialist', these professional organisations took up the challenge of reconciling medical care in a Christian tradition with developments in modern medicine, without losing sight of its moral grounding. This increasing emphasis on Catholic identity in healthcare initiatives can be illustrated via the histories of seaside vacation colonies for children. Every ideological pillar had its own homes, but the Catholic initiatives developed slightly more slowly (even though the Sisters of Charity of Jesus and Mary had been involved in the first seaside hospital in Wenduine that was created in 1881). Catholic involvement increased especially since the last year of the First World War with creation of 'Mont Thabor' (Berg Thabor) that helped children who were suffering from consumption. It had homes in Koksijde, Ostend and Middelkerke and employed religious women (Sisters of St Vincent de Paul and Dominican Sisters) alongside Catholic physicians.[29]

As for the Catholic involvement in healthcare in the colonies, that took a slow start too (see Chapter 3, pp. 113–6). Initially King Leopold II had little success in persuading Belgian Catholic orders to found missions in the Congo. They only started to arrive in the last decade of the nineteenth century (Scheutists in 1887 and Jesuits in 1893, other orders followed). From the 1920s onwards the numbers of religious and missionaries involved in Congo was on the rise. In 1908 there were still very few: 'only' 233 priest-missionaries and 102 religious, while between 1920 and the 1940s the numbers quadrupled from 895 in 1924 to 4,607 in 1959. This coincided with the feminisation of missionaries. In 1908, nuns made up one-third of the total of the missionary staff (102), in 1959 they were more or less half of the staff (2,130 out of 4,607).[30] So while the men saw the numbers rise primarily between 1908 and 1924, the women peaked a little later (278 per cent growth between 1924 and 1935).[31] Besides this feminisation of colonial healthcare, and similar to evolutions in the home country, a professionalisation took place. By the 1920s, nurses were required to follow a brief course at the School of Tropical Medicine (École de Médecine Tropicale) in Brussels. As in Belgium, the trend of replacing nuns with accredited nurses can be traced to the interwar period in the state hospitals in the colonies. There were, however, as Sokhieng Au has pointed out, exceptions: nuns remained active in certain types of palliative care (especially for leprosy) because of its close links to Christian theology and missionary work.[32]

After the Second World War, the challenge for religious orders to maintain their role in healthcare became ever more difficult, both in Belgium and the colonies. As the pace of secularisation increased since the 1960s, the number of (missionary) vocations declined and religious practice in Belgium diminished. In 1981, 72 per cent of Belgians declared themselves Catholics (a number that soon diminished: 65 per cent in 1990, 57 per cent in 1999 and 50 per cent in 2009). However, such a declaration of 'belonging' sometimes merely referred to the fact that they were baptised. At the same time, the development of the welfare state put pressure on the Christian ideal of *caritas*. With the introduction of mandatory health insurance in 1944, and the subsidising of new hospitals (public ones from 1949, and since 1953 also private – mostly Catholic – institutions), medical care was turned from a form of charity into a social right.[33] This policy of state support resulted in a rapid expansion of the number of hospital beds in Belgium, which reached a peak in the early 1980s. With such a rise in scale, in a society that was secularising at a rapid pace, the question of how to preserve the Christian identity of Catholic hospitals arose. As the community of women and men religious was aging and the participation of lay personnel grew – certainly after the Second Vatican Council, during which a more important role for laity in the church was discussed – the Christian nature of these institutions had to be rethought. Archbishop Leo Suenens and the League of Health Care Institutions took initiatives for the development of pastoral work in hospitals and for the creation of a 'humane approach' to healthcare.[34] During a conference organised by the League in 1972, the latter approach was regarded a counterweight to the growing technicality and bureaucratisation of healthcare. Four years later, a report on the role of religious personnel stated that their presence should act as 'yeast in the dough', reminding their colleagues of the Christian inspiration that lay at the basis of their medical work.[35] In 1976, when Suenens was succeeded by Godfried Danneels as archbishop of Mechelen, a letter by Jos De Saeger, president of Caritas Catholica at that time, captured the reform of Christian healthcare well:

> [Our hospitals] have made such efforts to humanize, for a humane welcoming, for the care of the dying ... the training of our staff, the renewal of our pastoral work ... ; in order for this last work not to form a separate 'service', left to the priest alone, but would integrate all those aspects in this so humane approach to man, as being ONE, in relation to what is beyond description ... to avoid all misunderstanding: I do not intend all of this as the obtrusiveness of the missionary work of half a century ago. We should make no pretensions to replace [God's] mercy, but we should be willing and prepared to assist when it calls upon us.[36]

In the last quarter of the twentieth century, a Christian tradition of medical care was thus recast in line with contemporary demands for the improvement of patient care. Religiously inspired caring, De Saeger believed, still had a role to play in easing the excesses of an all too radical medicalisation of society. As Liliane Voyé and Karel Dobbelaere have noted, in the last decades the importance of pastoral care has diminished. Yet, pastoral service is provided in all Catholic institutions (with the exception of some smaller houses) even if the priests and religious have been replaced by laymen with pastoral training. In fact, in all Belgian hospitals the sick can call upon the services of representatives of different religions or the Union of the Associations of Freethinkers.[37]

In spite of these evolutions, religious orders and the Christian Health Funds maintained their dominance: they still owned about 50 per cent of the general hospitals and 80 per cent of the psychiatric institutions in 1980.[38] Today, Catholic hospitals exist alongside the public system and other private initiatives. The League was split into two federations: the Fédération des Institutions Hospitalières (FIH, francophone) and the Verbond van Verzorgsinstellingen (VVI, Dutch-speaking), called Zorgnet since 2009[39] – both belong to Caritas Catholica. In 2007, 63 per cent of the beds of general hospitals in Flanders were in Catholic hospitals, in Wallonia the Catholic hospitals had 42 per cent of the beds. In psychiatric hospitals, they hold no less than 85 per cent of the beds in Flanders and 43 per cent in Wallonia. Caritas Catholica also comprises the federation 'Welzijnsverbond' that groups services that were initiated by the parents of the patients rather than religious orders and thus have a very pluralistic character (e.g. children with impairments or educational issues). The federation has its own ethical and pastoral service.[40]

Medical meanings of religious practice

A second level on which the fields of medicine and religion have interacted concerns therapeutic practices and the debates surrounding them. We focus more specifically on the use of religious rituals in relation to the (diseased) body. Rituals, religious phenomena and medical practices have historically been interconnected in different ways. Their use has inspired considerable debate in the Belgian medical community, triggering doctors to formulate an opinion and sometimes laying bare ideological divides between Catholic and liberal experts. In some cases, they have been considered sources of healing, and therefore as inspiring examples (e.g. in mental healthcare). In other cases, religious practice has been regarded as pathological of itself, that is causing or spreading illness rather than having a therapeutic effect.

The nineteenth-century belief in 'moral therapy' for psychiatric patients forms a telling example of the belief in the healing power of faith. This theory, attributed to the French physicians Philippe Pinel and Étienne Esquirol, was promoted in Belgium by the Ghent physician Joseph Guislain. It rested on a conception of mental illness as a lack of order, morality and self-discipline, which could be corrected through psychological influencing and the enforcement of a strict daily regime, similar to the structured lifestyle of men and women religious.[41] Guislain attributed many therapeutic benefits to religious influence. The stern appearance and solemn clothing of religious personnel, he argued, gave them an authority that was essential to the success of moral therapy. He also considered their soothing role as a form of treatment, an idea that matched well with a long-standing tradition of spiritual aid. By engaging in religious practices, patients could find a form of comfort, which could act therapeutically in particular when their mental illness was caused by feelings of sadness.[42] Patients, for example, participated in reading sessions of devotional texts, a religious practice that again resembled monastic life. Up until the 1960s, religious rituals (such as attending mass) constituted an obvious component of living in an asylum. Many institutions possessed their own chapel or cemetery, or even – as was the case at the asylum of Beau-Vallon – a grotto for the devotion of Our Lady of Lourdes.[43] At the Salve Mater Institute in Lovenjoel (1926), annual pilgrimages were organised at least up until the 1950s with different destinations according to patients' social class and medical condition (e.g. to the sites of Banneux, Beauraing or Koekelberg).[44]

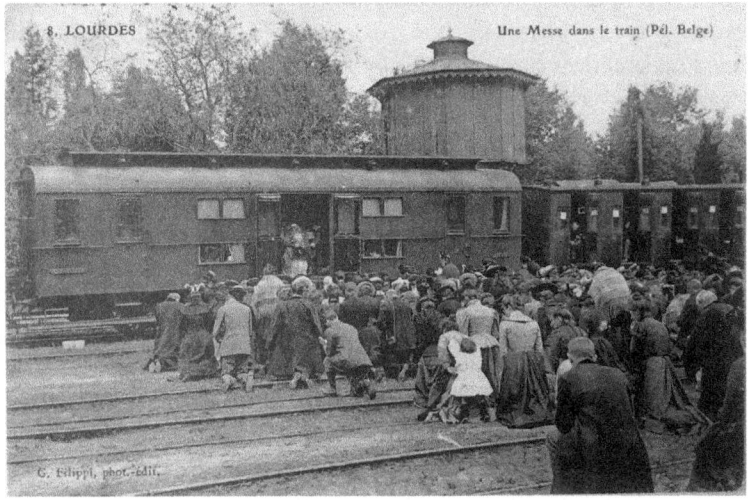

Figure 2.2 Postcard of Belgian pilgrims holding mass in a train.

Yet, religious practices have also been contested for medical reasons and these contestations were sometimes inspired by ideological motives. During the nineteenth-century cholera epidemics, public health specialists considered attending mass or holding a religious procession to be dangerous to spread the epidemic. On their advice, local authorities prohibited these events. For the Catholic population, however, the performance of religion (e.g. calling to a saint for help by holding procession) was a way to cope with the disease and the fears it generated. Here a medical and religious way of understanding disease clashed.[45] Similar tensions emerged surrounding the treatment of the deceased body. As the 'culture wars' between liberals and Catholics flared up in the late nineteenth century, funeral and burial rites became objects of intense conflict. The practice of cremation, which was promoted for being more sanitary, was opposed by Catholics who clung to the traditional burial out of respect for integrity of the body. Freethinkers embraced the civil burial – a burial without the interference of priests on newly founded civil, non-Catholic cemeteries. While such debates were of a wider ideological nature, they also impacted the medical field. Tinne Claes' and Jolien Gijbels' research on the use of the bodies of the poor for medical research and anatomical dissection has revealed the waning influence of the Catholic Church in Belgian public hospitals in the late nineteenth century. The unsanitary and disrespectful way in which the bodies of paupers were disposed, whose families could not afford to pay for a funeral and claim these bodies, led to the creation of both anticlerical and Catholic burial societies who took over these costs. As a result, not only did the (already existing) body shortage for dissections increase in the Brussels hospitals, but funeral rooms were also constructed, in addition to the existing chapels in hospitals, as spaces where non-Catholic funeral rites could be held.[46]

The relationship between devotion and medical expertise also worked the other way around and medical experts were summoned to make some religious activities run more smoothly. Devotional practices like the yearly Lourdes pilgrimage involved sick and invalid faithful and often required medical support. The number of sick pilgrims participating in the Lourdes trip grew steadily: in 1881, there were 60 of them; in 1895, 100 joined the pilgrimage (out of the more than 1,000 participants); and the following year they numbered 250 (out of 2,500 pilgrims).[47] To provide the pilgrimage participants with the care they needed, the organisers called upon the help of Catholic doctors. In 1895, a movement for the healthcare workers and the stretcher-bearers developed, called the Hospital Service of Our Lady of the Cross. They tried to have the necessary medical equipment at their disposal and used hospital wagons for their trip to Lourdes. Tellingly, the wagons had a double purpose for the Pope had granted a special permission to say Mass in these wagons and the organisers used every opportunity to stop in small villages, open the doors and allow everyone to participate in the Eucharist (Figure 2.2). The Belgian national pilgrimage seems to have been a forerunner in this perspective: the article of the movement's periodical introducing the wagon noted that if it was not needed by the Belgian pilgrims, the pilgrims from neighbouring countries could use it.[48]

The pilgrims of Lourdes also stimulated another type of medical involvement in the religious sphere. In particular, the 'miraculous' cures of sick pilgrims were carefully examined by a new office of the Catholic Church, the Bureau of Medical Verifications (1883). This 'medicalisation of the miracle', the call upon medical experts to examine exceptional cures,[49] can be traced in the Belgian context as well. The most well-known case is that of Pieter de Rudder whose injured leg healed suddenly at the replica Lourdes grotto of Oostakker in April 1875.[50] His cure, an 'organic' case of healing (devoid of the slightest hint of hysteria or suggestion) was the object of at least four medical examinations (some conducted after his death from pneumonia in 1898).[51] The church called for such thorough examinations since it was well aware that a well-examined case would be more difficult for its enemies to reject.[52] Not only world-famous Lourdes inspired medical interest; more local or national cases show a similar involvement. In Beauraing and Banneux, two Belgian apparition sites of the 1930s, miraculous cures were examined closely (and two of them were eventually used as proof for the official recognition of the Beauraing apparitions). However, medical experts were also present at these sites (and others) while the series of apparitions took place – studying and testing the ecstasy of the visionaries. In Beauraing, horror stories about those examinations (admittedly involving knives and candles) resulted in the visionaries' refusal to be tested again and the subsequent shift of focus of the medical experts from studying their bodies during the apparitions to their questioning after each episode (adopting interrogation techniques from criminal anthropology).[53]

Not all examinations reached the same conclusion however, and in Belgium, as in other countries, this difference in opinion was linked to anti-Catholic discourse. The most notorious case was that of the stigmatic from Bois-d'Haine, Louise Lateau. In the same year that she first displayed the (visible) wounds of Christ (1868) her bishop created a commission to examine her case and asked Dr Ferdinand Lefèbvre, professor of general pathology and therapeutics at the Catholic University of Leuven, to study her more closely. He concluded that no physical cause for her wounds could be detected and deemed a supernatural intervention at least possible.[54] It is unnecessary to state that his conclusion earned him not much more than mockery from his anticlerical colleagues. Hubert Boëns, a physician from Charleroi, presented his evaluation of Louise's case before the Royal Academy of Science in October 1874. He called her 'sick' and suffering under 'Christomanie' or 'stigmatic ecstasy' that had affected her nervous system and blood.[55] Still, Sofie Lachapelle notes, the Belgian setting of the discussion was quite different from

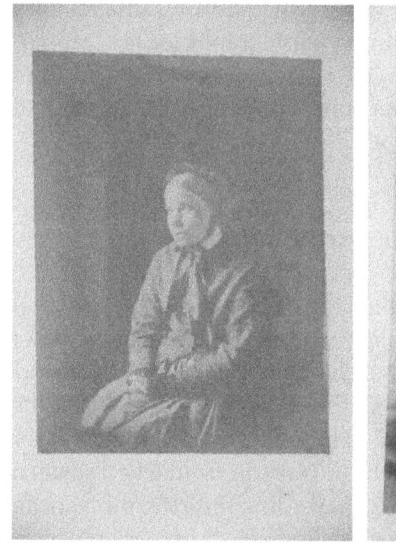
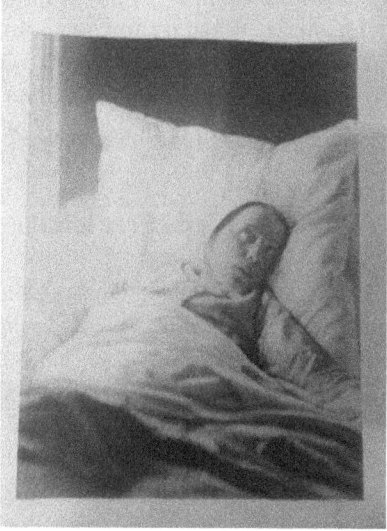

Figure 2.3 Louise in ecstasy (photograph by Lorleberg, October 1877).

that of polarised France where the 'pathologisation' of religious phenomena like stigmata and ecstasy and the redefinition of hysteria were a powerful weapon in the anti-Catholic struggle.[56] In Belgium, the 'collaboration between scientific and religious authorities was perhaps more amicable ... than elsewhere'. In France, Catholic universities were only allowed after 1875 'and never attained much recognition for their faculties of sciences' whereas the Belgian universities of Leuven and Liège were 'prestigious institutions'.[57] On the evaluation of such 'religious' phenomena by medical experts and the tensions and collaborations between the two knowledge systems, much work remains to be done. Scholars might take their cue from, for example, the work that has been done on German and Austrian asylums and its focus on religious mania, melancholia and the differentiation between, in the words of Ann Goldberg, excessive and rationalist religion.[58]

It is important to note that the faithful kept track of medical evolutions such as the redefinition of 'hysteria' and these also permeated Catholic discourses and images. In Lateau's case, for instance, the accusation of her being an 'hysteric' seems to have had an impact on her visual representation. Her supporters seem to have been well aware of her problematic reputation and the use of her case as exemplary for certain stages (e.g. 'passion', 'crucifixion') of hysteria. When it came to choosing photographs for her 'promotion', they selected what they called a 'saintly' image of Lateau in her 'natural state', rather than one of her ecstasy (that they also had at their disposal) (Figure 2.3).[59]

Catholic medical expertise and ethics

A third level on which we may gain new insights about the historical relation between medicine and religion is the level of Catholic views about reproduction and sexuality. The Italian historian Emmanuel Betta situates the emergence of 'Catholic biopolitics' between the mid nineteenth century and 1930, when the encyclical letter *Casti Connubii* was published, in which the Vatican definitely dismissed all kinds of birth control practices. According to Betta, the Vatican outlined its views on the reproductive body in this period not only as a reaction to an expanding medical discourse on the reproductive body in society, but also as an attempt to produce its own modern norms.[60] While the construction of Catholic biopolitical thinking was clearly a transnational process, to which Belgian Catholic doctors contributed, on the Belgian level as well bodily norms were debated. These debates, moreover, shaped the ways in which Catholic caregivers acted as professionals. Deontology, professional codes of conduct and guidelines for ethical decision making on medical interventions (e.g. abortion) were essential for the way they identified individually and collectively as Catholic practitioners. These norms allowed them to determine whether or not they performed medicine in ways that conformed to their religious beliefs. Recent research – discussed in this section – has turned to the ways in which Catholic medical views were debated and spread, with a particular focus on venues of sociability where Catholic doctors met with like-minded or ideologically opposed colleagues, or with religious actors such as priests and theologians.

During the nineteenth century, the Royal Academy of Medicine of Belgium (1841) acted as an important intellectual meeting place for outspoken Catholic professors of the Catholic University of Leuven, and their liberal counterparts of the Free University of Brussels. Jolien Gijbels has shown how questions surrounding medical interventions during difficult childbirths and the desire to baptise unborn foetuses (to save their souls) led to the weighing of religious and medical arguments in the academy, dividing members along ideological lines. Such debates treated the desirability of *in utero* baptism (1845), of medical abortion (and embryotomy) before and during difficult deliveries to save the lives of mothers with a small pelvis (1852) and of priests performing post-mortem caesarean sections (after the assumed death of the mother) to baptise foetuses (1845). Gijbels revealed a willingness to integrate religious concerns in medical debate, as long as such concerns were in line with physicians' codes of conduct.[61] Hence the widely spread custom of intrauterine baptisms in Belgium by means of a syringe filled with holy water – a practice, however, that was never fully approved by theologians who were uncertain about whether or not the water effectively reached the foetus's head. In general, academy members preferred to treat contentious matters as purely 'scientific questions' – a strategy that allowed them to avoid politicised debates and maintain professional unity. Only on rare occasions did Catholic physicians explicitly defend their religious beliefs in opposition to their professional viewpoints. When the Catholic professor of obstetrics Eugène Hubert stated in 1869 that priests had medical expertise (to recognise signs of death) and saved lives in their attempts to baptise foetuses by performing post-mortem caesarean sections, he took a rather exceptional position. His remarkable claim may also be explained by the political circumstances the time. In the late 1860s, the ideological conflict between Catholic and liberals reached a peak in Belgium. It seems no coincidence that in those same years a topic such as the post-mortem caesarean section caused a heated public debate.[62]

In the first decades of the twentieth century, the falling birth rate proved an important context to understand a growing Catholic influence in Belgium's biopolitical discourse.[63] Unlike in France, as Wannes Dupont has shown, the response to these changing demographics in Belgium was pervaded by Catholic reasoning and moral arguments. As elsewhere in Europe, Belgian intellectuals connected the country's declining natality to social problems and feared for a 'degeneration' and loss of national vitality. Yet, they also tied it to the rise of 'materialism' in Belgian society and the need for moral regeneration.[64] Such thinking played a crucial role in the development of a stricter general Catholic policy towards birth control. Joseph-Désiré Mercier, a Leuven professor who became archbishop of Mechelen and head of the Belgian church in 1906, took many initiatives in this regard, including a pastoral letter on the duties of conjugal life and stricter directions for priests on how to approach the matter of contraception during confession in 1909.[65] Mercier was also open to cooperation with Catholic physicians – gynaecologists in particular – to develop this new Catholic stance towards reproduction. In 1910, he initiated a meeting of Belgian Catholic physicians that led to the creation of the National League Against Depopulation.[66] Its president was the Leuven professor of obstetrics Rufin Schockaert (see Chapter 1, pp. 46–7). In his gynaecological clinic, Schockaert taught medical students about the social role of the gynaecologist. The latter had a moral role to play in fighting practices of birth control such as coitus interruptus, which Schockaert regarded as 'unhealthy' for women.[67] In the following decades, this reproductive message was spelled out for the Catholic laity in books like *The Christian Marriage*

(1918, by Canon Aloïs De Smet[68]) and mass gatherings like the Catholic congresses (the 1936 meeting featured a special section on the family).[69]

In addition to questions of sexual morality and birth control, the Catholic Action movement also exerted a strong influence on the Belgian medical profession. First coined by Pope Pius X, but narrowed down by his successor Pius XI in 1922 to a movement of Catholic laity designed to restore the Catholic grip on state and society, Catholic Action called upon Catholic physicians to take up a more visible social role. While new forms of Catholic medical sociability had emerged across Europe and the United States, for which the model of the first French Society of St Luc, St Cosmas and St Damian (1884) had acted as a source of inspiration, Reinout Vander Hulst and Joris Vandendriessche have shown how the Belgian Society of Saint-Luc (1922) was marked by a particular Catholic Action imprint. The society outlined a 'medical apostolate' for Catholic physicians in the form of a strict deontological code that was constructed at society meetings, at which Jesuit fathers acted as theological advisers, and that was spread through its journal *Saint-Luc Médical*.[70] Maarten Langhendries and Kaat Wils identified a similar notion of a 'lay apostolate' in the self-representations of Belgian doctors who were recruited by the Medical Missionary Aid Society (1925) to work in the Belgian Congo. In the latter society as well, both doctors and clergy were involved. Yet, they also conclude that this apostolate was above all a propagated ideal that was difficult to put into practice in the colonial context itself.[71]

In the 1930s, these new spaces of sociability testified of intense interactions between clergy and doctors, both on the national and the international level. Mercier's close colleague Arthur Vermeersch, for example, who became a professor at the Gregorian University in Rome, strongly influenced Pope Pius XI's encyclical letter *Casti Connubii* of 1930.[72] The Belgian bishops applauded the encyclical in a letter of 2 February 1931.[73] That same year, they discussed the usefulness of a medical examination of fiancées before their marriage. The moral theologian Arthur Janssen suggested in 1932 that the Catholic Action movement should propagate such premarital examinations to minimise the tensions and frustrations in marriage and diminish the number of divorces.[74] Both among clergy and doctors, there was less consensus about the desirability of periodic abstinence. In Janssen's opinion (and that of Pius XII), it was never acceptable when done out of selfish motives (e.g. material or physical concerns). However, it might be permitted when a couple already had some children and the physical and psychological strength of the mother (or both parents) were tested. Others, like Jean Dermine, the later chaplain ('proost') of the People's Movement for Families (Mouvement Populaire des Familles), were less open-minded.[75] In the Society of Saint-Luc as well, the question of whether physicians could recommend the method of periodic abstinence, and whether or not such information could be spread to the wider public was intensely debated.[76]

After the Second World War, the University of Leuven continued its role as a mediator between Catholic doctrine and new developments in the medical field. The 1950s formed a period of remarkable openness in this regard. Archbishop Leo Suenens played an important role in the redefinition of Catholic views on sexuality as part of the shaping of an 'intimate community of life and love' in marriage.[77] In 1958, at an international conference for Catholic physicians in Brussels, he pleaded for a closer collaboration between the medical world and the Catholic clergy – a message he repeated at an International Colloquium for Sexuality in Leuven a year later. Suenens acted as one of the strongest advocates of a more lenient position of the Catholic Church at the Second Vatican Council, where a committee was set up on the matter in which many Belgians participated.[78] In the same spirit of reform and collaboration, an Institute for Family and Sexuality Studies was opened at the University of Leuven in 1961. With the support of Suenens, the Institute was devoted to the scientific study of human sexuality. It focused on the use of contraceptive pills, and later also on questions of infertility, sterilisation and divorce, and hence fit in with wider attempts among Belgian Catholics in the post-war years to overcome the strict clerical guidelines regarding birth control.[79]

When Paul VI succeeded John XXIII in 1963, however, the Vatican again took a hard line concerning sexuality and family planning. The encyclical letter *Humanae Vitae* of 1968 strongly condemned 'artificial' forms of birth control.[80] The Belgian clergy were soon worried about those medical practices in Catholic hospitals that were at odds with the papal stance on the matter. In the Leuven academic hospitals, artificial insemination, sterilisation and abortion were effectively practised in strictly defined circumstances. Abortion, for example, was conducted in case of severe genetic defects.[81] In 1975, these medical practices were explained to the bishops on their request. To meet their objections, a Commission of Medical Ethics was established. The gynaecologist Marcel Renaer became its first president. Since the 1950s, Renaer had taught medical ethics to students and supported the use of contraceptive pills and the practice of sterilisation in certain cases, articulating the views of many Catholics who disagreed with the condemnation of such practices in *Humanae Vitae*. Together with the new commission, a chair of medical ethics was installed.[82] A need to rethink the relation between Catholic doctrine and medical practice thus led to a professionalisation of the field of medical ethics. In 1986, the Centre for Bioethics was founded, which was modelled after similar centres in the United States. Paul Schotsmans became its first director. Like Renaer, he was influenced by the personalist theories of the Leuven professor, priest and theologian Louis Janssens.[83]

Since the 1980s, ethical debates have sprung up from the field of human genetics. Liesbet Nys and Tinne Claes have shown that the technique of *in vitro* fertilisation (IVF) caused tensions within the Catholic medical world and the Leuven Faculty of Medicine. The conservative Catholic leadership of the faculty preferred keeping the birth of Belgium's first test-tube baby at the university hospital in 1983 quiet to avoid offending ecclesiastic authorities.[84] In particular, the fact that 'superfluous' fertilised egg cells were created during IVF raised questions about the start of human life. Prenatal genetic tests, which had been conducted for some time at the Leuven Centre for Human Genetics, similarly evoked ethical objections by the Belgian clergy. The rising number of these tests (e.g. amniocenteses during follow-up consultations of pregnancies) in the 1980s was feared to augment the number of abortions. After the publication of the encyclical letter *Donum Vitae* in 1987, Catholic ethicists such as Guido Maertens invested energy in the creation of an ethical framework for genetic counselling. *Donum Vitae* had stipulated that prenatal diagnoses could only be conducted if they were oriented towards healing and with respect to the 'integrity of the human foetus'. They were 'in opposition to moral laws' if they provoked abortions. In 1988, Roger Dillemans, rector of the

University of Leuven, and Maertens visited the Vatican as part of a delegation of Catholic universities to explain the medical procedures in Catholic academic hospitals. No conviction by the church followed.[85] Since 1994, every Belgian hospital is legally obliged to have an ethical commission; a national committee on bioethics was created in 1993 (as in other European countries). The committee has a double task: it advises on problems arising from biology and medicine and communicates these to the public and the authorities.[86]

In the last decades, debates on medical ethics have centred on questions of human suffering, particularly in regard to euthanasia. The death of the Flemish author Hugo Claus in 2008 from euthanasia brought the whole debate on the meaning of suffering in contemporary society to the fore again. Especially after Archbishop Danneels addressed the issue in his sermon on Holy Saturday:

> To leave one's life this way did not answer the problems of suffering and death. This way one only bypasses them. And to skirt around them is not an act of heroism and does not merit the front page of the newspapers ... Our society apparently does not know how to handle death and suffering. According to its own words, many taboos have been set aside. However, doing so, society has created new taboos, including one according to which death has no meaning and all suffering is absurd.[87]

The meaning of suffering is essential for understanding the different positions taken in this debate. As Voyé and Dobbelaere described in their article about the Catholic responses to the euthanasia debate in Belgium, 'suffering' can mean two things. For some, 'suffering is inhumane, useless, has no sense and it is immoral to let people suffer. For others, conversely, suffering may help to deepen the sense of one's own life ... suffering may also be of use to invite others to reflect on the sense of life.'[88] It is important to pause a moment to reflect on the meaning and history of 'suffering' from a religious point of view. In the previous centuries, for the religious, who were involved in healthcare and for the wealthy Catholic laymen who supported them (financially), illness and suffering were a 'gift' from God. They were meaningful and functioned either as a punishment or as a means to put the afflicted on the right track again.[89] This 'productive' view of pain (with its own salutary end) was criticised more and more in the nineteenth century as pain came to be regarded as something that needed to be controlled, eased (e.g. by anaesthetics) and treated.[90] Yet, one should be wary of presenting this story as a 'secularisation' of pain in the nineteenth century as this implies a rather oppositional view of the relationship between medicine and religion. Whereas 'philopassionism' was indeed a Catholic tradition and there was a revitalisation of this medieval idealisation of Christ's pain in the nineteenth century, this was certainly not the only Catholic view on pain of that time. As scholars as Richard Burton have emphasised, the idealised, voluntary, suffering was a minority calling and many Catholic women dedicated their lives to relieving suffering rather than seeking it out.[91] There is still much work that needs to be done on the interaction and coexistence of the two perspectives in the nineteenth and twentieth century (for the Catholic view on the beneficial effects of suffering continued up until the Second Vatican Council).[92] Studying the interaction between the views described above will at least better our understanding of the day-to-day interaction of the religious orders and the medical professionals in the hospital setting. In the euthanasia debate, for instance, religion was, according to Voyé and Dobbelaere, an important determinant for a negative attitude on the part of the nurses. The more religiously inspired they were (especially Catholics), the more they opposed euthanasia.[93]

As Voyé and Dobbelaere have amply illustrated, Belgium was one of the first Western European countries 'to introduce new legislation clashing head on with the prescriptions of the Catholic Church in these matters. In 1990, a law was passed de-penalising abortion, in 2002 a law authorising euthanasia and, in 2003, one legalising same-sex marriages.'[94] It is primarily on these occasions, when ethical questions arise, that we see the impact of Christian ideas on the debates (and voting behaviour of e.g. Christian Democrats). The aforementioned Law on Abortion stipulated that a pregnancy could henceforth be terminated within the first twelve weeks after conception. It was a piece of fairly liberal legislation, which neither the Christian Democrats nor the Belgian King Baudouin, a devoted Christian, supported. The latter would not sign the law and declared himself 'unfit to govern' for a single night, during which the law was signed by all ministers – a creative legislative solution.[95] As the country's politicians, following public opinion, further distanced themselves from a strict application of Catholic morality, the Catholic University of Leuven continued to struggle with the ethical implications of medical procedures. In forums such as the Platform for Christian Ethics (Overlegplatform Christelijke Ethiek) and in the organisation's journal *Ethical Perspectives* (*Ethische Perspectieven*), the technique of pre-implantation genetic diagnosis (PGD), which allowed genetic testing of embryos prior to implantation, was debated in the 1990s.[96] Research on stem cells generated a similar debate in the 2000s. In 2006, Archbishop Danneels and the rectors of the universities of Leuven and Louvain-la-Neuve again travelled to the Vatican to explain (with little success) the medical procedures in their academic hospitals.

Conclusions

Through the lens of Catholic thinkers and men and women religious, the historical relation between medicine and religion becomes a story of interaction, adaptation and mutual influencing. That is not to say of course that there were no conflicts. Debates over ethically contentious issues such as abortion, at least since the middle of the nineteenth century, were often fierce. But when we bypass the politicised representations of the downfall of religion in medical care in favour of scientific progress, we may better understand what was at stake in these intellectual debates and reveal more broadly how issues of sickness and health were tied to questions of identity and ideology. Here lies an agenda for future research, which may explore the history of the reception of medical technologies and techniques in the Catholic clerical and intellectual world, the everyday practices and rituals in Catholic hospitals and the often strikingly 'modern' responses of religious orders to the challenges of healthcare.

When it comes to the influence of religion on the medical field, the Belgian experience was quite particular. Religion was very much part of the 'politics' of Belgian medicine, meaning that shifts in the political power of the Catholic party shaped healthcare profoundly. The relative absence of the state in the organisation of healthcare in the nineteenth century, and the resulting dominance of religious orders, was a product of clerical–liberal compromises. The Catholic profiling of the interwar years was a reaction to the limited power of Catholic politicians in those days. In general, however, it seems fair to say that the relative comfort of Catholic healthcare, given its overall strong political support, allowed the sector to adapt itself to modern medicine without continuously being on the defensive. Future studies may find out whether or not this holds true for different aspects of the medical field. For a historiography seeking to balance collaborations and conflicts, the Belgian experience offers a fruitful test case.

Notes

1 Ghent, Archive of the Sisters of Charity of Jesus and Mary, 'Leuven: Spes Nostra', no. 3#1, *Memorial Book, 1928–71*. On the role of women religious in the Leuven academic hospitals, see J. Vandendriessche, *Zorg en wetenschap. Een geschiedenis van de Leuvense academische ziekenhuizen in de twintigste eeuw* (Leuven: Leuven University Press, 2019), 71–95.
2 On this topic, see H. Guillemain, *Diriger les consciences, guérir les âmes: une histoire comparée des pratiques thérapeutiques et religieuses (1830–1939)* (Paris: La Découverte, 2006).
3 K. Velle, *De nieuwe biechtvaders. De sociale geschiedenis van de arts in België* (Leuven: Kritak, 1991); K. Velle, 'De geneeskunde en de R.K. Kerk (1830–1940): een moeilijke verhouding?', *Trajecta: Tijdschrift voor de geschiedenis van het Katholiek leven in de Nederlanden*, 1:4 (1995), 1–21; K. Velle, 'Kerk, geneeskunde en gezondheidszorg in de 19de en het begin van de 20e eeuw', in *Het Verbond der Verzorgingsinstellingen 1938–1988. Vijftig jaar ten dienste van de Caritas-Verzorgingsinstellingen*, ed. J. Depuydt, L. Dhaene, K. Schutyser and K. Velle (Leuven: VVI/Kadoc, 1988), 35–59.
4 See, for example, J. Goldstein, 'The hysteria diagnosis and the politics of anticlericalism in late nineteenth-century France', *Journal of Modern History*, 54:2 (1982), 209–39.
5 See, for example, M. Pia Donato (ed.), *Médecine et religion: compétitions, collaborations, conflits (XIIe–XXe Siècles)* (Rome: École française de Rome, 2013); G. B. Ferngren, *Medicine and Religion: A Historical Introduction* (Baltimore, MD: Johns Hopkins University Press, 2014).
6 B. Mann Wall, *Unlikely Entrepreneurs: Catholic Sisters and the Hospital Marketplace, 1865–1925* (Columbus: Ohio State University

Press, 2005); K. Suenens, *Humble Women, Powerful Nuns: A Female Struggle for Autonomy in a Men's Church*. (Leuven: Leuven University Press, 2020).
7 The love for suffering fellow men is at the core of Christian teachings. According to Paul (1 Corinthians 13:13) it is the greatest of the Christian virtues. See C. Stiegemann, *Caritas: Nächstenliebe von den frühen Christen bis zur Gegenwart* (Petersberg: Michael Imhof Verlag, 2015); E. Baldas, 'Caritas', in *Lexikon für Theologie und Kirche*, vol. 2 (Freiburg: Herder, 1994), 947–51.
8 For a history of this first involvement of, for example, the Knights Hospitaller, see R. Stockman, *Pro Deo. De geschiedenis van de christelijke gezondheidszorg* (Leuven: Davidsfonds, 2008), 48–68.
9 The hospital sisters dated back to the twelfth and thirteenth centuries. See Stockman, *Pro Deo*, 94.
10 Velle, 'Kerk, geneeskunde en gezondheidszorg', 37–40.
11 For a brief discussion of the organisation of hospital care in France up until the early twentieth century, see B. M. Doyle, 'Healthcare before welfare states: hospitals in early twentieth-century England and France', *Canadian Bulletin of the History of Medicine*, 1:33 (2016), 174–204.
12 For an extensive overview, see Stockman, *Pro Deo*, 94–103; Ch. Vloeberghs, *Belgique Charitable* (Brussels: Librairie Nationale, 1904), 4.
13 Velle, 'Kerk, geneeskunde en gezondheidszorg', 48, 50.
14 Several institutional histories of medical institutes ran by the Sisters of Charity of Jesus and Mary have been published, but there is no synthesis of the congregation's work. See K. Leeman, F. Marysse and J. Demets, *Terug naar de toekomst: 1808–1908–2008: 100 jaar psychiatrisch centrum Caritas: 200 jaar psychiatrische zorg door de Zusters van Liefde* (Melle: Psychiatrisch centrum Caritas, 2008); A.-J. Billekens, *100 jaar psychiatrie in Venray: geschiedenis van de psychiatrische instellingen Sint Anna en Sint Servatius* (Zutphen: Walburg Pers, 2005); *150 Jaar Zusters van Liefde te Sint-Truiden* (Sint-Truiden: Psychiatrisch Ziekenhuis Sancta Maria, 1991); G. Deneckere, *Het Gentse Sint-Vincentiusziekenhuis: de zusters van liefde J.M. en de ziekenzorg te Gent, 1805 tot heden* (Ghent: Zusters van Liefde van Jezus en Maria, 1997); A. Roekens (ed.), *Des murs et des femmes: cent ans de psychiatrie et d'espoir au Beau-Vallon* (Namur: Presses Universitaires de Namur, 2014).
15 R. Stockman, 'De broeders van Liefde', in *Geen rede mee te rijmen*, ed. R. Stockman and P. Allegaert (Sint-Martens-Latem: Aurelia Books, 1989), 157.
16 Barbra Mann Wall has highlighted this feature of religious orders' involvement in American healthcare, see Wall, *Unlikely Entrepreneurs*.

17 J. Godderis, 'De geesteszieken: nieuwe inzichten en instellingszorg', in *Er is leven voor de dood: tweehonderd jaar gezondheidszorg in Vlaanderen*, ed. J. De Maeyer, L. Dhaene, G. Hertecant and K. Velle (Kapellen: Pelckmans, 1998), 65.
18 H. McLeod, 'New perspectives on the religious history of western and northern Europe 1815–1960', *Kyrkhistorisk Arsskrift*, 1:100 (2000), 135–45, at 137, 141. On the 'feminisation' of religion in this period and the role of female religious orders (disparate growth in comparison to male religious orders), see C. Langlois, 'Le Catholicisme au féminin', *Archives des Sciences Sociales des Religions*, 57:1 (1984), 29–53.
19 There were of course also orders combining activities in education and healthcare, these counted for 17.07 per cent in 1846, 20.48 per cent in 1900 and 16.47 per cent in 1947.
20 A. Tihon, 'Les religieuses en Belgique du XVIIIe au XXe siècle. Approche statistique', *Belgisch Tijdschrift voor Nieuwste Geschiedenis*, 1–2 (1976): 1–54, at 40–1 and fn 114. The French and Dutch periods of control over the Belgian territories had resulted in the high number of religious houses dedicated to healthcare (as these active congregations had often been deemed more useful than the contemplative orders that were suppressed).
21 'Die kirchliche Caritas trug ein weibliches Gesicht'; B. Schneider, 'Feminisierung der Religion im 19. Jahrhundert. Perspektiven einer These im Kontext des deutschen Katholizismus', *Trierer Theologische Zeitschrift*, 111 (2002), 126, 129.
22 The bourgeois laymen who joined the St Vincent de Paul movement, not only offered material support to the families they visited, but also advised them in matters of hygiene (well aware of its link with physical health). See S. Baré, *Het Wit-Gele Kruis, 1937–2007: 70 jaar thuis in verpleging aan huis* (Leuven: Kadoc, 2007), 21; J. Lory and J.-L. Soete, 'Implantation et affirmation (1845–1914)', in *Les Vincentiens en Belgique, 1842–1992*, ed. J. De Maeyer and P. Wynants (Leuven: Leuven University Press, 1992), 45–84.
23 J. De Maeyer, '"Les dames d'œuvres". 19de-eeuwse vrouwen van stand en hun zoektocht naar maatschappelijk engagement', in *Vrouwenzaken/Zakenvrouwen. Facetten van vrouwelijk zelfstandig ondernemerschap in Vlaanderen, 1800–2000*, ed. L. van Molle and P. Heyrman (Ghent: Provinciebestuur Oost-Vlaanderen, 2001), 108–27, references to Vloeberghs, *Belgique Charitable*.
24 K. Schultheiss, *Bodies and Souls: Politics and the Professionalization of Nursing in France, 1880–1922* (Cambridge, MA: Harvard University Press, 2001).
25 E. De Schampeleire, 'De socialist-geneesheer-vrijmetselaar Modeste Terwagne en zijn tijd' (Vrije Universiteit Brussel, unpublished licentiate

thesis, 1973); E. De Schampeleire, 'Modeste Terwagne: een vrijzinnige, sociaal bewogen arts', in De Maeyer et al., *Er is leven voor de dood*, 260–2; Velle, 'De geneeskunde en de R.K. Kerk', 11.
26 K. Velle, 'De opkomst van het verpleegkundig beroep in Belgie', *Geschiedenis der Geneeskunde*, 6 (1994), 17–26. See also the special issue 3 (1995) of *Sextant* on the secularisation of nursing. On the St Elizabeth Institute in Leuven, see A. Cousserier, *In goede handen: 75 jaar onderwijs verpleeg- en vroedkunde Leuven* (Leuven: Kadoc, 2004).
27 L. Dhaene, 'Stichting van Caritas Catholica en de eerste werkingsjaren', in Depuydt et al., *Het Verbond*, 63–84.
28 B. M. Wall, ' "Definite lines of influence": Catholic sisters and nurse training schools, 1890–1920', *Nursing Research*, 50:5 (2001), 314–21, at 319.
29 M. Constandt, Vakantiekolonies aan zee tussen 1885 en 1960. Voorgoed verdwenen zorginstellingen', *Tijd-Schrift*, 7:1 (2017), 58–75, at 60–1 and 66–7.
30 G. van Themsche, *Belgium and the Congo 1885–1980* (Cambridge, UK: Cambridge University Press, 2012), 66.
31 B. Cleys, J. De Maeyer, C. Dujardin and L. Vints, 'België in Congo, Congo in België. Weerslag van de missionering op de religieuze instituten', in *Congo in België. Koloniale cultuur in de metropool*, ed. V. Viaene, D. Van Reybrouck and B. Ceuppens (Leuven: Universitaire Pers, 2009), 147–65, at 153.
32 S. Au, 'Medical orders: Catholic and Protestant missionary medicine in the Belgian Congo 1880–1940', *Low Countries Historical Review*, 132:1 (2017), 62–82, at 66.
33 Dhaene, 'Stichting en uitbouw', 113–15.
34 Dhaene and Timmermans, 'De privé-ziekenhuizen', in De Maeyer et al., *Er is leven voor de dood*, 341–3; Stockman, *Pro Deo*, 126–7.
35 Dhaene and Timmermans, 'De privé-ziekenhuizen', 343.
36 KADOC, Private Archive of Jos De Saeger, 19.1.4.2., Letter of 26 December 1976 from J. De Saeger to G. Danneels.
37 L. Voyé and K. Dobbelaere, 'Portrait du Catholicisme en Belgique', in *Portraits du Catholicisme. Une comparaison européenne*, ed. A. Pérez-Agote (Rennes: Presses de Rennes, 2012), 11–61, 66.
38 Dhaene, 'Stichting en uitbouw', 118–22.
39 Voyé and Dobbelaere, 'Portrait du Catholicisme en Belgique', 46.
40 Ibid., 47–8.
41 J. E. Goldstein, *Console and Classify: The French Psychiatric Profession in the Nineteenth Century* (Chicago: University of Chicago Press, 2002).

42 E. van Staeyen, 'Guislain en de "traitement moral"', in Stockman and Allegaert, *Geen rede mee te rijmen*, 125–35.
43 B. Majerus and A. Roekens, 'Espaces psychiatriques, espaces religieux', in *Des murs et des femmes. Cent ans de psychiatrie et d'espoir au Beau-Vallon*, ed. A. Roekens (Namur: Presses Universitaires de Namur, 2014), 35–52.
44 Vandendriessche, *Zorg en wetenschap*, 92–3.
45 K. Velle, *Begraven of cremeren: de crematiekwestie in België* (Ghent: Stichting mens en kultuur, 1992).
46 J. Gijbels, 'Reassessing the pauper burial: the disposal of corpses in nineteenth-century Brussels', *Mortality* 23:2 (3 April 2018), 184–98; T. Claes, *Corpses in Belgian Anatomy, 1860–1914. Nobody's Dead* (Cham: Palgrave Macmillan, 2019), 237–251; T. Claes and P. Huistra, '"Il importe d'établir une distinction entre la dissection et l'autopsie." Lijken en medische disciplinevorming in laat negentiende-eeuws België', *Low Countries Historical Review)*, 131:3 (2016), 26–53; T. Claes, '"By what right does the scalpel enter the pauper's corpse?" Dissections and consent in late nineteenth-century Belgium', *Social History of Medicine*, 31:2 (2018), 258–77.
47 P.-G. Boissarie, *Les grandes guérisons de Lourdes* (Paris: Téqui, 1900), 488. The number of Belgian pilgrims was considerable: Belgium came in second place (after France) and in the years before the First World War Belgian pilgrims formed a quarter of the total of foreign pilgrims in Lourdes. See A. Kotulla, 'Lourdes und die deutschen Katholiken: Über die frühe Rezeption eines katholischen Kultes im deutschen Kaiserreich und die Anfänge der Wallfahrt bis zum ersten Weltkrieg', in *Maria und Lourdes. Wunder und Marienerscheinungen in theologischer und kulturwissenschaftlicher Perspektive*, ed. B. Schneider (Münster: Aschendorff, 2008), 139–65, at 154.
48 R. D'Hertefelt, 'Analyse van het Belgisch tijdschrift van Onze-Lieve-Vrouw van Lourdes (1895–1914)' (KU Leuven, unpublished licentiate thesis, 1989), 70.
49 J. Szabo, 'Seeing is believing? The form and substance of French medical debates over Lourdes', *Bulletin of the History of Medicine*, 76 (2002), 199–230, at 211; A. Desmazières, 'Psychology against medicine? Mysticism in the light of scientific apologetics', *Revue Belge de Philologie et d'Histoire*, 88 (2010), 1191–212, at 1192.
50 There were of course also Belgian miraculé(e)s healed in Lourdes, for example Joachime Dehante in September 1878. Boissarie, *Les grandes guérisons de Lourdes*, 162–83.

51 T. Van Osselaer, 'Introduction', in *Sign or Symptom? Exceptional Corporeal Phenomena in Religion and Medicine in the 19th and 20th Centuries*, ed. T. Van Osselaer, H. De Smaele and K. Wils (Leuven: Leuven University Press, 2017), 7–21; S. Kaufman, *Consuming Visions: Mass Culture and the Lourdes Shrine* (Ithaca, NY: Cornell University Press, 2005), 182.
52 N. Edelman, *Les métamorphoses de l'hystérique. Du début du XIXe siècle à la Grande Guerre* (Paris: Éditions La Découverte, 2003), 215; J. Maître, 'De Bourneville à nos jours: interprétations psychiatriques de la mystique', *L'Évolution Psychiatrique*, 64 (1999), 765–78, at 772.
53 Desmazières, 'Psychology against medicine'.
54 G. Klaniczay, 'Louise Lateau et les stigmatisées du XIXème siècle entre directeurs spirituels, dévots, psychologues et médecin', *Archivio Italiano per la storia della pietà*, 26 (2013), 279–319.
55 He published a book on the case, *Louise Lateau ou les mystères de Bois-d'Haine dévoilés* (second augmented and revised edition in 1875, Brussels). See S. Lachapelle, 'Between miracle and sickness: Louise Lateau and the experience of stigmata and ecstasy', *Configurations*, 12 (2004), 77–105, at 96; W. Dupont, 'Free-floating evils: a genealogy of homosexuality in Belgium' (PhD diss., University of Antwerp, 2015), 142.
56 Goldstein, 'The hysteria diagnosis'; Velle, 'Geneeskunde en de R.K. Kerk', 12.
57 Lachapelle, 'Between miracle and sickness', 88 fn 21.
58 A. Goldberg, *Sex, Religion and the Making of Modern Madness: The Eberbach Asylum and German Society, 1815–1849* (New York: Oxford University Press, 1999), 48; M. Heidegger, 'Religiöser Wahn, Identität und die psychiatrische Erzählung in der säkularisierten Antstalt (Tirol 1830–1850)', in *Identitäten verhandeln – Identitäten de/konstruieren*, ed. E. Appelt, E. Grabner-Niel, M. Jarosch and M. Ralser (Innsbruck: Innsbruck University Press 2015), 97–120; T. Van Osselaer and K. Smeyers, 'Divine hysteria: readings of the sacred disease in the late eighteenth and early nineteenth centuries', *Österreichische Zeitschrift für Geschichtswissenschaften*, 31:3 (2020), 54–75.
59 T. Van Osselaer, 'The affair of the photographs: controlling the public image of a nineteenth-century stigmatic', *Journal of Ecclesiastical History* 68:4 (2017), 784–806.
60 E. Betta, *Animare la vita: disciplina della nascita tra medicina e morale nell'Ottocento* (Bologna: Il mulino, 2006). See also L. Pozzi, 'The encyclical Casti Connubii (1930): the origin of the twentieth-century discourse of the Catholic Church on family and sexuality', in *La Sainte Famille: Sexualité, filiation et parentalité dans l'Église catholique*,

ed. Cecile Vanderpelen and Caroline Sägesser (Brussels: Editions de l'Université Libre de Bruxelles, 2017), 41–53.
61 Gijbels, 'Medical compromise'; J. Gijbels, 'Leve de foetus: liberale en katholieke artsen over de keizersnede in België (1840–1914)', *Handelingen der Koninklijke Zuid-Nederlandse Maatschappij voor Taal- en Letterkunde en Geschiedenis* 7:1 (2017), 85–98; J. Gijbels, 'L'omniprésence de la religion. Les médecins belges et le dilemme obstétrical (1840–1880)', *Annales de démographie historique*, 139:1 (2020), 207–35; P. Daled, 'Avortement médical, liberté de conscience et éthique utilitariste à l'université catholique de Louvain au XIXe siècle', *Le Figuier: Annales du Centre Interdisciplinaire d'Étude des Religions et de la Laïcité de l'Université Libre de Bruxelles*, 2 (2008), 97–110.
62 Gijbels, 'Medical compromise', 329–30.
63 On the discussion about birth rates in Belgium, see P. van Praag, *Het bevolkingsvraagstuk in België: ontwikkeling van standpunten en opvattingen (1900–1977)* (Antwerpen: De Sikkel, 1979).
64 On Belgian biopolitics, see Dupont, 'Free-floating evils', 259–60.
65 The Catholic Church's natalist policy was in tune with that of the Belgian government, which, alarmed by the drop in birth rates, had banned advertisement and the selling of contraceptives (1923) and created the National Work for Children's Well-Being (Nationaal Werk voor Kinderwelzijn, 1919). See E. Flour, E. Gubin, C. Marissal, L. van Molle and C. Wallemacq, *Jongens en meisjes .... bestemming bekend? België 1830–2000* (Brussels: AVG-Carhif, 2009), 17–19.
66 R. Christens, 'De orthodoxie van het zaad. Seksualiteit en sekse-identiteit in de Rooms-Katholieke traditie', in *Het lichaam m/v*, ed. K. Wils (Leuven: University Press Leuven, 2001), 241–2; L. Gevers, 'Gezin, religie en moderniteit. Visie en strategie van de Belgische bisschoppen (1830–1940)', *Trajecta*, 4 (1995), 103–21, at 113–14.
67 M. Derez, 'Rufin Schockaert: legendarisch vrouwenarts', in De Macycr et al., *Er is leven voor de dood*, 260–2; Christens, 'De orthodoxie', 241–3.
68 On neo-Malthusianism and contraceptives, see De Smet, *Het christelijk huwelijk* (Brugge: Beyaert, 1920), esp. 40.
69 The contacts between the Leuven theologian August-Joseph Lecomte, the University of Leuven and the Vatican in the 1870s are mentioned by Emmanuel Betta. See E. Betta, 'Le Saint-Officie et la fécondation artificielle (XIXe–XXe Siècle)', in *Médecine et religion: compétitions, collaborations, conflits (XIIe–XXe Siècles)*, ed. M. Pia Donato (Rome: École française de Rome, 2013), 279–303.
70 R. Vander Hulst and J. Vandendriessche, 'Physician-apostles for Christ: the Belgian Saint-Luc Society and the making of a Catholic

medical identity, 1900–1940', *Histoire, médecine, santé*, 17 (2020): 133–54.
71 M. Langhendries and K. Wils, 'When the physician becomes an apostle. The persona of the Catholic colonial doctor in interwar Belgium and the Belgian Congo', *Social Sciences and Missions* 33 (2021): 179–207.
72 Dupont, 'Free-floating evils', 285–9; Gevers, 'Gezin, religie en moderniteit', 117. *Casti Connubii* was written in an accessible language (not in other-worldly theological phrasing) to reach the whole church via the bishops (the first addressees). See J. Stengers, 'Les pratiques anticonceptionnelles dans le mariage au XIX et au XXe siècle: problèmes humains et attitudes religieuses', *Revue Belge de Philologie et d'Histoire*, 49:2 (1971), 403–81, at 425, and 49:4, 1119–74, at 1173.
73 Gevers, 'Gezin, religie en moderniteit', 117.
74 A. Janssen, *Het geneeskundig onderzoek voor het huwelijk* (Leuven: De Vlaamsche Drukkerij, 1932); J. De Maeyer, 'Relatie en huwelijk in de moderne tijd (ca.1800-ca.1950). Kerkelijke standpunten en strategieën', in *Levensrituelen. Het huwelijk*, ed. R. Burggraeve, M. Cloet and K. Dobbelaere (Leuven: Leuven University Press, 2000), 31–51, at 50.
75 De Maeyer, 'Relatie en huwelijk, 49–50.
76 Vander Hulst and Vandendriessche, 'Physician-apostles for Christ'.
77 Christens, 'De orthodoxie', 246–8.
78 W. Dupont, 'Catholics and sexual change in Flanders', in *Sexual Revolutions*, ed. G. Hekma and A. Giami (Basingstoke: Palgrave Macmillan, 2014), 81–98.
79 L. Nys, *Van mensen en muizen. Vijftig jaar Nederlandstalige Faculteit Geneeskunde aan de Leuvense universiteit* (Leuven: University Press Leuven, 2016); A.-S. Crosetti, 'The "converted unbelievers": Catholics in family planning in French-speaking Belgium (1953–1973)', *Medical History*, 64:2 (2020), 267–86; W. Dupont, 'In good faith: Belgian Catholics' attempts to overturn the ban on contraception (1945–1968)', in *'La Sainte Famille: sexualité, filiation et parentalité dans l'Église catholique': Problèmes d'histoire des religions* (Brussels: Bruxelles Editions de l'Univeresité de Bruxelles, 2017), 67–76.
80 A. Harris (ed.), *The schism of '68: Catholicism, Contraception and Humanae Vitae in Europe, 1945–1975* (Basingstoke: Palgrave Macmillan, 2018).
81 Vandendriessche, *Zorg en wetenschap*, 166–71.
82 Nys, *Van mensen en muizen*, 143–6.
83 J. Vermylen and P. Schotsmans (eds), *Ethiek in de kliniek. 25 jaar adviezen van de Commissie voor medische ethiek* (Leuven: Faculteit Geneeskunde, 2000).
84 Nys, *Van mensen en muizen*, 143–50; Tinne Claes, '"Catholic, but Not According to the Rules": Assisted Reproduction and Catholic Doctors

in Belgium, 1940s–1980s', *Journal of Religious History*, forthcoming; Ivo Brosens (ed.), *The Challenge of Reproductive Medicine at Catholic Universities: Time to Leave the Catacombs* (Leuven: Peeters, 2006).
85 J. Vandendriessche, 'Genetic counselling in Belgium: the Centre for Human Genetics at the University of Leuven, 1960–1990', in *History of Human Genetics: Aspects of Its Development and Global Perspectives*, ed. H. Petermann, P. Harper and S. Doetz (Heidelberg: Springer, 2017), 447–59.
86 L. Voyé and K. Dobbelaere, *Euthanasia and the Belgian Catholic World* (Leuven: Leuven University Press, 2015), 23.
87 Ibid., 15.
88 Ibid., 38.
89 J. Bourke, *The Story of Pain: From Prayer to Painkillers* (Oxford: Oxford University Press, 2014), 92.
90 J. Moscoso, *Pain: A Cultural History* (Basingstoke: Palgrave Macmillan, 2012), 2, 6; L. Bending, *The Representation of Bodily Pain in Late-Nineteenth-Century English Culture* (Oxford: Clarendon Press, 2000), 2.
91 R. Burton, *Holy Tears, Holy Blood: Women, Catholicism, and the Culture of Suffering in France, 1840–1970* (London: Cornell University Press, 2005), xiii; H. Roodenburg, 'Empathy in the making: crafting the believer's emotions in the late medieval Low Countries', *Low Countries Historical Review*, 129:2 (2014), 42–62.
92 P. Kane, '"She offered herself up": the victim soul and victim spirituality in Catholicism', *Church History*, 71:1 (2002), 80–119, at 82.
93 Voyé and Dobbelaere, *Euthanasia*, 33.
94 Ibid., 13, 21.
95 E. Witte, 'De liberalisering van de abortus-wetgeving in België (1970–1990)', in *Abortus*, ed. M. Scheys (Brussels: VUB Press, 1993), 21–102.
96 Vandendriessche, 'Genetic counselling in Belgium'.

Selected bibliography

Daled, P., 'Avortement médical, liberté de conscience et éthique utilitariste à l'Université Catholique de Louvain au XIXe siècle', *Le Figuier: Annales du Centre Interdisciplinaire d'Etude des Religions et de la Laïcité de l'Université Libre de Bruxelles*, 2 (2008), 97–110.
De Maeyer, J., Dhaene, L., Hertecant, G. and Velle, K. (eds), *Er is leven voor de dood: tweehonderd jaar gezondheidszorg in Vlaanderen* (Kapellen: Pelckmans, 1998).
Desmazières, A., 'Psychology against medicine? Mysticism in the light of scientific apologetics', *Revue Belge de Philologie et d'Histoire*, 88 (2010), 1191–212.

Dobbelaere, K. and Pérez-Agote, A. (eds), *The Intimate: Polity and the Catholic Church, Laws about Life, Death and the Family in So-Called Catholic Countries* (Leuven: Leuven University Press, 2015).

Gijbels, J., 'Medical compromise and its limits: religious concerns and the post-mortem caesarean section in nineteenth-century Belgium', *Bulletin of the History of Medicine*, 93:3 (2019), 305–34.

Labbeke, L., Poels, V. and Wolf, H. R. (eds), *Bezielde zorg: verpleging door katholieke religieuzen in Nederland en Vlaanderen (negentiende-twintigste eeuw)* (Hilversum: Verloren, 2008).

Lachapelle, S., 'Between miracle and sickness: Louise Lateau and the experience of stigmata and ecstasy', *Configurations*, 12 (2004), 77–105.

Langhendries, M. and Wils, K., 'When the physician becomes an apostle: the persona of the Catholic colonial doctor in interwar Belgium and the Belgian Congo', *Social Sciences and Missions* 34 (2021): 179–207.

Majerus, B. and Roekens, A., 'Espaces psychiatriques, espaces religieux', in A. Roekens (ed.), *Des murs et des femmes. Cent ans de psychiatrie et d'espoir au Beau-Vallon* (Namur: Presses universitaires de Namur, 2014), 35–52.

Stengers, J., 'Les pratiques anticonceptionnelles dans le mariage au XIX et au XXe siècle: problèmes humains et attitudes religieuses', *Revue Belge de Philologie et d'Histoire*, 49:2 (1971), 403–81 and 49:4, 1119–74.

Vandendriessche, J., 'Genetic counselling in Belgium: the Centre for Human Genetics at the University of Leuven, 1960–1990', in H. Petermann, P. Harper and S. Doetz (eds), *History of Human Genetics: Aspects of Its Development and Global Perspectives* (Heidelberg: Springer, 2017), 447–59.

Vander Hulst, R. and Vandendriessche, J., 'Physician-apostles for Christ: the Belgian Saint-Luc Society and the making of a Catholic medical identity, 1900–1940', *Histoire, médecine, santé*, 17 (2020): 133–54.

Van Osselaer, T., De Smaele, H. and Wils, K. (eds), *Sign or Symptom? Exceptional Corporeal Phenomena in Religion and Medicine in the 19th and 20th Centuries* (Leuven: Leuven University Press, 2017).

Velle, K., 'De geneeskunde en de R.K. Kerk (1830–40): een moeilijke verhouding?', *Trajecta: Tijdschrift voor de geschiedenis van het Katholiek leven in de Nederlanden* 1:4 (1995), 1–21.

Voyé, L. and Dobbelaere, K., *Euthanasia and the Belgian Catholic World* (Leuven: Leuven University Press, 2015).

3

Medicine and colonialism

Sokhieng Au and Anne Cornet

[Ethnographic description of a Bakongo medical ceremony:] On the day appointed the Nganga Nkosi, together with a troop of attendants furnished with drums and other musical instruments, starts for the village of the diseased. At the entrance to the village they pause and begin playing their instruments. The inhabitants go out to meet them and present the Nganga with a cock, a bunch of bananas and a basketful of groundnuts ... [various preparations are made at the house of the afflicted, at which point the Nganga chants]: O thou Nkosi who sheddest blood, Look upon this person. Thou hast laid hold of him, I have not seized him. But thou hast eaten thy snail long ago, Now vomit it forth. I shall rub thy vomitings upon his body, That he may become strong, that he may become vigorous. Do thou leave him – Let him sleep peacefully, Let him awaken when the sun is at its greatest height! (E ngeye, nkosi mbungu zi menga tala yuna nleke nge kunsimbidi, mono k'insimbidi ko. Kimpaka-mpaka udia mwaka, gana ubioka, kiad ye kia! bioko iziola mu nitu, kakala nkonso, kakala ngolo, Ngege unyambula, kaleka bwo, kasikama ntangu nlungu.)[1]

This chapter reviews the history of medicine in what were the Belgian colony of Congo and the administered territories of Ruanda-Urundi (now Rwanda and Burundi). A problem that many of the chapters in this book tackle, if sometimes indirectly, is what medicine is and who defines it. This question, while already difficult in the context of heterogenous communities in Belgium, is often the central problematic in studies of medicine in the colonies. The disciplinary lens of the scholar often delimits what medicine is. For example, ethnological recordings from the late nineteenth and early twentieth century on indigenous medicine and magic undertaken by men such as Reverends Joseph Van Wing and Karl Laman are often the reserve of scholars focused on anthropological and phenomenological analyses of human experience. Clinical records, as well as administrative records, newspaper reports and official correspondence are mined as more traditional historical data. Works of individuals such as John Janzen and Jan Vansina and, more recently Nancy Rose Hunt, have destabilised such divisions.[2] Further new methodologies such as the *histoire croisée* approach also suggest ways to encompass both the historicity and the culturally embedded nature of the object under study, as well as the cultural biases of the researcher.[3] Nonetheless, questions of interpretive frameworks, girded by often-unstated disagreements on what constitutes medicine, still vex the history of medicine in the colony. This tension is heightened when scholars of colonial medicine are in dialogue with more Europe-focused scholars of medicine. As observed by Waltraud Ernst, the history of science and medicine in the colony requires different historiographical and conceptual vantage points than 'Europe-based academics' to capture the indigenous perspective in the colonial exchange.[4] Further, because this collection is about Belgian medicine, we focus less here on indigenous medicine, particularly as we do not want to create facile comparisons between the changes in the medical domain occurring in Europe and those in the colony. In other words, to stay within the general theme of the collection (history of Belgian medicine), and to avoid reproducing Eurocentric assumptions about what counts as legitimate medicine to African populations, we limit our discussion to Western medicine, expanding beyond the political economical perspective to address some of the wider issues springing from such involvement, and leave the reader with further readings relating to issues of Congolese, Rwandan and Burundian medical practices. Some of these readings indicate how a shared history of a Belgian and African medicine in the colony has been written, but much more can still be done. This reflects in part the relatively light scholarship in Belgian colonial history in comparison to research in French and British Africa.

A history of medicine in the colony was, not too long ago, only the story of colonial medicine. But colonial medicine was and is often presumed to be many things: Western medicine, medicine of the state, missionary medicine, tropical medicine, public health, notions of hygiene and various imported concepts of disease and health. It is sometimes narrowly defined as the medical services administered by the colonial state, in this case Belgium. Under such a narrow definition, university research projects, missionary hospitals and private European medical care including that of major industries and the like are excluded. The discussion that follows includes medicine that is not specifically administered by the colonial government, in other words the more expansive domain of Western medicine in the Congo and Ruanda-Urundi, as they accompanied the imposition of Belgian colonial rule even if they were often not part of the colonial state. Thus, the following discussion presents what are often uncoordinated efforts by various actors to provide their versions of Western medicine in the Congo and Ruanda-Urundi. These actors had motivations and methods that sometimes overlapped, competed or even clashed. While the Belgian colonial state sometimes attempted to coordinate such efforts, it never truly controlled the heterogenous elements trying to 'heal' or 'sanitise' the region.

We also must keep in mind that no matter how inclusively we want to define colonial medicine, or even if we speak generally of European medicine, it was the medicine of a tiny minority. The vast majority of medicine practised in the Belgian Congo and Ruanda-Urundi would fall under the realm of what is now called traditional medicine, but what was at the time called 'sorcery', 'witchcraft', 'superstition', 'empiricism', 'quackery', 'fetishism' and the like. Some of the conflicts between popular medicine and state-approved medicine parallel those in the story of the professionalisation of medicine in Belgium, but certainly in degree if not kind, the differences here were much more substantial and wildly incommensurate on the political, social, economic and cultural level.

We have few studies tracing how these West and Central African medical practices were influenced in an epistemological sense by the importation of Western medicine distinct from colonialism more generally. We also know that there was a wilful dismissal of indigenous medical practices by Western medical practitioners. In this limited space, we cannot do justice to the complexities and issues in this domain, although we will briefly touch on 'where' indigenous medicine lies in relation to Western medicine. We also observe again that except for the research of a few individuals such as Maryinez Lyons, Nancy Rose Hunt and Jean-Luc Vellut, even Belgian *colonial* medicine is an underdeveloped field.

All cultures, including those of Central and West Africa, had thriving medical traditions before the arrival of the Europeans.[5] With the arrival of Europeans, most of this medicine was dismissively lumped into superstitions, witch doctors, fetishes and idols. While a great deal of work has been done in recovering the complexity of indigenous medical practices of the colonial and pre-colonial period, historians of medicine (particularly those who work primarily in the European context) sometimes reproduce in their analysis the historical relegation of such medical practices into the realm of culture. As such, one can imagine that real 'medicine' entered a healthcare vacuum. This is grossly incorrect. However, what we can say is that, as Vellut observed, it is really only in the field of medicine and healthcare that there exists 'so strict a division between the worlds of the colonized and the colonizers'.[6] Indigenous medicine continued to thrive and was little directly influenced by colonial medicine post-1885. To be clear, it would be strongly influenced by the changes wrought by colonialism writ large, but not by any direct competition with European medicine per se. For example, both the erosion of traditional political authority by new colonial administrations and the juridical abolition of trial by poison ordeal would reconfigure the possibilities for the exercise of traditional medicine.[7] As Nancy Hunt also reveals in her study of the Congo, a nuanced cultural history can be reconstructed from examining anxieties surrounding what are, in the West, squarely medical topics such as depopulation and infertility, through examination of 'therapeutic insurgency' from the Congolese as a response to a repressive biopolitics imposed by a 'nervous state'.[8]

This chapter focuses on both what is common and what is quite peculiar about the Belgian case in the history of medicine in the colonial context. Belgium was an imperial nation, but this fact was sometimes unnoticed during the colonial era and still is by many Belgians.[9] This in itself is part of the peculiarity of Belgian colonialism, and shaped Belgian colonial medicine. Political, economic and church interests vested in the Belgian colonies were in some instances freer to shape the colony as they saw fit, outside the interference of a general metropolitan public. The downside of such disinterest, however, included fewer resources from the metropole and a lack of checks on colonial abuses.

As noted in the opening pages of this book (see the Introduction), medical practice and discourse are implicated in identity formation, whether citizen or subject, gender or race. As other chapters in this book have demonstrated, in the metropole they interlinked questions of citizenship and the 'right' to health with notions of gender and class. One can debate whether colonial medicine exacerbated this differentiation, or simply followed the dictates of the state. As Shula Marks noted over twenty ago, biomedicine in the colonies 'played a major role in creating and reproducing racial and gendered discourses of difference' (see also Chapter 1, pp. 40–7).[10] The Belgian colonies were no exceptions to this general observation. In the Belgian Congo, one could even argue that such discourses of differences were more prevalent than in most other colonial situations. For example, while we have the stereotype of the Frenchman in Indochina or Algeria or Guinea proclaiming of his colonies, 'C'est la France!' we think a similar image, under a similar rhetorical imagining, cannot be conjured between Belgium and Ruanda-Urundi/the Belgian Congo. Colonial policies indicate that Rwandans, Burundians and Congolese were not meant to be assimilated as Belgians. Certainly this was true before the Second World War, but even the debut of indigenous identification cards in 1948 still explicitly delimited the non-Belgianness of its carriers: Africans were either colonial subjects or Belgians *of colonial status*. These lands would never become 'Greater Belgium', even if there existed some propaganda by pro-colonialists agitating for the Congo as Belgium's tenth province.[11]

The ever-contentious question of the colonial relationship confounds further an understanding of medicine's role in creating the citizen-subject. In other words, 'state' medicine could operate under similar justifications in Belgium or in the Congo, but the dynamic between the state and the subject was fundamentally different. Further, as illustrated in the opening quote, the conceptual gulf between state and subject as to what constituted medicine was also considerably greater. Even the term 'subject' attributed to the Congolese must be approached carefully. Congolese under Belgian rule were never citizens,[12] and it was often a stretch to view them as subjects. They were, most commonly, treated as objects. It is generally accepted that among 'colonial medicines', Belgium's version swung towards the more authoritarian and totalitarian end of the spectrum. Congolese, as medical consumers, were often coerced or cajoled rather than persuaded or served.

Belgian colonialism can be roughly divided into three stages: exploration and consolidation (1870–1908), expansion (1909–40) and relinquishment of control (1940–62).[13] The earliest stage coincides with the establishment of Leopold II's Congo Free State (CFS) (1885–1908), while expansion occurred during the period when Belgium took the CFS (and what was German Ruanda-Urundi in 1916) and implemented a territory-wide health administration. The period from 1940 onwards represented a sea change in the attitudes of both coloniser and colonised through all colonies in the globe as the assumptions of colonialism became increasingly untenable. In this period, colonial powers had to adjust both their message and their methods to justify control of entire other peoples. In some instances, colonising powers attempted to reestablish power after the disruptions of the Second World War, with widely varying success. Even those successful at maintaining their colonies, such as Belgium, were forced at minimum to appear to be 'preparing' their colonies for independence in the post-war epoch.

The beginnings of state medicine under the CFS

Western medicine in the Belgian colonies would ultimately be represented by four main activities: a state-organised medical service, missionary medicine, industrial medicine and research organisations and activities. The administrative structure of the CFS, recognised by the 1885 Treaty of Berlin, was a hasty conversion of a semi-private organisational presence on the ground, the Association Internationale du Congo.[14] These agents were multinational; the colonisation of the Congo forcibly a multinational and military enterprise due to Belgium's lack of direct colonial experience and insufficient resources at the moment of the creation of the CFS.[15] The CFS itself was not in fact a Belgian colony, but the personal fiefdom of Belgium's controversial monarch Leopold II. His treatment of this territory (almost eighty times larger than Belgium itself) as a personal domain to be ruthlessly commercially exploited led to some of the most notorious abuses of indigenous populations of the age of high colonialism (in a historical period where abuses were many and shocking). From 1885 until the end of the First World War, the state adopted measures drawn from the model of public health in Europe (sanitary cordons, lazarets, quarantines and so forth) but quickly realised that they were unsuited to the health situation in Central Africa.

State medicine, as introduced in the nineteenth century, overlapped considerably with military medicine. Medical doctors often served as integral parts of initial exploratory expeditions, mainly to ensure the health of expeditionary forces.[16] This reflects the fact that the history of medicine in the Congo, written from the perspective of Belgium, is a history of military conquest and commercial exploitation. When the CFS became the Belgian Congo, the structuring of the medical staff was still modelled on the military administration. Indeed, the health service was patterned on the military, with the grades of doctors corresponding to those of the notorious Force Publique.[17]

Not surprisingly, little was invested in medicine. In 1888, the health budget represented 2.24 per cent of the regular budget and dropped by 1906 to 1.9 per cent.[18] This was offset in part by special funding Leopold reserved for research on sleeping sickness, which was decimating the local populations.[19] The first two hospitals serving black populations were created to tackle the negative financial impact of sick workers on the two major railway projects in the region. In 1897, the Société du Chemin de fer des Cataractes created an indigenous hospital in Matadi and in 1903 the Compagnie des Chemins de fer du Congo supérieur created a hospital for workers in Stanleyville.[20] This also reflects the limited mandate of medicine, and the underlying rationale for healthcare provision. Health was not a public good but a commercial or military good – it was provided to improve military control and economic exploitation, thus only to those populations directly related to these aims.

Independent of the colonial state, missionaries and industrial concerns also developed substantial medical activities. Catholic and Protestant missions were significant Western medical care providers. Both were present from the founding of the CFS, although initially, Protestants outnumbered Catholics. The Catholics in large part participated through agreements signed with the Belgian State to be auxiliaries in the Native Medical Services (SAMI), or through agreements with the private industrial sector (e.g. the Sisters of St Marie of Namur were contracted to work with the Huileries du Congo belge). The Protestant denominations, many of whom were active in medical care, existed in uneasy, informal cooperation with the colonial state from the arrival of Henry Morton Stanley at Stanley Falls in 1877. Orders such as the British Baptist Missionary Society, the American Baptist Missionary Society and the Swedish Mission Society staffed their missions with accredited doctors and created hospitals and clinics throughout the territory.[21]

International agitation over the human tragedy of Leopold's CFS led to its annexation by Belgium in 1908. This did not fundamentally change the medical system, even if a department of health services was created in 1909 and a chief physician, Dr Heiberg, was appointed in 1911. Many services were simply carried over, and many agents of the CFS converted to agents of the Belgian Congo. In two years, the number of doctors doubled, reaching fifty-nine, still an insignificant number in a country with a population between ten and thirty million.[22] When the CFS was annexed by the Belgian state, state-supported discrimination against Protestant organisations continued, despite their presence being technically protected under the stipulation of religious freedom in the 1885 Berlin Act, which had created the CFS. In truth, the CFS and Belgium colonial state could more accurately be characterised as begrudgingly tolerating rather than protecting the Protestant presence in the region.[23] However, Belgium recognised the important contribution of the medical services provided by the Protestant Church. In fact, in Ruanda-Urundi, Protestant societies such as the Church Missionary Society or the Seventh-Day Adventists could only obtain entry into the mandated territories by creating modern hospitals.[24]

Expansion

Under the CFS, many doctors continued to be career soldiers, who seemed more willing to emigrate, on both the Belgian and Italian sides.[25] This trend would continue as the health services expanded. The health service also had a significant number of career military doctors placed at the disposal of the colony by the metropolitan army, and young graduates performing military service in the regions administered by Belgium.[26] In the interwar period, on average 42 per cent of doctors in Ruanda were doctors performing their military service through the colonial medical service. In total approximately 20 per cent of career military doctors served in the colonial medical service.[27]

The lack of investment in health characterises the entire period of the CFS, and lasted until the First World War. The expansion of the medical service, ostensibly to reach the entire indigenous population, was part of a wider global trend. The 1919 flu epidemic, which decimated populations across the globe, did not leave the Congo untouched. An estimated 4 per cent of the indigenous population succumbed to the murderous disease, as many as four hundred thousand individuals.[28] The shock of this wave of mortality may have also served to spur more organised and widespread action against epidemics. This change in policy can also be explained by other spreading epidemics – most notably sleeping sickness – and by the acceleration of economic exploitation in the colony, visible through the multiplication of major infrastructure projects and the development of the mining sector, all activities that were very labour-intensive. It became necessary to 'undertake a systematic, organised conquest of tropical environments' to allow 'penetration of industrial capitalism and its production methods' including ensuring a healthy workforce.[29] In French West Africa, medical assistance to the natives was launched in 1905, while the British colonial medical services grew out of the medical departments run by the Colonial Office at the turn of the century.[30] In the Belgian Congo, a native medical service (Service d'Assistance Médicale Indigène or SAMI) was launched in 1911. However, unlike the native medical services of Britain and France, its remit was much more limited, initially to the treatment of sleeping sickness, and later expanding to other communicable diseases.[31]

The medical services continued to have staffing shortages even as it tried to expand in the period of consolidation, for various reasons. In the Congo, state doctors were subordinate not only to administrative authorities, but also to Catholic Church authorities.[32] Further, state medical service was public health focused, with limited clinical practice and few chances to stay connected to an adjacent booming tropical medicine research network. Ambitious doctors desiring to finish their careers in the university or private practice would have few opportunities for advancement in the Congo. Low status, the conditions of life and the anti-liberal approach to medicine in the colony ultimately made recruitment difficult.[33] Thus the state frequently turned to foreigners, perpetuating the policy of the CFS.[34] The health service included a significant number of physicians from Italy (which had early on developed a naval medicine and worked at the forefront of the antimalarial fight).[35] However, during the interwar period, a nationalistic mood in Belgium translated to efforts to 'nationalise' staff in its colonies: regulations proliferated that adjusted the status of foreign physicians with temporary and limited term contracts, with a slightly higher salary but no right to a pension.[36]

In 1929, the colonial secretary Henri Jaspar noted in the House of Representatives that there were only 127 physicians in the Belgian Congo, roughly one doctor for every 94,500 Congolese. Shortly after, the Université de Bruxelles conducted a comparative survey, and noted that Cameroon in 1930 had one physician per 55,500 inhabitants, compared with one doctor per 350,000 inhabitants in the Belgian-administered Rwanda. This was perceived as a challenging gap, partially explained by the fact that the two territories had different population policies (economic exploitation versus settlement), and Cameroon had a higher Western population (which was always targeted as a priority by medical activity). As a comparison, the survey launched by the Université de Bruxelles reported on the basis of the statistics of the Bureau International Du Travail in Geneva that there was at that time one doctor per 2,344 inhabitants in Belgium, one per 832 in England and one per 1,509 in France.[37]

Rwanda, Burundi and the Belgian Congo followed the same basic administrative structure for their medical services, with an inspector general, several districts with medical officers, hospitals in the major colonial enclaves and lazarets run by religious orders. Under the orders of the *médecin en chef*, based in the capital, were the provincial doctors.[38] Secondary posts were entrusted to doctors of first and second class, who depended directly on local authorities to fulfil their mandates.[39] Medical assistants remained subordinate to Western staff. They were prohibited from performing certain medical procedures, except under the supervision of the Europeans. Their assignments were also decided by European staff. But European medical staff were ultimately too expensive and too sparse to ensure all the medical activity. African auxiliaries were imperative. The wages of the lowest paid European doctor were still six times higher than that of the highest-ranking medical African in the late 1920s; exactly the same ratio as Iliffe observed in British East Africa at the same time.[40] African employees, almost exclusively male, would remain socially, economically and technically subordinate to European staff. The Belgian Congo experimented with training programmes and schools for nurses and native auxiliaries from its creation in 1908, but largely failed in its efforts into the 1930s.[41] Indeed, the nursing schools created by Protestant missions initially met with more success. The state also attempted to train midwives and birth attendants, but like its nurse training schools, met with little success until the late 1950s, on the eve of independence.[42]

Sleeping sickness became the major problem of the colonial medical service. Its rapid spread, devastating effect on the populations of the region and the lack of real understanding of the disease or effective prophylaxis led to extensive efforts by the Belgian colonial government to experiment with various control methods. Sleeping sickness would spur early scientific research missions, experimental coercive public health measures and the implementation of a semi-military medical grid. Medical authorities of the CFS, and later the Belgian Congo, set up special itinerant missions to combat sleeping sickness. These units were responsible for regularly monitoring populations, detecting and isolating the ill. This eventually expanded to mobile teams that canvassed entire regions, village by village, screening and treating often unwilling native populations (Figure 3.1).

Both the British and the Belgian medical services strove for mass, decentralised medical treatment for sleeping sickness. However, the Belgian administration preferred to go to the patient and force him to submit to treatment, while the British expanded medical services through widespread dispensaries run by African nurses, encouraging local populations to receive treatment through their communities. They also developed several programmes to target the vector, the tsetse fly. Germany, with its strong expertise in laboratory medicine, focused on diagnosis. Ultimately, the three colonial powers wrestling with sleeping sickness – Germany, Britain and Belgium – each approached its eradication in different ways. While

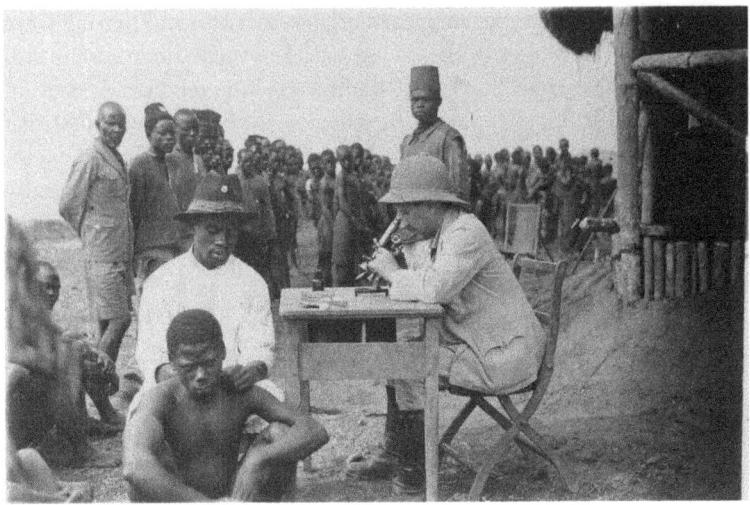

Figure 3.1 Health worker Ruyters visits patient, Beni, 1937 (Province of Costermansville).

the German East African solution was based on the microbiological model using widespread laboratory screening, British Uganda focused on an entymological solution and eradication of the tsetse fly and Belgium focused largely on policing and restricting human population movements.[43] The hubris of various African colonial governments around the treatment of sleeping sickness has been recently well documented by Guillaume Lachenal in his study of the development and use of the experimental drug Lomadine.[44]

In regions controlled by Belgium, systematic screening and treatment missions of sleeping sickness patients by mobile teams began in the interwar period (Schwetz in Kwango and Rodhain in Uele) between 1918 and 1920, in a context of concern over the widespread depopulation of the region.[45] The sleeping sickness campaigns would become *the* major public health and medical research intervention in the region. Europeans could not fail to notice that the Congolese who had the greatest interaction with European enclaves (workers, soldiers, catechists and African religious converts) were succumbing in alarming numbers to a variety of epidemics, sleeping sickness being the most noticeable. A state hospital construction programme was launched in 1921 for indigenous populations, followed by a new organisation of the medical service in 1922, which became autonomous and directly dependent on the governor general. The health service was organised in a network of fixed health facilities, supplemented by special missions against trypanosomiasis. The first efforts at medical surveillance would take place in Kwango in 1923–24, in a manner that 'seemed more a police operation than a public health operation'.[46] Kwango would also become a foil to later efforts at medical surveillance.

Major endemic and epidemic diseases were the focus of the interwar period. Parastatal organisations were formed in the interwar period, mostly focused on vertical programmes screening and treating specific diseases in circumscribed areas. These vertical programmes were the forerunners of today's public–private partnerships in global health. One of the first such programmes was the Queen Elizabeth Funds for Native Medical Assistance (Fonds Reine Elisabeth pour l'assistance médicale indigène or FOREAMI), created through a funding partnership between the Belgian state and the personal funds of Belgian Queen Elisabeth in 1930. The goal of FOREAMI, a semi-autonomous medical organisation, was to completely rehabilitate a delimited area by an organised comprehensive medical service. Its budget was substantial: the annual income of this capital accounted for more than 10 per cent of the total budget of health services.[47]

The Bas-Congo was selected as FOREAMI's first area of action, due to its proximity to major European enclaves, the relatively developed routes of transportation and the importance of the Congolese workers in this region, who were being decimated by sleeping sickness.[48] The sector was divided into subsectors run by doctors. Each subsector comprised a series of circles with a population of twenty-five to thirty thousand individuals, assigned a (European) doctor and a health worker and supported by African auxiliaries (nurses, nurse assistants, messengers, drivers, mechanics, etc.). At the circle level, a mix of SAMI, AMIB (also referred to as SADAMI/Service auxiliaire de l'Assistance Médicale Indigène) and FOREAMI doctors and health workers carry out mobile screening tours, accompanied by African auxiliaries. FOREAMI intended to fully canvas selected regions and 'turn around' the health situation, then defer medical responsibility to the colonial health service. This would not be as straightforward as assumed. FOREAMI's initial activities in the Lower Congo affected around 600,000 people, involving 26 doctors, 23 health workers, 4 medical officers, 40 missionary nurses and nearly 500 Congolese auxiliaries. Expansion of the FOREAMI model was planned for Kwango and eventually other territories. Between 1932 and 1935 FOREAMI was also active in the Ruandan territory of Tanganika-Ruzizi. Here it was focused solely on sleeping sickness, following what its director referred to as a purely 'nosological' programme rather than the integral programme of Bas-Congo.[49] The attempt to move into the Kwango in 1935 with a concomitant decrease in activity in the Bas-Congo was aborted, in part due to the perceived primitive conditions in the Kwango, but also due to a recrudescence of epidemics in the Bas-Congo. Budget cuts, resistant 'native mentalities' and geopolitical events ultimately delayed further expansion of the FOREAMI until after the Second World War.[50]

In many ways, the medical model of FOREAMI was new, even as it built upon the experience and frustrations of Belgian medical officials in effectively reaching a wider population. It put into practice a new approach to the SAMI that grew from previous mobile sleeping sickness treatment units, namely a relatively thorough medical census of a region carried out methodically by mobile teams.[51] Doctors working in the Congo and Ruanda-Urundi were aware of the specificity of their health system. For Janssens, mobile teams practising a full medical population census constituted one of the most striking and original features of the Congolese health organisation.[52] A similar system existed since 1916 in French Equatorial and Western Africa, led by Dr Eugène Jamot, but it was a largely vertical programme targeting only sleeping sickness.[53] The originality of FOREAMI lay in its objectives: not only to eradicate all diseases in a specific area but also to improve public health.

While FOREAMI was broader in its ambitions than SAMI, it was limited in its geographic reach. Other programmes, targeting specific diseases, could be highly invasive but likely had little effect on overall population morbidity and mortality. For example, nearly five million Congolese were examined each year on the eve of the Second World War for diseases such as yaws and leprosy.[54] It should be noted that both diseases, while aesthetically unpleasing, were not terribly mortal. Vellut considered such medical grids as 'totalitarian fantasies that crossed the history of the relationship between colonial bureaucracies and African peasantries', adding that they sought in fact to 'guarantee a complete mastery over the transition between two models of health, that inherited by the Old Regime which was more or less degraded or impacted depending on regions, and that which corresponded to the demands of a new era. They were transitioning from a primitive colonial regime to an advanced colonial economy' and the response to these growing demands.[55] FOREAMI was inspired by this new philosophy.

The medical services continued to have a military character in the interwar period, as young physicians coming out of universities could perform compulsory military service (one to three years) in the territories under Belgian colonial administration, either in the service of the state, the Fondation médicale de l'Université de Louvain (FOMULAC) or national missions.[56] Further, the significant proportion of career military doctors was also partly due to the fact that lieutenant doctors could get ahead by working a few years in the colonial service.[57] Ultimately, all the chief medical officers of the colony of the interwar period had worked in the health services of the colonial troops during the First World War, encouraging the continued military character of Belgian state medicine. The rigid, authoritarian bias of colonial social medicine would compromise its efficacy, because it was ultimately maladapted to the struggle in conditions of rural poverty, despite the fact that the authorities 'had the intention to practice a "constructive imperialism" '.[58]

As the colonial medical services expanded, it attempted to bring religious and charitable health providers under its loose direction through a constellation designated the Charitable Native Medical Services (Assistance Médicale Indigène Bénévole or AMIB, also later referred to in reports as SADAMI – see above). The AMIB, a unique configuration of public and private medical services in the Belgian Congo, was created after the governor general observed in 1920 the lack of coordination among the various charitable medical organisations working in the Congo. Its creation was in part an effort to co-opt the medical capacity of the Protestant medical missions, which represented an important contribution to Western medicine in the region, and a continuation of the historical legacy of the 1906 Concordat between the Vatican and Leopold II for Catholic missionary services in the CFS.[59] Through the AMIB, the government supplied drugs and equipment and supplemented funding for salaries and expenses to missions. In exchange, these missionaries provided services for the colonial health services, including basic medical care in rural areas and collection/reporting of medical statistics.

After completing a basic course at the School of Tropical Medicine, missionaries were charged with prophylaxis and treatment of specific endemic and epidemic diseases (particularly sleeping sickness). Moreover, Protestant societies, like some Catholic societies, also committed some doctors, nurses and health workers to the goals of the state, including the work of FOREAMI. The AMIB, and the heavy and extended formal involvement of religious orders in state medicine, was a uniquely Belgian phenomenon. This was in part a reflection of the heavy and sometimes controversial involvement of Catholics more generally in colonial governance (see Chapter 2, pp. 72–3).[60]

Both Catholic and Protestant missions, for their part, realised the value of medical care to their proselytisation efforts. Medical care could draw indigenous populations. Protestant missions in particular easily framed the provision of medicine within their more general mission of caring for the afflicted. Thus, medical care was often provided with a heavy dose of religious ministering. For example, patient families could be required to attend prayer services while the patient was being treated, and patients' ministrations could be simultaneously spiritual and physical, as, for example, when prayer services were conducted in recovery wards.[61] Baby clinics and milk distribution could take place immediately after church services, or 'rewards' for regular infant consultations would be given on Christmas Eve (Figure 3.2). Ultimately, medical provision increased the visibility and attractiveness of the missions' work.[62]

It could be argued that the unique atmosphere at missionary dispensaries made their offer of Western medicine more attractive than that of a secular health centre. The integration of Christian symbolic gestures into medical activities (blessing of the sick, sign of the cross, prayers) and the social support available in missions may have aligned their practices more closely with Congolese therapeutic systems, which largely recognised disease as signs of individual and community imbalance most effectively treated by including the entire social body. Congolese medicine involved the ritual action of many members of the community beyond the immediately

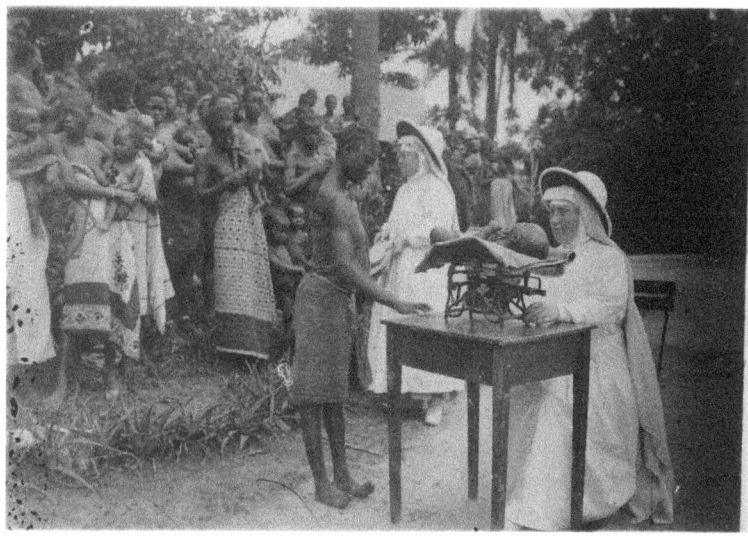

Figure 3.2 Leopoldville. Milk depot and baby clinic, n.d.

afflicted. Therefore, missionaries could be perceived, like their peers elsewhere in Africa, as healers with mystic abilities, because they combined ritual prayer with medical care. The similarity between the two created church distrust of native medicine because missionaries were aware that it linked health and sacred action.

Dispensaries, antenatal care and baby clinics, maternity hospitals and hospitals, leper houses, nurseries, homes for disabled and elderly people, labour occupational medicine, surgery, lazarets for sleeping sickness patients, tuberculosis or sanatoriums for incurable patients, camps for infectious patients, insane asylums and *Goutte de lait*[63] were some components of the missionary health services. Christian networks of villages and outposts run by African evangelists provided rural bases for the organisation of vaccination or medical screening campaigns. Thus, similar to Europe a century earlier, priests, nuns, ministers and deaconesses were key to expanding new sorts of health services to rural areas and dispersed populations (see Chapter 2, pp. 68–71).

Indeed, missionary societies largely practised what Dr Schweitzer has called a 'sentimental medicine',[64] in contrast to the 'combat medicine' disseminated by government mobile health teams that adopted an army-inspired organisation to align, order, sort and treat the masses. A variety of Protestant missions (largely foreign) and Roman Catholic orders (almost exclusively Belgian) would ultimately provide medical care in the region. Women's congregations were predominant in healthcare on the Roman Catholic side, as nuns provided care in most colonial hospitals and clinics (see Chapter 1, p. 40). Catholic fathers also ran some lazarets and dispensaries. The Protestant medical teams were more internationally mixed, and were composed of licensed doctors, nurses and lay staff mainly of British, American, Swedish and South African origin. Broadly speaking, Catholics worked in the domain of palliative care while Protestants provided more acute medical services. For instance, before the Second World War, Protestant missions in the Congo performed a substantial number of surgeries annual, and Catholic missions none.[65]

However, as in many other fields, Roman Catholics and Protestants were often fiercely competitive with each other in their offer of medical care. Indeed, in part to avoid conflict, colonial authorities limited the presence of several health centres in the same region. Spiritual influence (and first arrival) at times de facto determined who would be assigned to what geographic region. A relatively sophisticated Protestant medical apparatus arrived early in the region, independent of colonial control. Catholics, however, were formally and extensively involved in the colonial state medical apparatus, although the church would attempt with middling success to provide medical services linked more tightly with Catholic missions beginning in the interwar period. This included luring licensed doctors to work in Catholic missions and sending mission staff for accreditation in nursing and tropical medicine in Belgium. Protestant missions quickly experimented with local schooling of African auxiliaries in medicine, successfully opening a state-recognised medical auxiliary school in 1932.[66] The rancorous competition between the two religious groups led to several instances of accusations, denouncements and legal proceedings relating to medical practice, among other issues.

Parallel to the establishment of colonial state and missionary care provision, the private sector would also launch medical programmes for the industrial workforce. A dual medical system worked in parallel: that of the government, on the one hand, and that of religious missions or trading and agro-industrial companies, on the other. Even while it was still in its formative stages in 1905, the Union Minière du Haut Katanga (UMHK) assessed the risk of sleeping sickness in Katanga during a prospecting mission. In 1914, it appointed a doctor to organise a medical service that, with the help of the colonial government and the Comité spécial du Katanga,[67] included in its remit displacement of villages (from locations deemed unhealthy), deforestation and monitoring of population movements and the establishment of disease screening and healthcare facilities. This accompanied an explosion in labour recruitment, with the union's mining workforce increasing from 2,500 African workers in 1914 to 12,000 in 1920, with an average mortality of almost 12 per cent. The union would develop a comprehensive pyramidal medical structure for early detection, isolation and prevention of diseases through medical action at all levels. It instituted a sprawling health apparatus to assure the health of the workforce through dispensaries in mines, factories and camps, hospitals with several hundred beds in the various operating sites and a central hospital well equipped with all modern medical technology. This policy yielded impressive results, as morbidity would drop from 3.85 per cent in 1926 to 0.91 per cent in 1955, and mortality per thousand workers from 37.8 in 1920 to 3.55 in 1959.[68]

The union's comprehensive health policy would become the archetype for large-scale enterprises in the Belgian Congo. Other major companies followed suit, such as the Compagnie du Kasaï, the Forminière (particularly active in the fight against sleeping sickness), the Huileries du Congo belge, the Kilo-Moto gold mines, the Minière des Grands Lacs, Symétain, Otraco, etc. Such occupational medicine was dictated by both the economic imperatives of a healthy workforce and by legislation on labour protection requiring a medical check for those entering into the service of any private company. The colonial government also demanded that large companies invest in the campaigns against endemic diseases, vaccinations and curative care for populations neighbouring these worksites.[69]

Rather late, in the 1920s, Belgian universities became involved with the other heterogenous sectors involved in healthcare in the Congo. The Catholic University of Leuven partnered with the Jesuit Catholic order in Kisantu province to create the Medical

Foundation of Leuven University (la Fondation médicale de l'Université de Louvain or FOMULAC)[70] in 1926. Intended as both a research and medical foundation, it had three main goals: research on tropical medicine, medical provision through hospital service and training of African nurses and medical assistants. It worked in Kisantu in 1925, Katana in Kivu province in 1929 (after a government request) and Kalenda in the Kasai in the 1950s. The colonial state treated FOMULAC much like other parastatal and religious organisations: it requested that the organisation assist in the work of FOREAMI for the rural sector of Kisantu, where a FOMULAC hospital and nurse training school were constructed in 1928. It also requested that FOMULAC take over the hospital complex constructed by the government after the Second World War (through the FBEI, discussed later). Similar to FOMULAC, in 1936 the Free University of Brussels created the Medical and Scientific Centre of the Free University of Brussels (Centre scientifique et médical de l'Université Libre de Bruxelles or CEMUBAC) to carry out combined scientific research and medical care provisioning, focusing on tuberculosis.[71]

The model of CEMUBAC revealed the ties between university health research and the private sector, as it collaborated with the Lomami and Lualaba Company (a subsidiary of the Compagnie du Congo pour le commerce et l'industrie, a holding owned by the Société générale), while FOMULAC worked more on a university–government partnership model (Figure 3.3). Collaboration between Belgian metropolitan universities and European health actors in the Congo would continue after the Second World War, with increasing numbers of universities involved, including the University of Liège and the University of Ghent.[72] These links between metropolitan universities, European public health actors and private industry have in some cases endured through independence, civil war, dictatorship and into the current fragile state of the Democratic Republic of Congo.

Even as state, charitable and industrial medical services expanded in this period, the exposure different Congolese populations had to Western medicine would remain wildly uneven, with many Congolese never seeing a Western doctor. Most Congolese who received Western medicine were those central to colonial enclaves: military, workers, prisoners, religious converts and, to a lesser extent and at

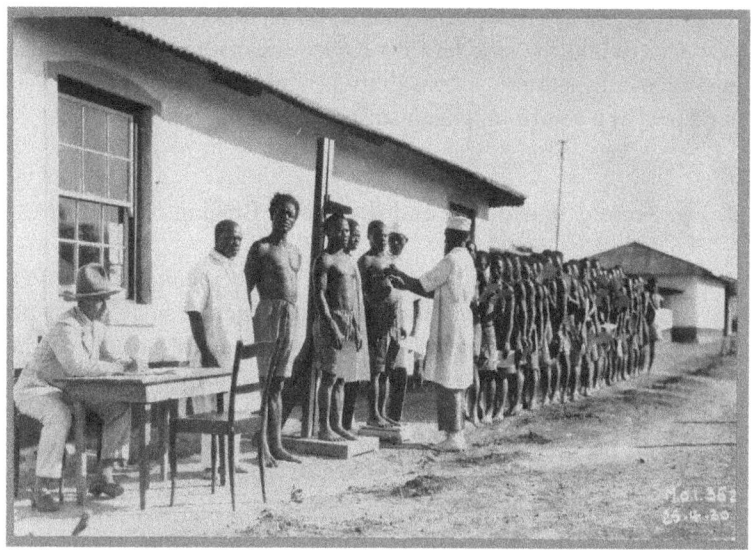

Figure 3.3 Lomami Recruitment Mission (MOI) for the UMHK, 1930. The doctor carefully examines each native at the preparation camp and thus establishes his robustness index (index of Pignet).

a later period, colonial functionaries. It should be observed that, with the partial exception of religious converts, these categories were largely male and of working age. Women, children and elderly people were thus exposed to Western medicine to a much lesser degree, often as 'dependants' of their male counterpart. Such populations were often separated from their original communities and had to adhere to a new model of social life, including a different medical domain. Soldiers or mine workers and their families were automatically exposed to preventive and curative measures dictated by the standards of Western medicine. Even after death, their bodies remained embedded in this other medical logic, as, for example, all of the deceased at Lubumbashi hospital (of the UMHK) were systematically autopsied for medical research until at least 1918.[73] The people attending the missions entered for their part a Christian space and were enclosed in a net of educational, religious, sanitary, economic and social activities aimed at separating them from their 'pagan' past and creating a good Christian. Converted mothers were strongly urged to attend baby clinics and abandon former childcare practices, while the sick had no choice but to get treatment in a missionary dispensary as consultation with traditional healers was perceived as a return to 'paganism'.

The Second World War and the end of Belgian colonialism

After the disruptions and devastations of the Second World War, all colonial powers, including Belgian, reached a crisis point. The recently created United Nations was openly hostile to the assumptions of colonialism. In this context, reform was necessary. Belgium launched a ten-year plan (*Plan décennal*) intended to forward both the economic and social development of the Congo. The social aspect had a strong medical component: it aimed to improve living standards and prevent rural depopulation, as indigenous well-being became perceived as 'the best guarantee to ensure and keep the friendship of the Congolese population',[74] preventing impoverished populations from establishing 'a dangerous revolutionary potential'.[75] State medical and health budgets and activities thus exploded after the war. At first glance, it may seem paradoxical to align such activities with the increasing likelihood of colonial independence, but in fact, such interest was in part inspired by a concern to appease an increasingly vocal indigenous elite about the benefits of the colonial relationship. The comprehensive medical networks developed during the interwar period in limited regions of the Congo by FOREAMI were applied to entire populations, both urban and rural. In 1947, the Fund for Indigenous Well-Being (Fonds du bien-être indigène or FBEI) was set up to ensure social investments in the rural areas of the Congo. Its funding came 'from the reimbursement by Belgium of the expenses of sovereignty assumed on its behalf by the Congo during the war 1940–1945'.[76] This capital was increased thereafter by grants from the National Lottery and the Colonial Lottery. The FBEI financed the construction and equipping of medical and surgical centres and rural hospitals, maternity wards, infant clinics, medical schools and sanatoriums as part of the ten-year development plan. The fund also financed programmes for leprosy, tuberculosis screening and disinfestation.

A medical school in Congo would be created at the very late date of 1954, on the eve of independence, when a private partnership between the Jesuits of the Lower Congo and the Catholic University of Leuven created the Faculty of Medicine of Lovanium. Lovanium's first two doctors would not graduate until the independence of the Congo, in 1961. The colonial state for its part did not open a Faculty of Medicine until 1956, within the University of the Belgian Congo and Ruanda-Urundi in Elisabethville.

Nonetheless, the ten-year plan and the creation of the Congolese universities could not stop the direction of history. The Second World War had broken the illusion of European superiority and power. The thinness of the 'white line' that kept subjected populations in check had been made apparent for both imperialists and colonised populations.[77] The rise of communism and the Cold War further weakened the position of pro-colonialism. In 1960, the Belgian Congo became the independent Republic of Congo; Ruanda-Urundi followed suit to become the independent countries of Rwanda and Burundi in 1961–62.

For much of the population, and for a majority of afflictions, medical authorities would ultimately have little interaction with the sick. Indeed, similar to French or Belgian farmers of the nineteenth century, colonised populations continued to use both traditional and Western medicine 'to satisfy their physical well-being, as well their social well-being', in the words of Jean-Marie Bouron, utilising a medical pluralism that still marks the therapeutic regime in the region.[78] In short, African patients did not consider that Western doctors held the monopoly in remedies for physical and mental problems.

Conclusion

In many ways, Belgian colonial medicine was very much typical of its time. The state medical system was strongly influenced by other colonialisms. The colonial administration made explicit comparisons and research into how its peers were running their medical administrations. France was particularly influential. But the British colonies, protectorates and mandates also offered some models that occasionally inspired practitioners and administrators.

The colonisation of Central Africa in the late nineteenth century coincided with the birth of tropical medicine as a recognised medical research speciality. Medical research expeditions in some senses grew out of geographical exploratory expeditions. While early research expeditions were largely foreign organised, as the Belgian colonial medical service grew, so too did its research capacities. The first medical laboratory in the CFS was set up in 1899 in Leopoldville. Not surprisingly, many research expeditions were focused on sleeping sickness, including the well-known 1903–05 Dutton Todd Christy expedition conducted by the Liverpool School of Tropical Medicine. Medical officers could serve as part of wider imperial networks of scientific research, particularly in relation to sleeping sickness.[79] However, the majority of medical doctors in the Congo were ancillary to these networks, working in difficult conditions in the bush, often in a public health surveillance role, with limited autonomy and low status. Colonial possessions enabled tropical medicine. They provided the resources, the rationale and the legitimacy for tropical medical research. African bodies were important source materials for such research.[80]

Certain other global trends in colonial medicine are repeated in Belgian Africa. Services dedicated to indigenous populations beyond colonial enclaves were created (sometimes only at first on paper) in Africa, South East Asia and Latin America in the first decade of the twentieth century, so-called native health services or assistances médicales indigènes. In the Congo, this would be called the SAMI, but its remit was much narrower than that of other contemporary medical services for indigenous populations. Further, as in other colonies, private charitable and religious institutions provided medical care, although this phenomenon was comparatively more pronounced and more enduring in the Congo. Professionalisation in the interwar period in Europe was also followed by pushes to professionalise medical staff in colonies around the globe, with more stringent accreditation and training requirements and the phasing out of lay health workers in state institutions. Again, in the Congo, this was done to a lesser extent. The use of certain metrics, such as under-five mortality, would come into vogue in the interwar period as a synecdoche for both the health of the general population and the effectiveness of the civilising mission of the coloniser.

The Belgian case is also marked with several distinct peculiarities. The Belgian colonial endeavour began through the ambitions of the Belgian King Leopold II and would become influenced by his excesses. When Belgium acquired the CFS, the blueprint for medical care laid down during Leopold's abusive personal fiefdom continued in some fashion. For example, the military doctors who oversaw care of the Europeans working in the exploitative CFS became the 'civilian doctors' overseeing care of Europeans working in the ostensibly more enlightened Belgian Congo. The conservation of an entire cadre of men (and they were all men initially) complicit in a violent, oppressive system offers an interesting historical lens to view how care evolved in the 1910s and 1920s. As Belgians in the metropole had little say in Leopold's endeavours in Africa, so too did most continue to have little interest in a Belgian colonialism, unlike in neighbouring countries such as France and the Netherlands, where large swaths of the population had a vested interest in overseas ventures that extended beyond economic gain.[81] The metropole's indifference is one of the striking distinctions of Belgian colonialism, as are its more restrictive immigration and emigration policies.[82] Further, as Vellut has argued, the state was essentially hamstrung by a very strong industrial coalition that confined, if not dictated, its functioning.[83]

Medical training for indigenous personnel, usually planned in conjunction with the creation of a native medical service in colonies globally,[84] was largely aborted in the Congo. While many colonies had difficulty creating such a cadre of workers, Belgium's efforts were particularly ineffective. This was in part due to the thinness of resources from the metropole, but was also strongly influenced by the Catholic monopoly on primary school education in the region. Such education, critics argued, emphasised moral and social training rather than technical or administrative skills.[85] Further, as in most colonies in the world, colonial officials in the Congo and Ruanda-Urundi repeatedly expressed their fear of educated Africans wishing to emancipate themselves from European tutorship, and who would be disconnected from local people. Like France's Instituts Pasteur, parastatal research institutes tightly connected to the metropole, such as Lovanium, began providing specialised education to so-called *évolués*, but this would be after the Second World War.[86] Thus, unlike in colonies such as Algeria or

Indochina, such training would not be offered until what would be labelled the period of 'decolonisation'. Was this development at this late date an effort at 'catch-up' by Belgium to what other colonial powers offered, or was it also an effort to meet the growing vocal demands of indigenous populations for education, a political voice and socio-economic opportunities? It was likely both.

As in other colonies around the globe, the Second World War heralded the beginning of the end of Belgian colonialism. Populations in both Ruanda-Urundi and the Belgian Congo began to agitate for independence in the 1950s. Medical care slowly passed into the hands of the *évolués*, and, indeed, medical doctors such as Gaston Diomi Ndongala and Pierre Canon would become prominent in the independence movement.[87]

Belgian colonial medicine, in the end, left strong traces in the current field of international humanitarian aid. In some ways, the public–private cooperation for healthcare pioneered by movements such as FOREAMI and FOMULAC have become the template for providing care in current, so-called fragile states. In such fragile states, because a robust political administration is lacking, public services are arranged through public–private partnerships that are largely independent of political processes. Bureaucratic and administrative authority was always weak in the Congo, arguably more so than in many other colonies.[88] The indifference of the general metropole to the colony in the pre-Second World War era likely further weakened such authority. In addition, the disproportionate power of the Catholic Church subtracted from the administrative legitimacy of the colonial state. As Vellut observed, the power bloc of colonial companies and the administrators of the colonial state (and we would include the Catholic Church in this formulation), excluded effective political control.[89] We could even, provocatively, call the Belgian Congo a hybrid of a colonial state and the modern fragile state.

The Belgian Congo's answer to the call for a population-level health service was thus fundamentally different than that of other colonies. The colonial bloc would forcibly partner with private industries and charitable groups to achieve wider health action, bypassing the lack of political will. This is currently how international humanitarian organisations often approach provision of care in instable regions. Further, vertical programmes such as the massive campaigns for sleeping sickness that begin in the first and second decade of the twentieth century could be seen as templates for later programmes such the hookworm eradication programmes of the 1930s and the mass vaccination programmes against smallpox in the 1950s. Belgium, starting a bit 'behind the curve' as a colonial power, had to innovate solutions for health problems in a colony that was poor in resources and political will.

Notes

1 J. van Wing, 'Bakongo magic', *Journal of the Royal Anthropological Institute of Great Britain and Ireland*, 71:1/2 (1941), 85–97, at 89.
2 N. R. Hunt, *A Nervous State: Violence, Remedies, and Reverie in the Belgian Congo* (Durham, NC: Duke University Press, 2016); J. M. Janzen, *Lemba, 1650–1930: A Drum of Affliction in Africa and the New World*, Critical Studies on Black Life and Culture 11 (New York: Garland, 1982); D. Newbury, 'Contradictions at the heart of the canon: Jan Vansina and the debate over oral historiography in Africa, 1960–1985', *History in Africa*, 34 (2007), 213–54; J. Vansina, *The Tio Kingdom of the Middle Congo, 1880–1892* (Oxford: Oxford University Press for the International African Institute, 1973).
3 M. Werner and B. Zimmermann, 'Beyond comparison: *histoire croisée* and the challenge of reflexivity', *History and Theory*, 45:1 (2006), 30–50.
4 W. Ernst, 'Beyond East and West: From the history of colonial medicine to a social history of medicine(s) in South Asia', *Social History of Medicine*, 20:3 (December 2007), 505–24, at 507.
5 For traditional medicine in Rwanda and Burundi, see, for the precolonial period, I. Berger, *Religion and Resistance: East African Kingdoms in the Precolonial Period* (Tervuren: RMCA, 1961); and C. Taylor, *Milk, Honey, and Money: Changing Concepts in Rwanda Healing* (Washington, DC: Smithsonian Institution Press, 1992). John Janzen's work on the drums of Lemba straddles the precolonial and early colonial period, see Janzen, *Lemba, 1650–1930*. There are also studies about these practices during the colonial period, including many interested in the pharmaceutical value of traditional medicines: A. Lestrade, *La médecine indigène au Ruanda et Lexique des termes médicaux français urunyarwanda* (Brussels: Académie royale des sciences coloniales, 1955); J.-M. Durand, *Les plantes bienfaisantes du Ruanda et de l'Urundi* (Butare: Groupe scolaire,

1966), annotated edition with review of articles appearing between 1955 and 1959; E. Viaene and F. Bernard, *L'Art de guérir chez les peuplades congolaises, extrait du Bulletin de la Société Royale Belge de Géographie* (Brussels: Lith. Alex. Berqueman, 1911). For the postcolonial period in Rwanda, see P. C. Rwangabo, esp. *La médecine traditionnelle au Rwanda* (Paris: Karthala, 1993). For Zaire, see the research of Mahaniah Kimpianga, the extensive canon of John Janzen, the anthropology of Wyatt McGaffey, as well as works that usually intersect politics and health, such as F. Hagenbucher-Sacripanti, *Santé et rédemption par les génies au Congo. La 'médecine traditionnelle' selon le Mvulusi* (Paris: Publisud, 1990); N. Eggers, 'Mukombozi and the Monganga: the violence of healing in the 1944 Kitawalist uprising', *Africa*, 85:3 (2015), 417–36.

6 J. L. Vellut, 'La médecine européenne dans l'Etat Indépendant du Congo (1885–1908)', in *Médecine et hygiène en Afrique centrale de 1885 à nos jours*, ed. P. G. Janssens, M. Kivits and J. Vuylsteke (Brussels: Fondation Roi Baudouin, 1992), 61–81, at 67.

7 See J. M. Janzen, 'Science and spirit in postcolonial North Kongo health and healing', *African Studies Quarterly*, 15:3 (June 2015), 47–63. Perhaps the most detailed work has been done by Peter Geschiere, exploring how colonial intrusions continue to impact Central African society today, through its disruptions of witchcraft, political authority and healing practices. See P. Geschiere, 'Chiefs and the problem of witchcraft: varying patterns in South and West Cameroon', *Journal of Legal Pluralism and Unofficial Law*, 28:37–8 (1996), 307–27; P. Geschiere and J. Roitman, *The Modernity of Witchcraft: Politics and the Occult in Postcolonial Africa* (Charlottesville: University of Virginia Press, 1997); P. Geschiere, *Witchcraft, Intimacy, and Trust: Africa in Comparison* (Chicago: University of Chicago Press, 2013).

8 Hunt, *A Nervous State*.

9 While there was a spike of interest in the colony after the Second World War, when the Parti libéral belge and the Parti socialiste belge coalitions attempted to reshape the relationship between the state and the Catholic Church in Belgium and the Congo, this was a late and ultimately ephemeral phenomenon.

10 S. Marks, 'What is colonial about colonial medicine? And what has happened to imperialism and health?', *Social History of Medicine*, 10:2 (1997), 205–19, at 210.

11 M. G. Stanard, *Selling the Congo: A History of European pro-Empire Propaganda and the Making of Belgian Imperialism* (Lincoln: University of Nebraska Press, 2012).

12 For example, as Matthew Stanard notes, Congolese subjects never had any right to political representation. See M. G. Stanard, 'Belgium, the Congo, and imperial immobility: a singular empire and the historiography of the single analytic field', *French Colonial History*, 15:1 (2014), 87–110, at 95.
13 This kind of division is convenient for the age of high colonialism generally. See, for example, C. Young, *The African Colonial State in Comparative Perspective* (New Haven, CT: Yale University Press, 1994); N. Tarling, *The Cambridge History of Southeast Asia. Volume 2 Part One: From c.1800 to the 1930s* (Cambridge, UK: Cambridge University Press, 1992); N. Tarling, *The Cambridge History of Southeast Asia. Volume 2 Part Two: From World War II to the Present* (Cambridge, UK: Cambridge University Press, 1992).
14 L. De Clerck, 'L'administration coloniale belge sur le terrain au Congo (1908–1960) et au Ruanda-Urundi (1925–1962)', *Annuaire d'Histoire administrative européenne*, 18 (2006), 187–210.
15 Vellut, 'La médecine européenne', 64.
16 Some notable examples include Lucien Donny, Sidney Langford Hinde, and Leslie Wolfe.
17 The Force Publique was the army/militia of the Belgian Congo, consisting initially of largely foreign European officers, mercenaries and conscripted African soldiers. Its role was internal pacification and policing rather than the traditional role of an army as defence against foreign threats.
18 Vellut, 'La médecine européenne', 66.
19 Ibid.
20 Fédération pour la Défense des Intérêts Belges à l'Etranger, *L'assistance Médicale Indigène Au Congo* (Brussels: A&G Bulens Frères, 1907).
21 C. C. Chesterman, 'The contribution of Protestant missions to the health services of the Congo', *Annales de la Société Belge de Médecine Tropicale*, 27 (1947), 37–46; S. Au, 'Medical orders: Catholic and Protestant missionary medicine in the Belgian Congo 1880–1940', *BMGN: Low Countries Historical Review*, 132:1 (2017), 62–82.
22 J.-L. Vellut, *La mémoire du Congo: le temps colonial* (Gand: Snoeck, 2008), 8; A. H. M. Kirk-Greene, 'The thin white line: the size of the British colonial service in Africa', *African Affairs*, 79:314 (1980), 25–44, at 38.
23 See, for example, M. D. Markowitz, *Cross and Sword: The Political Role of Christian Missions in the Belgian Congo, 1908–1960* (Stanford, CA: Hoover Institution Press, 1973).
24 A. Cornet, *Politiques de santé et contrôle social au Rwanda 1920–1940* (Paris: Karthala Editions, 2011); A. Cornet, 'L'ère de du soupçon.

Missionnaires anglicans et fonctionnaires belges entre défiance et tensions. Rwanda, 1916–1940', *Outre-Mers*, 380–1 (2013), 143–62.
25 Vellut, 'La médecine européenne', 72.
26 However, the proportion of military physicians or militiamen employed by the Belgian colonial health administration was lower than that observed by Iliffe for German East Africa on the eve of the First World War (80 per cent). See J. Iliffe, *East African Doctors: A History of the Modern Profession* (Cambridge, UK: Cambridge University Press, 1998), 28. See also J. Koponen, *Development for Exploitation: German Colonial Policies in Mainland Tanzania, 1884–1914* (Helsinki: LIT Verlag, 1994).
27 Cornet, *Politiques de santé et contrôle social au Rwanda*, 46.
28 J. P. Sanderson, *Démographie coloniale congolaise. Entre spéculation, idéologie et reconstruction historique* (Louvain-la-Neuve: Presses universitaires de Louvain, 2019).
29 Vellut, 'La médecine européenne', 72.
30 A. Crozier, *Practising Colonial Medicine: The Colonial Medical Service in British East Africa* (London: I. B. Tauris, 2007).
31 J. André, J. Burke, J. Vuylsteke and H. van Balen, 'Evolution of health services', in *Health in Central Africa Since 1885: Past, Present and Future* (Brussels: King Baudouin Foundation, 1997), 59–158, at 106.
32 African Archives, Ministry of Foreign Affairs, Belgium, collection on Missions and Medicine, file 594. An administrative note to staff observes that according to the Convention of 26 March 1906, religious staff outranks the lay staff in all administrative categories. This ranking was of key importance in any ceremonial proceedings.
33 G. Trolli, 'Le service médical au Congo belge depuis sa création jusqu'en 1925', *Congo*, 8:1 (1927), 187–204, at 193: 'Le service colonial du Gouvernement ne semble présenter aucun attrait pour les médecins belges'.
34 L. Armani, *Diciotto mesi al Congo* (Milan: Fratelli Treves, 1907), 119, quoted by Vellut, 'La médecine européenne', 64.
35 Vellut, 'La médecine européenne', 64 and 71.
36 This statute was created in 1923. See Trolli, 'Le service médical', 193.
37 'Les médecins et la colonie. Résultats de l'enquête de la Commission coloniale de l'Université libre de Bruxelles', *Congo*, 2:1 (August 1931), 83–132.
38 Trolli, 'Le service médical', 190.
39 Ibid.
40 Iliffe, *East African Doctors*, 78. In the British colonies, however, there was an intermediate level between the highest-ranking African and the lowest European doctor: the Indian assistant surgeon, who earned between one-third and one-half of the European doctor.

41 See the Annual Medical Reports for the Belgian Congo from 1908 to 1940. See also Belgian Ministry of Foreign Affairs, African Archives, Collection Hygiene 4555 ter, folder entitled 'Ecole infirmiers noirs et assistants médicaux indigènes'.
42 N. Hunt, 'Colonial maternities', in *A Colonial Lexicon of Birth Ritual, Medicalization, and Mobility in the Congo* (Durham, NC: Duke University Press, 1999), 237–80.
43 M. Worboys, 'The comparative history of sleeping sickness in East and Central Africa, 1900–1914', *History of Science*, 32:1 (1994), 89–102.
44 G. Lachenal, *Le médicament qui devait sauver l'Afrique: un scandale pharmaceutique aux colonies* (Paris: La Découverte, 2014).
45 A society-wide fear of depopulation was a common motif in metropolitan France and Belgium as well in the interwar period. See Chapter 2 in this volume, and, for France, see R. A. Nye, *Crime, Madness, and Politics in Modern France: The Medical Concept of National Decline* (Princeton, NJ: Princeton University Press, 1984); W. Schneider, *Quality and Quantity: The Quest for Biological Regeneration in Twentieth-Century France* (New York: Cambridge University Press, 1990).
46 J.-L. Vellut, *Congo: Ambitions et désenchantements, 1885–1960* (Paris: Karthala Editions, 2017), 231.
47 A. André and J. Burke, 'Développement des services de santé', in P. G. Janssens et al., *Médecine et hygiène en Afrique centrale*, 83–160, at 107.
48 FOREAMI, *Rapport annuel sur l'Exercice 1931* (Brussels: Marcel Hayez, 1932).
49 FOREAMI, *Rapport annuel 1932* (Brussels: Imifi, 1933).
50 See the FOREAMI annual reports for 1935–47; and André et al., 'Evolution of health services'.
51 M. Lyons, 'Public health in colonial Africa: the Belgian Congo', in *The History of Public Health and the Modern State*, ed. D. Porter (Amsterdam: Rodopi, 1994), 356–84, at 372.
52 P. G. Janssens, 'Comparative aspects: I. The Belgian Congo', in *Health in Tropical Africa during the Colonial Period. Based on the Proceedings of a Symposium held at New College, Oxford, 21–23 March 1977*, ed. E. E. Sabben-Clare, D. J. Bradley and K. Kirkwood (Oxford: Clarendon Press, 1980), 209–27, at 221.
53 On the role and methods of colonial physician Eugène Jamot (1879–1937), see, in particular, J.-P. Bado, *Médecine coloniale et grandes endémies. Lèpre, trypanosomiase humaine et onchocerchose* (Paris: Karthala Editions, 1996).
54 A. Dubois and A. Duren, 'Soixante ans d'organisation médicale au Congo belge', *Annales de la Société belge de Médecine Tropicale*, 27,

supplément. Liber Jubilaris J. Rodhain à l'occasion de son soixante-dizième anniversaire (1947), 1–36, at 8.
55 Vellut, *Congo*, 237.
56 Capt. Vandevelde, 'Le recrutement des médecins du Congo', *Courier Médico-Pharmaceutique*, 3 (March 1932), 124–5; Séance du 20 mars 1929 du *Conseil supérieur d'hygiène coloniale* (AA, Brussels, Hyg 4437 no. 692).
57 Royal decree no. 15366 (26 May 1923).
58 Vellut, *Congo*, 239.
59 Markowitz, *Cross and Sword*, 7.
60 D. Northrup, 'A church in search of a state: Catholic missions in eastern Zaire, 1879–1930', *Journal of Church and State*, 30:2 (1988), 309–19.
61 Au, 'Medical orders'; A. Cornet, 'Politiques sanitaires, État et missions religieuses au Rwanda (1920–1940). Une conception autoritaire de la médecine coloniale?', *Studium: Tijdschrift voor Wetenschaps- en Universiteits-Geschiedenis*, 2:2 (2009), 57–67.
62 J.-M. Bouron, 'Le paradigme médical en milieu catholique: offre sanitaire missionnaire et demande de santé en Haute-Volta', *Histoire et missions chrétiennes*, 21 (Missions religieuses, missions médicales et 'mission civilisatrice', XIXe et XXe siècles, issue led by Olivier Faure) (March 2012), 103–36, at 114.
63 *Goutte de lait* was a service providing assistance to mothers with problems breastfeeding, derived from the long-standing Catholic tradition of praying to the Virgin Mary for ample breastmilk for newborns.
64 Graham Greene reporting a conversation with Schweitzer in his essay, 'The victor and the victim' (1988), in *Collected Essays, Part 3* (London: Penguin, 1993), n.p. (quoted by Vellut, 'La médecine européenne', 76).
65 See Archives Africaines of the Minister of Foreign Affairs, Belgium, collection RACB, Annual Medical Reports for the Belgian Congo.
66 The school was opened in 1932 and its diploma recognised by the state in 1935. See Au, 'Medical orders'.
67 The Comité spécial du Katanga (CSK) was a private enterprise that took over the Compagnie du Katanga (created in 1891), which had been granted ownership of approximately a third of the land of the province of Katanga. In 1900 the CFS and the Compagnie signed an agreement for joint state–industry management of the region through the newly created CSK.
68 R. Coosemans, 'Hygiène et santé des travailleurs', in P. G. Janssens et al., *Médecine et hygiène en Afrique centrale*, 531–48, at 538.
69 André and Burke, 'Développement des services de santé', 123.

70 F. Malengreau, *Une fondation médicale au Congo belge, la Fomulac (1926–1940)* (Louvain: Aucam, 1941); André and Burke, 'Développement des services de santé', 122.
71 André and Burke, 'Développement des services de santé', 122.
72 The Fondation de l'Université de Liège pour la recherche scientifique au Congo et au Ruanda-Urundi (FULREAC) was created in Elisabethville after the Second World War to work in nutrition. The University of Gand planned a foundation 'Ganda Congo' to do medical work in the Congo, but independence cut those plans short. André and Burke, 'Développement des services de santé', 123.
73 R. Mouchet, 'Documents anatomo-pathologiques sur la nosologie de la main-d'oeuvre indigène à Elisabethville de 1915 à 1921', *Bulletin des Séances de l'Institut Royal Colonial Belge*, 14:2 (1943), 422–52.
74 Quoted by G. Vanthemsche, *Genèse et portée du 'Plan décennal' du Congo belge (1949–1959)* (Brussels: Arsom, 1994), 32–3.
75 Ibid.
76 André et Burke, 'Développement des services de santé', 120.
77 Kirk-Greene, 'The thin white line'.
78 Bouron, 'Le paradigme médical', 105.
79 M. Mertens and G. Lachenal, 'The history of "Belgian" tropical medicine from a cross-border perspective', *Revue Belge de Philologie et d'histoire*, 90:4 (2012), 1249–71; H. Tilley, *Africa as a Living Laboratory: Empire, Development and the Problem of Scientific Knowledge 1870–1950* (Chicago: University of Chicago Press, 2011). See also Chapter 4, this volume.
80 S. Au, 'Anatomical collecting and tropical medicine in the Belgian Congo', in *Bodies Beyond Borders: Moving Anatomies 1750–1950*, ed. K. Wils, R. De Bont and S. Au (Leuven: Leuven University Press, 2017), 91–111.
81 This disinterest is not for lack of trying on the part of pro-colonialists. See V. Viaene, 'King Leopold's imperialism and the origins of the Belgian Colonial Party, 1860–1905', *Journal of Modern History*, 80:4 (2008), 741–90.
82 See, for example, S. Demart, 'Congolese migration to Belgium and postcolonial perspectives', *African Diaspora*, 6:1 (1 January 2013), 1–20; Stanard, 'Belgium, the Congo, and imperial immobility'.
83 J.-L. Vellut, 'Hégémonies en construction: Articulations entre Etat et Entreprises dans le bloc colonial belge (1908–1960)', *Canadian Journal of African Studies / Revue Canadienne des Études Africaines*, 16:2 (1982), 313–30.
84 France began to train African doctors in Madagascar in 1896, in West Africa in 1905 and in 1918 the Dakar School of Medicine was opened.

The British opened high schools for Africans after the First World War, most in Uganda and Sudan. One of the main objectives was to prepare auxiliary doctors. Iliffe, *East African Doctors*, 60–90; H. Brunschwig, *Noirs et Blancs dans l'Afrique noire française* (Paris: Flammarion,1983), 198–200.
85 P. M. Boyle, 'School wars: church, state, and the death of the Congo', *Journal of Modern African Studies*, 33:3 (1995), 451–68.
86 The '*évolués*' (or evolved) were a status of Congolese created by the Belgians, to denote those who were Christian, monogamous and educated.
87 Mutamba Makombo, *Du Congo belge au Congo indépendant: émergence des 'évolués' et genèse du nationalisme* (Kinshasa: Publications de l'institut de formation et d'études politiques, 1998), 317.
88 As has been argued by other scholars, many colonial states existed through a sort of 'will to power', more than actual power. A pithy explanation of this can be found in Kirk-Greene, 'The thin white line'.
89 Vellut, 'Hégémonies en construction'.

Selected bibliography

Cornet, A., *Politiques de santé et contrôle social au Rwanda 1920–1940* (Paris: Karthala Editions, 2011).

Feierman, S. and Janzen, J. M., *The Social Basis of Health and Healing in Africa* (Berkeley: University of California Press, 1992).

Hunt, N. R., *A Nervous State: Violence, Remedies, and Reverie in the Belgian Congo* (Durham, NC: Duke University Press, 2016).

Janssens, P. G., Kivits, M. and Vuylsteke, J. (eds), *Médecine et hygiène en Afrique Centrale de 1885 à nos jours* (Brussels: Fondation Roi Baudouin, 1992).

Janzen, J. M., *Lemba, 1650–1930: A Drum of Affliction in Africa and the New World. Critical Studies on Black Life and Culture 11* (New York: Garland, 1982).

Janzen, J. M., *The Quest for Therapy in Lower Zaire* (Berkeley: University of California Press, 1978).

Lachenal, G., *The Lomidine Files: The Untold Story of a Medical Disaster in Colonial Africa.* (Baltimore, MD: Johns Hopkins University Press, 2017). Translated from *Le médicament qui devait sauver l'Afrique: un scandale pharmaceutique aux colonies* (Paris: La Découverte, 2014).

Lyons, M., *The Colonial Disease: A Social History of Sleeping Sickness in Northern Zaire, 1900–1940* (Cambridge, UK: Cambridge University Press, 1992).

Taylor, C., *Milk, Honey and Money: Changing Concepts in Rwandan Healing* (Washington, DC: Smithsonian Institute, 1992).

Tilley, H., *Africa as a Living Laboratory: Empire, Development and the Problem of Scientific Knowledge 1870–1950* (Chicago: University of Chicago Press, 2011).

Vansina, J., *Being Colonized: The Kuba Experience in Rural Congo, 1880– 1960* (Madison: University of Wisconsin Press, 2010).

Vaughan, M., *Curing Their Ills: Colonial Power and African Illness* (Palo Alto, CA: Stanford University Press, 1991).

Vellut, J. L., 'La médecine européenne dans l'Etat Indépendant du Congo (1885–1908)', in P. G. Janssens, M. Kivits and J. Vuylsteke (eds), *Médecine et hygiène en Afrique centrale de 1885 à nos jours* (Brussels: Fondation Roi Baudouin, 1992), 61–81.

4

Public health, hygiene and social activism

Thomas D'haeninck, Jan Vandersmissen, Gita Deneckere and Christophe Verbruggen

In 1910, the Dutch physician Pieter Eijkman published *L'internationalisme médical*.[1] In his introduction he referred to the German-born British physician August Schuster, who one year earlier, at the XVIe Congrès international de Médecine in Budapest (1909), strongly expressed the need for a coordination of the almost countless and often competing international efforts in the field of medical science and healthcare.[2] Based on a typology of 30 categories, Eijkman listed 199 medical organisations and saw his extensive overview as a first step towards the establishment of an organisation of international organisations. In his overview, Eijkman praised three initiatives taken or supported by Belgians. The first was the Union internationale des Patronages, founded in Belgium by Henri Jaspar, secretary of the Commission royale des Patronages de Belgique. The union stressed the importance of health and hygiene, but went beyond purely medico-scientific practices by widening its scope to child protection, patronage of detained prisoners and ways of helping beggars and vagabonds. The second was the Concours pour un Remède contre la Maladie du Sommeil, an international prize installed in 1906 by King Leopold II, until 1908 sovereign of the Congo Free State (CFS). Sleeping sickness (human trypanosomiasis) was a devastating epidemic that in the first decade of the twentieth century ravaged entire populations, in particular in British Uganda and the CFS. King Leopold II turned to researchers of the Liverpool School of Tropical Medicine and awakened wider medical attention to sleeping sickness with the installation of a two hundred thousand franc prize for the discovery of a cure, thus cunningly presenting himself on the world stage as a humanist and philanthropist, not as the aggressive exploiter he really was (see Chapter 3, p. 104).³ The third initiative was the Association générale des Ingénieurs, Architectes et Hygiénistes municipaux de France, Algérie-Tunisie, Belgique, Suisse et Grand-Duché de Luxembourg, of which the main objectives were to link the engineer's 'art' to the precious skills of the municipal hygienist and to enhance international dissemination of knowledge about sanitary techniques and public works through, among other things, the journal *La technique sanitaire et municipale*.⁴

L'internationalisme médical hints at the importance of international influences on Belgian medicine and the intertwinement of Belgian social and medical initiatives in transnational dynamics. The (partially) Belgian contributions to medical internationalism mentioned by Eijkman connect to the leitmotivs of this chapter. We argue that the emergence of public healthcare in Belgium cannot be seen apart from cross-border exchanges, scientific innovations, social reform ambitions but also inter- and intra-imperial dynamics. Although Belgian history of medicine and public health is clearly intertwined with dynamics that go beyond the borders of states, it has, however, often been studied within a national framework, focusing on an urban context⁵ and on processes of institutionalisation and professionalisation.⁶ Recent research also emphasises that physicians were involved in transnational dynamics that went beyond their professional discipline.⁷ Cross-border dynamics between physicians and medical associations were part of a wider trend of transnational circulation of intellectual and cultural goods in the second half of the nineteenth century. The emergence of so-called transnational spheres can be seen as a catalyst for the formation of many scientific disciplines, expertise and ideological frameworks.⁸ Thorough research into cross-border dynamics on public health policies and practices is lacking for the Belgian case, which is striking since scholars have been indicating the strong intertwinement of Belgian history with international dynamics in the nineteenth and twentieth century.⁹ Sources such as *L'internationalisme médical* are an ideal point of departure to include them.

At the end of the eighteenth century a modern view on public health and social medicine emerged. Due to the growing awareness that many diseases had socio-economic origins, physicians started to collect information on the (urban) environment, searched for measures for the improvement of living conditions and advised policymakers on medical campaigns, prevention strategies and healthcare initiatives. In that way, physicians were drawn into a dynamic that seems to go beyond the scope of the individual body.[10] They increasingly felt the urge to advocate for better living conditions and social change too.[11] This process is referred to as the medicalisation of society. During the nineteenth century self-proclaimed experts with medical backgrounds perceived, diagnosed and declared social problems as if they were illnesses.[12] Historians therefore share the view that physicians must be considered as a driving force for social change in the nineteenth and twentieth centuries. The formation of medical professions and related scientific specialisms had wider repercussions, which also influenced society in general.

Physicians, however, were not the only advocates for social change and progress. Their growing social commitment cannot be dissociated from upcoming philanthropic and reformist advocacy networks.[13] The medicalisation of society was strongly intertwined with both the overall scientification of society and the rationalisation of dealing with the social question on a pan-European scale.[14] Medical internationalism as described by Eijkman and Schuster and the medicalisation of society coincided with the formation of transnational reformist networks and the internationalisation of the social question.[15] Hence, in this contribution we look at the social activism of medical doctors and hygienists in a twofold manner: first, as part of scientific and intellectual movements from which emerges the field of social medicine; second, as an essential formative element in the construction of expertise within reformist and social movements. We consider it impossible to make a rigid a priori distinction between science, knowledge and expertise. Whether knowledge is classified as expertise is ultimately premised on recognition as such by other actors in the field. We define expertise as forms of knowledge that are based on scientific ways of reasoning, while contributing to political and societal discussion and activism. Also, methodologically social and scientific movements can be addressed in a single manner, as both are constituted through collective action beyond borders.[16] We therefore do not investigate social reformers and experts in local or national isolation, but we consider them as

Public health, hygiene and social activism 137

actors in a global field of discourse and practice. Such an actor-oriented approach reveals the ways in which experts set in motion global processes of knowledge exchange and transformation, which ultimately fuelled processes of scientific discipline formation based on relationships of mutual recognition, support and mobility across boundaries. With regard to the nineteenth- and twentieth-century colonial empires (including Belgium) these dynamics manifested themselves on an inter- and intra-imperial scale. In this chapter we therefore widen the scope by including public health measures implemented in Congo.

This chapter consists of four parts, which will be structured in a chronological way. The first part starts in the late eighteenth century and focuses on the emergence of 'scientific medicine' and the growing awareness that the study of many diseases could not be separated from the socio-economic context in which they originated. The second part discusses the impact of new bacteriological theories and insights on public health questions in the 1870s, linking social medicine more profoundly to applied sciences and preventive healthcare; social medicine became increasingly entangled with other reformist movements. The third part deals with the further development of social hygiene and the rise of eugenics, national health protection and the improvement policies in the interwar period. Finally, the fourth part re-evaluates the period after 1960 when national public health systems were strongly questioned, local community health centres emerged in the wake of 1968 and medical activism went increasingly beyond borders.

These four periods strongly overlap with what Pierre-Yves Saunier calls four different 'circulatory regimes' in the field of social reform and social policy. Saunier identified a first regime in the early nineteenth century, when the social question is defined in different places by observation of local conditions in relation to urbanisation and industrialisation processes.[17] A second regime emerged at the end of the nineteenth century, when processes of specialisation in social knowledge led to the emergence of institutions and disciplines, as exemplified by the typology given by Eijkman in *L'internationalisme médical*. Cross-border dynamics and transnational circulation of knowledge became essential features of the process of discipline formation.[18] In the interwar period, a third regime arrived when (new) institutions ambitiously searched for universal norms and standards for social policies, professions and practices, which were believed to lead to the 'well-being of humanity throughout the world'.[19] The League of Nations became an important actor within this field of social policy and many pre-war epistemic communities became further institutionalised.[20] The fourth and last period is characterised by the presence of influential global players such as the World Health Organization (WHO), the emergence of new social movements and new international non-governmental organisations (INGOs) devoted to social medicine and global public health, on the one hand, and advocates of more efficiency and privatisation, on the other.[21]

The physician and the social question

The emergence of a modern view on public health and social medicine dates back to the end of the eighteenth century. At the turn of the century, the interest in epidemiological research boomed.[22] There was a growing awareness that many diseases were caused by bad living conditions and baleful socio-economic influences, urging physicians to plea for the improvement of the urban environment. Also, it was a widely held view that illnesses caused disasters and poverty and therefore undermined the (physical) strength and viability of both the individual and the state. In that way, physicians were drawn into a dynamic that went beyond the scope of the individual body[23] and strongly stimulated a professional sense of belonging.[24] In addition to the growing 'professional' interest physicians showed for social determinants, the ratio of physicians per capita increased in the course of time. Between 1831 and 1940 the number of physicians in Belgium more than tripled in proportion to the population.[25] All of these factors lead to the enhanced social position of physicians[26] and stimulated a process that is often referred to as the 'medicalisation of society': during the nineteenth century self-proclaimed experts coming from medical backgrounds perceived, diagnosed and declared social problems as if they were illnesses.[27]

Medical doctors in Belgium – as in other countries in Western Europe – became more and more convinced that the improvement of public health could not only be achieved via medico-technical and infrastructural innovations or scientific discoveries, but also by initiating, developing and steering social policies. A number of physicians pleaded for sanitation measures to be taken on a wide scale, and suggested actions that had to encourage personal and public hygiene and prevent epidemics. They reached an audience of fellow medical professionals, policymakers, but also members of the working class. Their ambitions strongly overlapped with initiatives taken by philanthropists and social reformers. Until the 1870s, these groups must be seen as strongly intertwined because they fought for the same social causes, met each other in learned societies such as the Académie royale des Sciences, des Lettres et des Beaux-Arts de Belgique and wrote for and/or read the same journals (e.g. *Le Progrès*).[28] However, medical societies had emerged already in the 1820s in urban centres such as Brussels (Société des Sciences médicales et naturelles de Bruxelles, 1822), Ghent (Société de Médecine de Gand, 1834) and Antwerp (Société de Médecine d'Anvers, 1834).[29] The differences between these private associations and newly founded public institutions such as the Académie royale de Médecine de Belgique (1841) were minimal, both with regard to their membership and the recommendations they made to the Belgian government and local authorities.[30]

The case of Adolphe Burggraeve, a practising surgeon and professor of anatomy and surgery at the State University of Ghent, illustrates the emergence of a modern type of professionalised physician who used his medical training in his search for social reform measures (Figure 4.1). Burggraeve was renowned for his innovative treatment of wounds and fractures. His elegant style of presenting preparations appealed both to a scientific and a wider audience.[31] In 1835 he was appointed as professor of anatomy at his alma mater in Ghent, where in 1828 he had obtained a degree in medicine with a thesis on syphilis. Burggraeve belonged to an engaged urban elite. As a member the Académie royale de Médecine de Belgique and the Société Huet,[32] and as a co-founder of both the Société de Médecine de Gand (1834) and the Société royale d'Histoire naturelle de Gand (1851), he was rooted in several associations that incarnated the changing spirit of the time.

Especially the Société de Médecine de Gand offered a platform where Burggraeve and fellow academics, hospital staff and military physicians discussed both medical innovations and measures

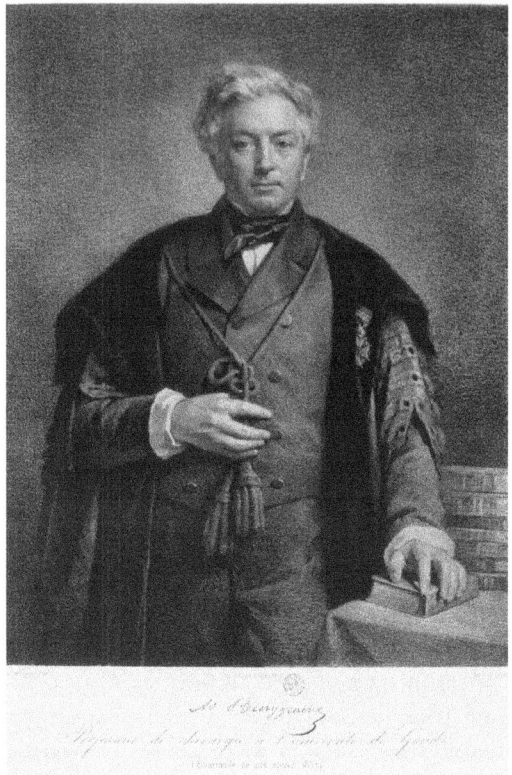

Figure 4.1 Portrait of Adolphe Burggraeve.

to improve urban living conditions.[33] They collected and published leaflets and handbooks on infections, epidemics and venereal diseases and on social issues such as food provision, the installation of public toilets or the softening of sickening smells. Moreover, they advised the Belgian government and local authorities on health policies and made suggestions for the improvement of the industrial environment. One of the most prominent studies in this field was written in 1845 by Daniel Mareska and Jean-Julien Heyman. Their investigation of the labour conditions and moral and physical situation of the workers employed in Ghent's cotton mills[34] stimulated further inquiries but also initiated social policies.[35] In the 1860s, plagues of cholera struck several neighbourhoods in Ghent. Relying on the recommendations he found in the old report of Mareska and Heyman, Burggraeve took action with a drastic sanitation of the Batavia quarter. This working-class neighbourhood, known as an 'urban furuncle', was demolished and rebuilt.[36] The reuse of urban space would also shape new opportunities: the university reached an agreement with city authorities to build a prestigious Institut des Sciences (1883) on terrain that had been cleared.[37]

Burggraeve and his fellows at the Société de Médecine de Gand illustrate that the role physicians played in the development of public healthcare went beyond the scope of the individual body or the neutrality of their scientific training. The rise of public health resulted directly from the growing social commitment of physicians. By advocating social change and progress, their medical expertise could hardly be dissociated from upcoming philanthropic and reformist advocacy networks or political movements. Physicians in Belgium are therefore not to be regarded as neutral: they claimed a social position and influenced decision-making processes. Especially the upcoming progressive wing[38] within the Belgian Liberal Party functioned as an ally for social physicians: the political programme proposed by the '*progressisten*' for tackling the bad living conditions of the working class focused on improved housing, better nutrition and accessible education.[39] Hence, the fact that Adolphe Burggraeve participated in the elections for Ghent City Council in 1858 and got elected for the Liberal Party was by no means an exception.[40] Physicians of Burggraeve's kind were embedded in contemporary ideological discussions and as a group of expert professionals they became both an instrument for and a force behind the gradual expansion of the state and its social policies.[41] In consequence, the rise of public healthcare was a process of negotiation between medical professionals and state officials, whereby the difference between the physician and the politician was sometimes paper-thin.[42]

It must be stressed that in nineteenth-century Belgium the development of public health initiatives was first and foremost entrusted to local medical societies, authorities and institutions. The image of the Belgian night-watch state is related to the relative absence of interventions by the national state itself, at least up till the 1890s. However, the growing social engagements of physicians were limited to the local context. Many transnational connections between reform-minded citizens were established. The increased transnational interlinking between learned societies, where the social question is defined in different places by observation of local conditions in relation to the urbanisation and industrialisation processes, has been identified by Pierre-Yves Saunier as the first circulatory regime. Clergy, political activists, entrepreneurs, academics and politicians exchanged words and experiences in the North Atlantic space.[43] In absence of INGOs, international congresses became the most important form of 'scientific internationalisation' in the early and mid nineteenth century.[44] They were the venues par excellence for scientists, administrators, politicians, artists and others to meet and exchange ideas. Several Belgian physicians took leading roles at these events, but none as prominent as Adolphe Burggraeve. At the second meeting of the Association internationale pour le Progrès des Sciences sociales, held in Ghent in 1863, he presented his model for the ideal working-class quarter: a clean and healthy neighbourhood with many hygienic facilities and infrastructure for childcare and education.[45] His plans were influenced by models in London and Mulhouse, which were also discussed at the association's events. In a similar vein, these models linked the housing question of the working class to savings, mutual support and popular education. In his speech, Burggraeve grasped the opportunity to highlight the information on the situation in Ghent collected by his colleagues and himself and to criticise the small progress made by local politicians when it came to improving the workers' living environment. The 'battalions of disease and death' in Ghent were believed to contrast strongly with the situation in Mulhouse.[46] These international gatherings were not just fructifying meeting places for fellow socio-medical experts to exchange new ideas and practices. More so, here, an *epistemic community* was in the making. However, the congresses also offered a platform that strengthened the expert's image and offered him an opportunity to build personal networks with fellow reform-minded elites. Burggraeve's international engagements made sure that his voice was heard on a local and national level. His reputation as a leading man within the international scientific elite increased his influence in policymaking processes: by reporting facts (information politics) he fostered change and by relying on his cross-border network while evoking foreign best practices, he had a considerable impact on the ways like-minded people would lobby for and advocate social change.[47]

Applied sciences and preventive healthcare

The establishment of the Ghent Institut des Sciences was a direct result of the growing sociopolitical role physicians claimed, but the construction of modern scientific laboratories inspired by the German polytechnical schools in several Belgian university cities also marked changing views on medical knowledge, the physician's professional identity and public healthcare. In Liège, Leuven and Brussels similar institutions were built, inspired by model institutes in Heidelberg, Bonn and Berlin. In this new infrastructure experience and education were linked together (see Chapter 5, p. 185).[48] This maelstrom of building works was strongly supported by the first Belgian minister for education, the liberal Pierre van Humbeeck, who provided government funding for universities to modernise their scientific infrastructure. The investments of the state in modern science and laboratories indicate the shift from the local to the national level, which the Belgian liberals were trying to carry through, at least in the educational field, during the (short) period they were in power (1879–84). The models of the polytechnic schools of Dresden and Berlin were widely discussed at the Congrès international de l'Enseignement held in Brussels in 1880 and inspired the present elite educators and policymakers and certainly also members of the Ligue de l'Enseignement belge such as Van Humbeeck.[49] The influence went beyond architecture: the German scientific innovations were fiercely discussed in Belgian magazines, many Belgian professors like Héger and Frédéricq established firm ties with German colleagues and German scientific journals became important models.[50]

The new insights obtained between 1870 and 1890 are part of what is generally called the Pasteurian or bacteriological revolution. They stimulated the physician's training and interdisciplinary research, which resulted in several scientific innovations, the improvement of diagnostics, cures and prevention strategies and the establishment of the laboratory as part of the physician's infrastructure.[51] The new university infrastructures not only left their mark on academic achievements, in Ghent, Leuven and Liège they were also used by the provincial authorities. In the absence of a Ministry of Public Health and given the local fragmentation of hygienic initiatives, these provincial authorities would, from the

1890s onwards, develop public laboratories for bacteriology. By the turn of the century provincial institutes were established in Liège, Mons, Namur and Brussels. Both the academic and the provincial laboratories would provide public services such as the inspection of potable water, the distribution of sera against infectious diseases and bacteriological diagnosis of cholera, diphtheria, tuberculosis and rabies. Local authorities, physicians, medical societies and veterinarians could make use of the services of these laboratories free of charge. An imagery of commitment to public service was cultivated by the medical professionals operating these laboratories, such as Ernest Malvos, Martin Herman or Achille Haibe.[52]

The bacteriological revolution had a strong impact on the social role of physicians and public health questions too, linking social medicine more profoundly to applied sciences. More than merely advising policymakers on healthcare issues, physicians were employed by the government to implement hygienic measures. The private elite practitioners of the 1850s, rooted in philanthropic circles, slowly made space for public healthcare professionals. By the 1880s, local Belgian governments had taken over many of the medical services that were traditionally provided by private practitioners, denominations and beneficence houses. The number of physicians working in governmental service significantly rose and they provided medical service in working-class districts, prisons, schools, etc.[53] This was of major influence for the professional development of physicians in general and healthcare experts and hygienists in particular.[54] The institutionalisation of medical professions went hand in hand with the centralisation of social policies and healthcare provision. Due to the foundation of the Superior Health Council (Conseil supérieur de la santé) (1849), the Royal Society of Public Health (Société royale de médecine publique) (1876) and medical journals such as *Le Scalpel* or *Le Mouvement hygiènique*, local public medical services and the national healthcare agenda became more aligned and coordinated. The campaigns and measures to improve public health became more extensive and no longer focused solely on problem solving but also on prevention. Public spaces with a high risk for raising epidemics or infections were closed and disinfected when possible. Medical checks were made mandatory for risk groups such as prostitutes, children, miners, etc. Nevertheless, the degree of state intervention in public health remained a contentious political issue, which divided the liberal party between hesitant conservative liberals – advocates of the nightwatchman state – and their more interventionist progressive colleagues.[55]

Hence, the most far-reaching preventive health measures, such as the establishment of medical inspection services for public schools, occurred in the liberal strongholds of Brussels (1874), Antwerp (1882) and Ghent (1896).[56] Here school hygiene was brought to the attention of policymakers due to the alliance of progressive (liberal) politicians and politically active physicians. The physician Eugène Janssens played a vital role in the development of Brussels' health services,[57] and his pioneering work in the 1870s was presented as a successful example by like-minded physicians in Antwerp, Ghent, Liège and Charleroi. Soon after, Janssens founded a service of medical inspection in public schools in Brussels as part of the city's centralised health service (1874); the Antwerp physician Victor Desguin presented Janssens's model and ideas to the Société de Médécine d'Anvers. Moreover, as a member of Antwerp City Council and later also as alderman for education, Desguin would plead for the improvement and modernisation of the local healthcare system, with special attention for children and education. The networks of these physicians went beyond the borders of the Belgian nation state. Both Desguin and Janssens participated in the Congrès international de l'Enseignement (Brussels, 1880) where a section was dedicated to the matter of school hygiene. Two years later, Desguin established a medical school inspection in Antwerp, which he considered a model to be promoted actively abroad.[58] At the sixth international hygiene and demography congress (Vienna, 1887), Desguin presented the Antwerp model.[59] The medical school inspection had to highlight the city's modern, science-based educational policy. In general, these services came about when liberals were in power and were used as propaganda against the Catholics. The medical school inspection only had the authority to medically check the children of public schools. Catholic schools did not benefit from these centralised medical services and were therefore framed as unhealthy and unhygienic.[60]

Preventive medical campaigns were also initiated by private activists and organisations. The fight against alcohol was fought by (army) physicians, clergymen and teachers (rather than by local or national authorities), who joined forces and founded private temperance societies in the late 1870s. Until 1889 no licence was needed for opening drinking establishments in Belgium. The first restrictive laws were voted only around 1900, and the Comité national antialcoolique was founded in 1912. The majority of anti-alcohol campaigners were rooted in urban progressive Catholic milieus, while a minority was socialist or claimed to be apolitical.[61] The anti-alcohol movement found an ally in the women's rights movement. The Ligue belge du Droit des Femmes strongly believed that women could play a role in solving the problem of alcohol abuse. Wives were direct victims of the drunkenness of their husbands. Hence, feminists such as Marie Parent claimed that women had the important task to stop men from excessive drinking.[62]

More than a pure medical issue caused by social factors, alcoholism was perceived in Belgium as a problem of the individual resulting from a lack of awareness and willpower. The Ligue patriotique contre l'Alcoolisme was founded in 1879 by three physicians, Louis Martin, Hippolyte Barella and Théodore Belval. Their main focus was to spread anti-alcohol propaganda and establish local temperance societies throughout the country. The Ligue was successful. After the violent strikes of 1886, the number of societies rapidly increased.[63] They campaigned, among other things, via physicians who published both scientific works as well as practical leaflets that informed the population about the dangers of alcoholism and countered prejudices and superstitions with scientific facts. One key work was *De alcohol in't licht der wetenschap*, written by the physician Alfred De Vaucleroy, in which he disaffirmed with scientific experiments the popular beliefs that alcohol stimulates the digestive system or has healing properties (see Chapter 9, p. 339). He was actively involved in the transnational networks of the temperance movements and discussed his views at many of the Congrès internationaux contre l'abus des boissons alcooliques. Although his thoughts were well perceived by the international audience of alcohol experts, *De alcohol in't licht der wetenschap* was illustrative for the particular position of Belgium in the fight against alcohol. In contrast to protestant countries, many Belgian reformers were not in favour of total abstinence. They rather plea for moderation, by raising awareness and banning distilled drinks in general and absinthe in particular.

Public health, hygiene and social activism 147

In the Congo, preventive medicine followed the same dynamics of specialisation enhanced by transnational exchange of knowledge (see Chapter 3, p. 104). However, this occurred with some delay in comparison with things happening in Belgium. Understandably, this has to do with the fact that participation of Belgians in expansionist projects in Africa started only in 1876. The CFS, founded by King Leopold II in 1885 in the margins of the Berlin Conference, was a one-man business in many ways, in which the Belgian state did not participate officially. No wonder that it mobilised but a small body of medical experts and provided scanty means for the development of a *service médical* (founded in 1888).[64] The Leopoldian exploitation economy was dependent on private concessionary companies, investing, inter alia, in the construction of railways. These companies recruited no more than a few doctors, mainly to keep their white staff healthy. They undertook little action to protect the health of African and Asian labour forces, and certainly did not take prevention measures involving the rest of the population. In Belgium, the development of tropical hygiene and healthcare came late and one may say that it happened in an unstructured way, certainly when compared with countries with a much older imperial past such as France, where 'colonial' hygiene was shaped by provincial military institutions belonging to the navy; or the United Kingdom, which took advantage of its maritime medical tradition while at the same time relying on experience in combating epidemics in colonial India and the rest of the empire, thus leading, at the end of the nineteenth century, to the creation of schools for tropical hygiene and medicine in Liverpool and London.[65]

Nevertheless, in Belgium during the last quarter of the nineteenth century there was a gradual professionalisation in tropical hygiene and healthcare. In this respect, we should emphasise the importance of transnational knowledge exchanges through four channels: first, the international congresses on colonial hygiene and acclimatisation, where Belgians matched their experiences in Congo against those of other empires; second, a new intellectual 'colonial' sociability, comprising the geographical societies of Brussels and Antwerp, the Institut national de Géographie and the Société (royale) belge d'Etudes coloniales, which popularised and distributed knowledge in the fields of colonial hygiene and healthcare via lectures, courses, journals and books, thereby using information accumulated through an extensive network of relationships with similar societies abroad; third, the CFS's medical apparatus, consisting of Belgian and foreign staff, who initially managed a few poorly equipped sanatoria in the Lower Congo and focused exclusively on white state officials, but eventually also had a medical laboratory in Leopoldville, and from 1906 onwards, received support from a school of tropical medicine in Brussels, equipped with a bacteriological laboratory; fourth, inter-imperial knowledge exchange in combating major epidemics such as sleeping sickness, smallpox, leprosy and malaria, leading to prevention and vaccination campaigns, which initially focused on the white coloniser, but later on, when the human catastrophe was at its height and could no longer be ignored, became also oriented towards the African population.[66]

To understand Belgian appreciation of hygiene in an African context during the 'installation' phase of Leopoldian rule, one has to split up the concept into two complementary types: 'travel hygiene' and 'residential hygiene'. However, in the early years of Belgian presence, the first type prevailed, as exploration was at the heart of the African enterprise. The literature produced in the 1870s and 1880s primarily aimed at making European explorers survive the 'hostile' environment they had to cross, focusing on 'healthy' rules of conduct for white males while cruising the African rivers, the Maxim gun in hand ... As more and more people were faced with death – especially when the Free State's first, unprepared agents were establishing stations for permanent residence – attention shifted to 'residential hygiene'. This included health education for state officials, guidelines for building houses, laying emphasis on good aeration of the premises, inspired by studies that highlighted the impact of climate on the health of Europeans in Africa. The explorer Jérôme Becker illustrates this shift at a Berlin congress on colonial hygiene in 1886. In his speech he stressed the importance of physical training, clothing, balanced food and drinks and taking precautions against heat, cold and humidity.[67] From the 1890s onwards the discussion became more emphatically medical, with an increased participation of physicians in public debate and more pronounced attention given to linking fieldwork to laboratory research, and ultimately to prevention campaigns. Gustave Dryepondt's career illustrates the various aspects of this transition period in a tropical context very well.

Born in Bruges in 1866, Dryepondt graduated in medicine at the University of Brussels in 1890. The very same year he was recruited as physician to join the Van Kerckhoven expedition, initially destined to 'pacify' the eastern part of the Congo Basin, but known in later years as a violent imperialist attempt by the Leopoldian regime to gain access to the Nile Basin. During a stop in Leopoldville, Dryepondt was instructed to give medical aid to the white agents in this increasingly important station that gave direct access to the Upper Congo. Health reasons withheld him from continuing his work for the expedition, but in Leopoldville he lay the foundations of a small hospital. After a three-year stay in Congo, Dryepondt returned to Belgium in 1893 to recuperate. He immediately valorised his newly acquired medical knowledge, becoming an energetic speaker at learned societies, in particular the Société belge d'Etudes coloniales, where in 1894 he started the first medical courses for Belgians destined for a career in Congo. The content of his lessons was integrated in a *Guide pratique hygiénique et médical du voyageur au Congo*, issued by the administration of the CFS, on behalf of which Dryepondt served as *conseiller médical*. Dryepondt paid particular attention to climatic conditions. For many years Dryepondt's guide had a major impact on the life of Belgian agents in Congo. In fact, the guide became the second part of the collective work *Manuel du voyageur et du résident au Congo*, published by the Société belge d'Etudes coloniales in 1897. Every 'colonist' was expected to read this book.[68] Dryepondt returned to Africa several times, both as a physician and as an administrator of colonial companies. Eventually he started pleading in favour of creating a Belgian school for tropical medicine following the British example. For this purpose, he established contacts with foreign experts, mainly at international congresses. Dryepondt shifted his attention to a more medical approach of tropical hygiene and healthcare. He became an advocate of introducing a professionalised organisation of the medical services in Congo as well as of establishing a medical laboratory in Leopoldville. It should be stressed that only in the post-Leopoldian period did he become really interested in the hygienic conditions of the African populations, supporting large-scale prevention campaigns.[69] As Mertens and Lachenal have stressed, with the Belgian takeover of Congo the international significance of the sleeping sickness in particular served as a leverage, at the national level, for the profession of tropical medicine to obtain support within the state. Moreover, in the interwar period physicians such as Jérôme Rodhain and Jean E. van Campenhout contributed to the embedding of Belgian knowledge in an international sphere of expertise, taking a prominent role in the coordination of the fight against sleeping sickness and other epidemics through the League of Nations Health Organization (LNHO).[70] Several contributions stress the international dimension of medical care, highlighting the growing influence of pharmaceutical multinationals and international health organisations. Such internationalism, moreover, was not limited to the European mainland. Medicine in the Belgian Congo, as Sokhieng Au makes clear, cannot be understood without acknowledging the competing presence and influence of American Protestant missions in the region.[71]

National health protection and the well-being of the state and its citizens

At the turn of the twentieth century and especially after the First World War, medicine became the social science par excellence. The Polish-French medical doctor Petre Trisca wrote in 1923 that 'there is no one better than the doctor to observe society, the physician is urged by his professional training to penetrate into all environments and to see everything. He truly understands the economic state of the country, the psychology of the various social classes, the moral diseases that use the energies, the physical diseases that destroy the body.'[72] Trisca's words reflected the growing awareness that there was a close relation between social and economic progress and public health. Therefore, physicians and policymakers were convinced that social medicine should be more than providing public healthcare, it should also be searching for ways to protect and improve national health. This resulted in the emergence of new scientific medical disciplines, domains and practices like eugenics, craniology, pre-marital check-ups, birth control for disabled people, periodic medical examination, the sterilisation of abnormalities and social prophylaxis in order to prevent venereal diseases and 'racial hygiene' (see Chapter 8, p. 287).[73]

Public health, hygiene and social activism 151

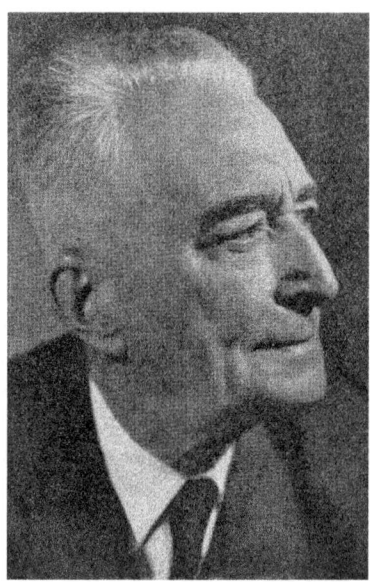

Figure 4.2 Portrait of René Sand. From an obituary notice connected with the International Congress of Social Work, 1953.

'*Pour prospérer, la nation a besoin de toutes ses forces*'.[74] This precept of the Belgian journal *Revue d'eugénique* reveals how social medicine was regarded as the solution to many problems and being healthy was turned into a moral duty. Physicians therefore felt the urge to claim a greater role in defining social/health policies and protective laws.[75] Indicative for the important role physicians played in Belgian society was the *loi de défense sociale* (9 April 1930), which allowed medical professionals to decide whether perpetrators of crimes were (ir)responsible because of their mental state. The purpose of this law was twofold: to provide those deemed insane with appropriate care and to protect society. In the first half of the twentieth century, social medicine further institutionalised, which resulted in a professionalisation of the healthcare system. In 1913, the *Bulletin de l'Association belge de Médecine sociale* was founded by the physician René Sand (Figure 4.2), providing a platform for knowledge exchange on social questions within the field of medicine and advocacy for civil servants, members of various medical boards, 'hygienist physicians' – in 1908, a one-year postgraduate training for physicians to obtain the degree of *médecin hygiéniste* was installed at the State Universities of Ghent and Liège – and other medical professionals. The journal responded to the urgency of coordinating the proliferation of measures, initiatives, councils and (often local) semi-public and private medical associations dealing with public healthcare and social medicine. A major influence was the growing importance of labour legislation for which physicians played both an advising as well as an executing role.[76]

Historians have argued that during the twentieth century the domain of industrial medicine and industrial diseases has been a scene of crucial struggles at the transnational level.[77] Although Belgium, like France and the Netherlands, was sometimes left out of major discussions in the industrial hygiene section of the International Labour Organisation (ILO), it was strongly involved in many transnational social medical exchanges.[78] Already near the end of the First World War, in spring 1918, the Belgian government sent a mission to the United States to study the organisation of labour, industrial production, social services and American society as a whole. The mission included the physician, social worker and internationalist René Sand.[79] In 1919 René Sand published his views on the methods and aims of social work in the United States and Britain in order to stimulate the professionalisation of social work in Belgium.[80] In the same year, together with Marie Derscheid, he started building the first Belgian school for the education of social workers (Ecole temporale de service social). In 1927, Sand translated and spread the work of Mary Richmond (*What is Social Casework? An Introductory Description*), which can be seen as a milestone in the professionalisation of social work.[81]

Professional social work stems from cognate scientific fields as social medicine and hygiene but also from a transnational knowledge exchange and the development of international organisations such as the Red Cross and platforms like the International Conferences of Social Work.[82] Sand, who contributed to the resurgence of the Red Cross in Belgium after the First World War, was in 1921 appointed as general secretary of the Ligue des Sociétés de la Croix-Rouge, which stimulated the international cooperation in social work. Together with Alice Masarykova, Sand would play an important role in the establishment of the first Conférence internationale de Service social (Paris, 1928).[83] He also contributed to the international exchange of socio-medical knowledge as he travelled all over the world to lecture on social medicine. Already in the early 1920s, Sand belonged to a group of socio-medical professionals including Alfred Grotjahn, Ludwig Teleky, Alfons Fischer, Adolf Gottstein and Andrija Stampar who gave social medicine a scientific underpinning, stimulating the emergence of several university chairs for social medicine and the foundation of social hygienic academies.[84]

Sand's initiatives are marked by a strong international scope, making him part of a wider trend identified by Saunier as the third circulatory regime, when social experts searched for universal norms and standards for social policies, professions and practices. They were strongly convinced that the universal spread of scientific social knowledge in general, and social medicine in particular, would lead to the 'well-being of humanity throughout the world'. The third regime was marked by the emergence of new international players with worldwide responsibilities such as the Office international d'Hygiène publique (OIHP, founded in 1907) and the aforementioned LNHO (founded in 1922). The League of Nations became an important actor in this field of social policy and many pre-war epistemic communities became further institutionalised.[85] Collectively, they formed the diverse landscape of the international health work of the interwar period.[86] Among these newly found international players, the Rockefeller groups particularly distinguished themselves with their contribution to the circulation of technical knowledge in the field of social hygiene and social medicine and financing of several new initiatives.[87] With the support of the Rockefeller Foundation, Sand managed to create the first academic chair for history of medicine and social medicine at the Université Libre de Bruxelles (1945).[88]

New activism, new public health systems?

As it has been stipulated throughout this book, the medical history of Belgium in the twentieth century has been to some extent underexposed and this has also been the case with the history of social medicine and the public healthcare system. The public healthcare system was expanded and became more regularised and institutionalised in the wake of the Second World War. The Belgian government initiated an obligatory health insurance (*Ziekte en Invaliditeitsvoorziening*, ZIV 1944) which came into the hands of a new central government agency, the Rijksdienst voor Ziekte- en Invaliditeitsverzekering. The national unity government also launched the so-called social pact, which bundled legislation on sickness and invalidity insurance, unemployment, pensions, child benefit and annual holiday for employees with the aim of improving the social security system and implementing the measures more efficiently (see Chapter 6, p. 224).[89]

Physicians were integrated in the system as mediators between the state, the patient and the health insurance agencies. They determined whether someone needed medical care (financial) support, but they were also expected to act as financial watchdogs to prevent abuse. Already from the start, ZIV caused a lot of problems. On the one hand, the law was full of gaps, leading to serious financial deficits.[90] On the other hand, ZIV caused political controversy. The public healthcare system became politicised to a far greater extent than before. In Belgium several attempts were made to control the constantly expanding healthcare budget.[91] As it had been the case everywhere in Europe in the period after 1960, the Belgian public health system was strongly questioned, leading to continuous political debate about the healthcare system's sustainability.[92] Western healthcare systems were facing spiralling costs that needed to be kept within reasonable limits without losing the principle of distributive justice in the welfare state.[93] But also the relation between the physicians as a professional group and the government became at times tense due to debates on the efficiency of medical service, savings in costs or the negations of the physicians' fees.

The postcolonial period is characterised by policies of efficiency and privatisation. At the same time, the field of social medicine took a global dimension thanks to initiatives launched by WHO, and planetary debates and actions concerning public health ignited by social movements and INGOs.[94] Global health implies the consideration of the health needs of people of the whole planet above the concerns of particular nations. The term 'global' is also associated with the growing importance of actors beyond governmental or intergovernmental organisations and agencies, for example the media, internationally influential foundations, non-governmental organisations (NGOs) and transnational corporations.[95] The work of contemporary players of 'global' stature such as the microbiologist Peter Piot, who discovered the Ebola virus in the 1970s, or the world-renowned fertility expert Marleen Temmerman, is clearly rooted in the 'Belgian' context of social activism, although both soon widened the scope of their scholarly and social commitments, first to Africa and its most vulnerable citizens, and finally to the entire planet.

The Institute of Tropical Medicine in Antwerp in particular gave the children of May 1968 wings to support their solidarity with what was then called the 'Third World'. Their engagement was embedded in the broader activism of the emerging 'new' social movements of the 1970s, the Third World movement in particular. Development work meant exercising social commitment. In the Belgian medicine faculties of the 1970s, this was certainly not a central concern. The number of initiatives was rather limited and they were not really 'carried' by the corps of professors, only by a minority of socially driven scholars within the faculties. In the fall of 1976, Peter Piot moved to the village of Yambuku on the Congo River to investigate the outbreak of an unknown disease that caused high fever, diarrhoea and severe bleeding. Piot had joined the Institute of Tropical Medicine in Antwerp two years after graduating and he specialised in microbiology.[96]

In September 1976, a blue thermos flask from Kinshasa arrived at the Antwerp laboratory for microbiology, containing blood samples from a Flemish missionary sister. An electron microscope survey showed that the deadly disease was not a normal virus, but a giant worm structure that had never been observed before. The then twenty-seven-year-old Peter Piot, who had never visited Africa before, boarded a C-130 aircraft, and flew from the capital of Congo/Zaire to the rainforest. His mission was to diagnose the mysterious virus in its local context and stop the epidemic. After three months of improvising on the spot, he succeeded in observing how the virus was transferred. The virus was named after a neighbouring river, the Ebola. Forty years later, the sociopolitical circumstances in which the Ebola virus thrives has hardly changed. Political destabilisation, a dysfunctional health system, superstition, denial, poverty: the classical curative approach with vaccines, medication, isolation and quarantine is not enough if political, social and cultural factors are not taken into account. In addition, international organisations such as WHO fail to safeguard universal human rights. When in the summer of 2014 a very serious Ebola epidemic again broke out in West Africa, WHO was only seriously alerted after two American citizens had been flown home in alarming conditions. Meanwhile, more than a thousand dead victims were counted in Africa. At that moment Peter Piot had acquired the moral authority to denounce this scandalous fact worldwide.[97] In Piot's opinion, science cannot be separated from activism and politics.

In October 1983, six years after the discovery of the Ebola virus, Piot discovered more than fifty acquired immune deficiency syndrome (AIDS) victims – men and women – in the Mama Yemo Hospital in Kinshasa. This confirmed the hypothesis that the infection was also transmitted through heterosexual contacts. For Piot this was a eureka moment of tremendous importance. Project SIDA in Zaire – an American–Belgian–Zairian research mission – became the world's first international AIDS campaign. In the 1990s Piot made the move from medicine to international institutions 'to change the world'. He took leading positions in the International AIDS Society, the AIDS programmes of WHO and UNAIDS, of which he was the founding executive director, combining his work with the position of assistant secretary-general of the United Nations. In Belgium itself, AIDS had initially appeared as an 'imported' disease, which was thought to be limited to (American) homosexuals and Africans. As a result of this, as Hans Neefs has shown, AIDS policy first developed largely outside the established public health structures. It was a new terrain of public health that developed from below through the work of medical experts such as Piot and Jan Desmyter. These medical experts developed policies of testing (surveillance), AIDS education, contact tracing, etc. In the second half of the 1980s, grass-roots AIDS organisations succeeded in reframing AIDS as a wider public health problem, not limited to gay people. Politicians now followed in setting up campaigns on safe sex, tackling ideologically difficult questions of sexual morality.[98]

Marleen Temmerman, a gynaecologist, women's rights activist and professor at Ghent University, followed a similar course. In 1987 she went to Kenya in the context of an AIDS research project set up by Peter Piot at the Kenyatta National Hospital in Nairobi. There she examined if and how women and children could be infected with human immunodeficiency virus (HIV). In 1992, the year she returned to Ghent, she received 2.4 million ECU from the European Commission to build an institute. It was seed money for starting up the International Centre for Reproductive Health (ICRH), founded in 1994. The ICRH was anchored in Ghent, with branches in Kenya and Mozambique. More than twenty-five years later it has grown into one of the largest centres of excellence in the field of reproductive health in the world. It has projects on a range of issues such as AIDS, sexually transmitted diseases, contraception, abortion, family planning, maternal mortality, genital mutilation, women's and children's health and sexual violence. The centre's strength is the dynamic interaction between multidisciplinary science and development cooperation and the implementation of research results into policy. It is no coincidence that Temmerman has been involved in politics. She was a senator for the Flemish Socialist Party from 2007 to 2012. She believes that scholars have the moral duty of giving politicians a language to speak and ask the right questions about public health. The UN Sustainable Development Goals provide a good guideline. From 2012 to 2015 Temmerman was a director at WHO. Since 2015 she has returned to Kenya, where she is leading the Department of Obstetrics and Gynaecology at Aga Khan University and continues to address women's health issues through the Aga Khan Development Network.[99]

In conclusion, it is clear that Piot and Temmerman are part of a long-standing tradition of social and medical activism. The history of public health and social medicine was a dynamic process of interaction between policymakers, physicians, medical and other professionals (civil servants, teachers, publicists, etc.), on the one hand, and social activists and reform movements, on the other. Moreover, public health is also a process of negotiation between various medical professionals and other experts on the issues of what public health was supposed to be, how it could be studied and how it needed to be improved. Both Adolph Burggraeve and Victor Desguin illustrated that in this process of negotiation no clear distinction could be made between the state, private practitioners and physicians who were never neutral and did not only influence decision-making processes but also became politically engaged, as they conducted policies and became a cog in the machinery of government. Many early local urban initiatives were launched by both medical professionals (in the making) and statisticians, thus trying to identify and explore socio-economic determinants for disease outbreaks.[100] Regarding the late nineteenth century, it has been observed that these local dynamics evolved towards more centralised actions targeting the containment of epidemics, thus resulting, in the course of the twentieth century, in the emergence of national medical policies that aimed at improving public health.[101]

At the same time, social and medical activists negotiated their theories and policies and exchanged their thoughts and practices in an increasingly globalising world. As Eijkman had already noticed, these dynamics in the nineteenth and twentieth century were barely restricted by the borders of the (Belgian) nation state. Therefore, we have argued that the emergence of public healthcare in Belgium cannot be seen apart from cross-border exchanges, scientific innovations, social reform ambitions, but also inter- and intra-imperial dynamics. A similar story can be told in regard to social reform, starting with the initiatives taken by urban philanthropic circles. These initiatives contributed to the institutionalisation of social action, the emergence of national social policies and the development of social legislation. With the rise of the modern welfare states in the course of the twentieth century and the internationalisation of social politics, the entanglement of social and medical policies became even stronger. The role the physician René Sand played in the professionalisation of social work clearly illustrated that in the early twentieth century no strict distinction between medicine, public healthcare and social welfare could be made. The changing circulatory regimes, scientific development and sociopolitical circumstances had a profound influence on the evolving concept of social medicine, but in essence public health and hygiene initiatives and locally rooted social activism remained closely intertwined. In this chapter we have shown that in Belgium sociopolitical interventions were more coordinated than argued before. Nineteenth-century Belgium has indeed predominantly been described as a nightwatchman state. But when hygienists and the like are approached as part of a (transnational) movement, we should nuance and even doubt this. Historians have shown that already in the early nineteenth century private and public actors tried to improve public hygiene and living conditions, increasingly seeking government support from the second half of the nineteenth century onwards. Especially at the local level, many social interventions and actions took place in nineteenth-century Belgium. Furthermore, recent studies have shown that locally active physicians and the like belonged to a wider (transnational) movement, transcending their professional and disciplinary borders.[102] This is similar to the upcoming labour unions and health insurance funds, which were also firmly rooted in international epistemic communities.[103]

Notes

1 Pieter Hendrik Eijkman, *L'internationalisme médical* (Amsterdam: F. van Rossen, 1910); Warden Boyd Rayward, *Information Beyond Borders: International Cultural and Intellectual Exchange in the Belle Epoque* (London: Ashgate, 2014), 204.
2 François de Torday, *Compte rendu du XVIe Congrès international de Médecine* (Budapest: Franklin-Tarsulat, 1909).
3 Maryinez Lyons, *The Colonial Disease: A Social History of Sleeping Sickness in Northern Zaire, 1900–1940* (Cambridge, UK: Cambridge University Press, 1992), 76–136, 281; Myriam Mertens and Guillaume Lachenal, 'The history of "Belgian" tropical medicine from a cross-border perspective', *Revue belge de Philologie et d'Histoire*, 90 (2012), 1249–72.
4 Stéphane Frioux, 'Sanitizing the city: the transnational work and networks of French sanitary engineers, 1890s–1930s', in *Shaping the Transnational Sphere: Experts, Networks and Issues from the 1840s to the 1930s*, ed. Davide Rodogno, Bernhard Struck and Jakob Vogel (New York: Berghahn, 2015), 44–59; Viviane Claude, 'Technique sanitaire et réforme urbaine: l'Association Générale des Hygiénistes et Techniciens Municipaux 1905–1920', in *Laboratoires du nouveau siècle. La 'nébuleuse réformatrice' et ses réseaux en France 1880–1914*, ed. Christian Topalov (Paris: EHESS, 1999), 269–98.
5 Joris Vandendriessche, *Medical Societies and Scientific Culture in Nineteenth-Century Belgium* (Manchester: Manchester University Press, 2018).
6 Hans Neefs, *Between Sin and Disease: The Social Fight against Syphilis and AIDS in Belgium (1880–2000)* (Saarbrücken: LAP Lambert, 2010).
7 Dorothy Porter, 'Stratification and its discontents: professionalization and conflict in the British public health service, 1848–1914', in *A History of Education in Public Health: Health That Mocks the Doctors' Rules*, ed. Elisabeth Fee and Roy M. Acheson (Oxford: Oxford University Press, 1991), 83–113.

8 Christophe Charle, Jürgen Schriewer and Peter Wagner, *Transnational Intellectual Networks: Forms of Academic Knowledge and the Search for Cultural Identities* (Frankfurt: Campus, 2004); Davide Rodogno, Bernhard Struck and Jakob Vogel (eds), *Shaping the Transnational Sphere: Experts, Networks, and Issues the 1840s to the 1930s* (New York: Berghahn, 2015).

9 Daniel Laqua, Christophe Verbruggen, Gita Deneckere, Pierre-Yves Saunier, Timothy Baycroft and Martin Conway, 'Beyond Belgium: encounters, exchanges and entanglements, 1900–1925', *Journal of Belgian History-Revue belge d'Histoire contemporaine-Belgisch Tijdschrift voor Nieuwste Geschiedenis*, 43:4 (2013), 148–63.

10 Porter, 'Stratification and its discontents'.

11 Karel Velle, *De nieuwe biechtvaders: de sociale geschiedenis van de arts in België* (Leuven-Amsterdam: Kritak-Meulenhof, 1991).

12 Liesbet Nys, Henk De Smaele, Jo Tollebeek and Kaat Wils (eds), *De zieke natie: over de medicalisering van de samenleving, 1860–1914* (Groningen: Historische Uitgeverij, 2002); Peter Conrad and Valerie Leiter (eds), *Health and Health Care as Social Problems* (Lanham, MD: Rowman & Littlefield, 2003); Peter Conrad, *The Medicalization of Society: On the Transformation of Human Conditions into Treatable Disorders* (Baltimore, MD: Johns Hopkins University Press, 2008); Frank Huisman and Harry Oosterhuis (eds), *Health and Citizenship: Political Cultures of Health in Modern Europe* (London: Routledge, 2016).

13 Heidi Rimke and Alan Hunt, 'From sinners to degenerates: the medicalization of morality in the 19th century', *History of the Human Sciences*, 15:1 (2002), 59–88.

14 Lutz Raphael, 'Die Verwissenschaftlichung des Sozialen als methodische und konzeptionelle Herausforderung für eine Sozialgeschichte des 20. Jahrhunderts', *Geschichte und Gesellschaft*, 22:2 (1996), 165–93.

15 Jasmien van Daele and Christian Müller, 'Peaks of internationalism in social engineering: a transnational history of international social reform associations and Belgian agency, 1860–1925', *Revue belge de Philologie et d'Histoire*, 90:4 (2012), 1297–319; Thomas D'haeninck, Nico Randeraad and Christophe Verbruggen, 'Visualizing longitudinal data: rooted cosmopolitans in the Low Countries, 1850–1914', *CEUR Workshop Proceedings*, 1399 (2015), 116–21 (First Conference on Biographical Data in a Digital World, CEUR WS, 2015).

16 Scott Frickel and Neil Gross, 'A general theory of scientific/intellectual movements', *American Sociological Review*, 70:2 (2005), 204–32.

17 Pierre-Yves Saunier, 'Les régimes circulatoires du domaine social 1800–1940: projets et ingénierie de la convergence et de la différence', *Genèses*, 71:2 (2008), 4–25.

18 Charle et al., *Transnational Intellectual Networks*; Rodogno et al., *Shaping the Transnational Sphere*.
19 Saunier, 'Les régimes circulatoires', 20.
20 Eckhardt Fuchs, 'The creation of new international networks in education: the League of Nations and educational organizations in the 1920s', *Paedagogica Historica*, 43:2 (2007), 199–209; Van Daele and Müller, 'Peaks of internationalism in social engineering', 1311–15.
21 As argued by Hu and Manning, a new global model of privatisation emerged the 1980s. Aiqun Hu and Patrick Manning, 'The global social insurance movement since the 1880s', *Journal of Global History*, 5:1 (2010), 125–48.
22 Jean-Pierre Goubert, '1770–1830: La première croisade médicale', *Historical Reflections/Réflexions Historiques*, 9:1–2 (1982), 3–13; Karel Velle, 'Medisch-topografisch en epidemiologisch onderzoek in België sinds het laatste kwart van de 18de eeuw tot ca. 1850: een bijdrage tot de sociale geschiedenis', *Handelingen van de Koninklijke Zuid-Nederlansche Maatschappij voor Taal- en Letterkunde en Geschiedenis*, 38 (1984), 209–29.
23 Porter, 'Stratification and its discontents'.
24 Michel Foucault, Anne Thalamy and Blandine Barret-Kriegel, *Les machines à guérir: aux origines de l'hôpital moderne* (Brussels: Mardaga, 1979), 7–18.
25 Karel Velle, 'Arts, geneeskunde en samenleving: medicalisering in België in de 19de en de 20ste eeuw' (PhD diss. Rijksuniversiteit Gent, 1987–88), 1047.
26 Ibid., 61–85. Velle also refers to Foucault et al., *Les machines à guérir*.
27 Velle, 'De misdaad als kwaal', 332–55; Conrad and Leiter, *Health and Health Care as Social Problems*; Conrad, *The Medicalization of Society*.
28 Joris Vandendriessche, 'Arbiters of science: expertise in public health in nineteenth-century Belgian medical societies', in *Scientists' Expertise as Performance: Between State and Society, 1860–1960*, ed. Joris Vandendriessche, Evert Peeters and Kaat Wils (London: Pickering & Chatto, 2015), 31–48, at 33–6.
29 Karel Velle, 'Het verenigingsleven van de Belgische geneesheer', *Annales de la Société belge d'histoire des hôpitaux et de la santé publique*, 26–7 (1988–89), 47–118; Joris Vandendriessche and Kaat Wils, 'Een traject van onderhandeling. Hygiënisme als wetenschap, Antwerpen 1880–1900', *BMGN: Low Countries Historical Review*, 128:3 (2013), 3–28.
30 Vandendriessche, 'Arbiters of science', 34.
31 Veronique Deblon and Pieter Huistra, 'Het geheim van de anatoom: Adolphe Burggraeve en de ontwikkeling van de Belgische anatomie

in de negentiende eeuw', *Studium*, 9:4 (2017), 202–16; Veronique Deblon, 'Adolphe Burggraeve en de schoonheid van de dood', in *Post-Mortem. Vesalius tussen kunst en wetenschap*, ed. Marjan Doom (Ghent: Gents Universiteitsmuseum, 2015), 63–5; Marjan Doom, *Het museum van de twijfel. Een bescheiden manifest van een wetenschapscurator* (Ghent: Academia Press, 2020), 77–84.
32 This association was named after the charismatic professor François Huet. For a short period it was the meeting place in Ghent for freethinkers to discuss philosophical, political and social problems. E. C. Coppens, 'La Société Huet. Tussen revolutie en reaktie', *Handelingen der Maatschappij voor Geschiedenis en Oudheidkunde te Gent*, 26:1 (1972), 131–51.
33 Vandendriessche, 'Arbiters of science', 33–6.
34 Daniel Mareska and Jean-Julien Heyman, *Enquête sur le travail et la condition physique et morale des ouvriers employés dans les manufactures de coton, à Gand* (Gand: Gyselynck, 1845).
35 Vandendriessche, 'Arbiters of science', 34–5.
36 Bart Vos, 'De Bataviawijk: studie van een arbeidersbuurt in de eerste generatie (1836–1914)' (Master's diss., Rijksuniversiteit Gent, 1985).
37 Adolphe Pauli and Auguste Wagener, *Le nouvel Institut des sciences à Gand* (Gand: Hoste, 1892).
38 Doreen Gaublomme, 'Doctrinairen en progressisten tijdens de 19de eeuw', in *Het Liberalisme in België. Tweehonderd jaar geschiedenis*, ed. Hervé Hasquin and Adriaan Verhulst (Brussels: Uitgeverij Delta, 1989), 201–8.
39 Joris Vandendriessche, 'Medische expertise en politieke strijd. De dienst medisch schooltoezicht in Antwerpen, 1860–1900', *Stadsgeschiedenis*, 6:2 (2011), 113–28.
40 Kathleen Devolder, *Gij die door 't volk gekozen zijt ... De Gentse gemeenteraad en haar leden 1830–1914* (Ghent: Maatschappij voor Geschiedenis en Oudheidkunde, 1994).
41 Oliver MacDonagh, 'IV. The nineteenth-century revolution in government: a reappraisal', *Historical Journal*, 1:1 (1958), 52–67; Roy MacLeod, *Government and Expertise: Specialists, Administrators, and Professionals* (Cambridge, UK: Cambridge University Press, 1988); David S. Barnes, *The Great Stink of Paris and the Nineteenth-Century Struggle against Filth and Germs* (Baltimore, MD: Johns Hopkins University Press, 2006).
42 Vandendriessche and Wils, 'Een traject van onderhandeling'.
43 Saunier, 'Les régimes circulatoires', 4–25.
44 Eckhardt Fuchs, 'Educational sciences, morality and politics: international educational congresses in the early twentieth century', *Paedagogica Historica*, 40:5–6 (2004), 758.

45 Carmen van Praet, 'Liberale hommes-orchestres en de sociale kwestie in de negentiende eeuw. Tussen lokaal en internationaal' (PhD thesis, Ghent University, 2015), 141–6.
46 Ibid., 144.
47 Margaret E. Keck and Kathryn Sikkink, 'Transnational advocacy networks in international and regional politics', *International Social Science Journal*, 51:159 (1999), 88–101.
48 Robert Halleux, Geneviève Xhayet, Pascal Pirot, Jan Vandersmissen and Rik Raedschelders, *Tant qu'il y aura des chercheurs. Science et politique en Belgique de 1772 à 2015* (Liège: Luc Pire, 2015), 44–8; Robert Halleux, Jan Vandersmissen, Andrée Despy-Meyer and Geert Vanpaemel (eds), *Geschiedenis van de wetenschappen in België 1815–2000* (Brussels: Dexia Bank-La Renaissance du Livre, 2001), 289–305.
49 Halleux et al., *Tant qu'il y aura des chercheurs*, 44–8.
50 Alan J. Rocke, *Image and Reality: Kekulé, Kopp, and the Scientific Imagination* (Chicago: University of Chicago Press, 2010); Halleux et al., *Geschiedenis van de wetenschappen in België 1815–2000*, 289–305.
51 Velle, 'Arts, geneeskunde en samenleving', 57; Halleux et al., *Tant qu'il y aura des chercheurs*.
52 Sofie Onghena, 'Altruïstisch ambtenaar of heroïsch genie? Het gepropageerde beeld van provinciale en academische directeurs van bacteriologische laboratoria in België (ca. 1900–1940)', *Studium*, 2:4 (2009). On government laboratories in Belgium, see Lyvia Diser, *Wetenschap op de proef. Laboratoria in het Belgisch overheidsbeleid, 1870–1940* (Leuven: Leuven University Press, 2016).
53 About prison doctors, see chap. 3 in Amandine Thiry's forthcoming doctoral thesis (UCLouvain/UGent). Her research project is entitled: 'Confinement as social utopia. "Belgian" reformers and transnational ideas on prison'.
54 Vandendriessche, *Medical Societies and Scientific Culture*, 181–96; Liesbet Nys, 'Nationale plagen. Hygiënisten over het maatschappelijk lichaam', in Nys et al., *De zieke natie*, 220–41.
55 Evert Peeters and Kaat Wils, 'Ambivalences of liberal health policy: lebensreform and self-help medicine in Belgium, 1890–1914', in Huisman and Oosterhuis, *Health and Citizenship*, 101–17.
56 Ilse De Buyser, 'Bijdrage tot de geschiedenis van het medisch schooltoezicht in België. Van de eerste initiatieven tot de inrichting van het verplicht MST, 1874–1914' (master's diss., KU Leuven, 1995); Karel Velle, 'De schoolgeneeskunde in België (1850–1940)', *Geschiedenis der Geneeskunde*, 5 (1998), 354–66.

57 Karel Velle, 'Eugène Dorothé Janssens: ambtenaar en medisch-statisticus', in *Er is leven voor de dood. Tweehonderd jaar gezondheidszorg in Vlaanderen*, ed. Jan De Maeyer, Lieve Dhaene, Karel Velle and Gilbert Hertecant (Kapellen: Pelckmans, 1998), 111–13.

58 Joris Vandendriessche, 'Medische expertise en politieke strijd. De dienst medisch schooltoezicht in Antwerpen, 1860–1900', *Stadsgeschiedenis*, 6:2 (2011), 113–28.

59 Nico Randeraad, 'Triggers of mobility: international congresses (1840–1914) and their visitors', in *Mobility and Biography*, ed. Sarah Panter (Berlin: De Gruyter, 2015), 69–71.

60 Vandendriessche, 'Medische expertise en politieke strijd', 124–6.

61 Liesbet Nys, 'De grote school van de natie. Legerartsen over drankmisbruik en geslachtsziekten in het leger (circa 1850–1950), *BMGN: Low Countries Historical Review*, 115:3 (2000), 392–425.

62 Marie Parent, *Le rôle de la femme dans la lutte contre l'alcoolisme* (Brussels: Ligue patriotique contre l'alcoolisme, 1892).

63 Martine Timmerman, 'De sociale ernst van het alkoholisme en de mobilisatie voor drankbestrijding vanaf het laatste kwart van de 19de eeuw' (master's diss., Ghent University, 1981); Maurice De Vroede, 'Primary education and the fight against alcoholism in Belgium at the turn of the century', *History of Education Quarterly*, 25:4 (1985), 483–97.

64 Albert Duchesne, 'Premier centre médical de l'Afrique noire: le 'sanitarium' du Docteur Allart à Boma (1883)', in *Le Centenaire de l'Etat Indépendant du Congo: recueil d'études = Bijdragen over de honderdste verjaring van de Onafhankelijke Kongostaat* (Brussels: Académie royale des Sciences d'Outre-Mer-Koninklijke Academie voor Overzeese Wetenschappen, 1988), 313–22; J. André, J. Burke, J. Vuylsteke and H. van Balen, 'Evolution of health services', in *Health in Central Africa since 1885: Past, Present and Future*, ed. P. G. Janssens, M. Kivits and J. Vuylsteke (Brussels: King Baudouin Foundation, 1997), vol. 1, 89–158.

65 Michael A. Osborne, *The Emergence of Tropical Medicine in France* (Chicago: University of Chicago Press, 2014); Ryan Johnson, *Tropical Medicine and Imperial Power: Science, Hygiene and Health in the Late British Empire* (London: I. B. Tauris, 2014).

66 Deborah J. Neill, *Networks in Tropical Medicine: Internationalism, Colonialism, and the Rise of a Medical Specialty, 1890–1930* (Palo Alto, CA: Stanford University Press, 2012), 1–43; Jan Vandersmissen, *Koningen van de wereld: Leopold II en de aardrijkskundige beweging* (Leuven: Acco, 2009), 251–84; Pieter G. Janssens, Maurice Kivits and Jacques Vuylsteke (eds), *Médecine et hygiène en Afrique Centrale: de 1885 à nos jours* (Brussels: Fondation Roi Baudouin, 1992), 1–61.

67 Jérôme Becker, 'Gymnases d'exploration et de colonisation. Projet présenté par l'auteur au Congrès d'Hygiène et d'acclimatement de Berlin (1886)', in *La vie en Afrique ou trois ans dans l'Afrique centrale*, ed. Jérôme Becker (Paris: J. Lebègue & Cie, 1887), vol. 2, 489–500.

68 Jan Vandersmissen, 'De "Manuel du voyageur et du résident au Congo" en de voorbereiding op het dagelijkse leven in de Onafhankelijke Congostaat op het einde van de 19de eeuw', in *Quotidiana. Huldealbum Dr. Frank Daelemans*, ed. Ria Jansen-Sieben, Marc Libert and André Vanrie (Brussels: Archief-en bibliotheekwezen in België, 2012), 413–36.

69 Pedro Monaville, '"Conseils aux partants": Une lecture politique des manuels d'hygiène coloniale publiés en Belgique (1895–1950)', *Journal of Belgian History: Revue belge d'Histoire contemporaine-Belgisch Tijdschrift voor Nieuwste Geschiedenis*, 36:1–2 (2012), 97–125.

70 Mertens and Lachenal, 'The history of "Belgian" tropical medicine', 1262–9.

71 Sokhieng Au, 'Medical orders: Catholic and Protestant missionary medicine in the Belgian Congo (1880–1940)', *BMGN: Low Countries Historical Review*, 132:1 (2017), 62–82.

72 Translation from French, see Petre Trisca, *Les médecins sociologues et hommes d'Etat* (Paris: Alcan, 1923), 14–15.

73 Velle, 'Arts, geneeskunde en samenleving', 1054; Raf De Bont, 'Meten en verzoenen. Louis Vervaeck en de Belgische criminele antropologie (circa 1900–1940)', *Cahiers d'histoire du temps présent*, 9 (2001), 63–104.

74 The *Revue d'eugénique* was founded in 1921 by the physicians René Sand, George Boulenger, Albert Govaerts, Rulot and the judge Wets: Velle, 'Arts, geneeskunde en samenleving', 49.

75 Velle, 'Arts, geneeskunde en samenleving', 1057.

76 Ibid., 1087.

77 Thomas Cayet, Paul-André Rosental and Marie Thébaud-Sorger, 'How international organisations compete: occupational safety and health at the ILO, a diplomacy of expertise', *Journal of Modern European History*, 7:2 (2009), 195.

78 Ibid., 179.

79 Michaël Amara, 'La propagande belge et l'image de la Belgique aux Etats-Unis pendant la Première Guerre mondiale', *Journal of Belgian History-Revue belge d'Histoire contemporaine-Belgisch Tijdschrift voor Nieuwste Geschiedenis*, 30:1–2 (2000), 173–226, at 200–2.

80 René Sand, *La bienfaisance d'hier et la bienfaisance de demain* (Brussels: Impr. L. Vogels, 1919); Kerstin Eilers, 'René Sand (1877–1953) and his contribution to international social work, IASSW-president 1946–1953', *Social Work and Society*, 5:1 (2007), 102–9.

81 Alain Anciaux, *Le docteur René Sand ou la culture des valeurs humaines* (Brussels: Université Libre de Bruxelles, 1988); Alain Anciaux, *René Sand: un médecin belge humaniste ou la vocation de la médecine sociale* (Brussels: Université Libre de Bruxelles, 1988).
82 Eilers, 'René Sand'.
83 Ibid.; Sabine Hering-Calfin and Berteke Waaldijk, *History of Social Work in Europe (1900–1960): Female Pioneers and Their Influence on the Development of International Social Organizations* (New York: Springer Science and Business Media, 2012), 119–28.
84 Iris Borowy, *Coming to Terms with World Health: The League of Nations Health Organisation 1921–1946* (Frankfurt am Main: Peter Lang, 2009), 21; Patrick Zylberman, 'Fewer parallels than antitheses: René Sand and Andrija Stampar on social medicine, 1919–1955', *Social History of Medicine*, 17:1 (2004), 77–92.
85 Fuchs, 'The creation of new international networks in education'; Van Daele and Müller, 'Peaks of internationalism in social engineering'.
86 Iris Borowy, 'The League of Nations Health Organization: from European to global health concerns', in *International and Local Approaches to Health and Health Care, Bergen, University of Bergen*, ed. Astri Andresen, William H. Hubbard and Teemu Ryymin (Oslo: Novus Press, 2010), 11–30.
87 Saunier, 'Les régimes circulatoires'; John Farley, *To Cast Out Disease: A History of the International Health Division of the Rockefeller Foundation (1913–1951)* (New York: Oxford University Press, 2004).
88 Eilers, 'René Sand'.
89 Karel Veraghtert and Brigitte Widdershoven, *Twee eeuwen solidariteit. De Nederlandse, Belgische en Duitse ziekenfondsen tijdens de negentiende en twintigste eeuw* (Amsterdam: Aksant, 2002); Ineke Meul, 'De professionalisering van het medisch-specialistisch beroep in het kader van de verplichte Ziekte-en invaliditeitsverzekering in België (1944–2014)' (PhD thesis, Universiteit Antwerpen, 2016).
90 Meul, 'De professionalisering', 111.
91 Ibid.
92 Huisman and Oosterhuis, *Health and Citizenship*.
93 Frank Huisman, Joris Vandendriessche and Kaat Wils, 'Blurring boundaries: towards a medical history of the twentieth century', *BMGN: Low Countries Historical Review* 132:1 (2017), 11.
94 See Hu and Manning, 'The global social insurance movement since the 1880s'.
95 Theodore M. Brown, Marcos Cueto and Elizabeth Fee, 'The World Health Organization and the transition from "international" to "global" public health', *American Journal of Public Health*, 96:1 (2006), 62–72.

96 Gita Deneckere, *Uit de ivoren toren: 200 jaar Universiteit Gent* (Ghent: Tijdsbeeld, 2017), 277–9.
97 Peter Piot, *No Time to Lose: A Life in Pursuit of Deadly Viruses* (New York: W. W. Norton & Company, 2012).
98 Neefs, *Between Sin and Disease*, 219–96.
99 Deneckere, *Uit de ivoren toren*, 286–7.
100 Vandendriessche and Wils, 'Een traject van onderhandeling'.
101 Velle, *De nieuwe biechtvaders*; Elisabeth Bruyneel, *De Hoge Gezondheidsraad (1849–2009): Schakel tussen wetenschap en volksgezondheid* (Leuven: Peeters, 2009).
102 Van Praet, 'Liberale hommes-orchestres'.
103 Van Daele and Müller, 'Peaks of internationalism in social engineering', 1311–15.

Selected bibliography

Cayet, Thomas, Rosental, Paul-André and Thébaud-Sorger, Marie, 'How international organisations compete: occupational safety and health at the ILO, a diplomacy of expertise', *Journal of Modern European History*, 7:2 (2009), 174–96.

Neefs, Hans, *Between Sin and Disease: The Social Fight against Syphilis and AIDS in Belgium (1880–2000)* (Saarbrücken: LAP Lambert, 2010).

Neill, Deborah J., *Networks in Tropical Medicine: Internationalism, Colonialism, and the Rise of a Medical Specialty, 1890–1930* (Palo Alto, CA: Stanford University Press, 2012).

Nys, Liesbet, De Smaele, Henk, Tollebeek Jo and Wils, Kaat (eds), *De zieke natie: over de medicalisering van de samenleving, 1860–1914* (Groningen: Historische Uitgeverij, 2002).

Peeters, Evert and Wils, Kaat, 'Ambivalences of liberal health policy: lebensreform and self-help medicine in Belgium, 1890–1914', in Frank Huisman and Harry Oosterhuis (eds), *Health and Citizenship. Political Cultures of Health in Modern Europe* (London: Pickering & Chatto, 2015), 101–17.

Saunier, Pierre-Yves, 'Les régimes circulatoires du domaine social 1800–1940: projets et ingénierie de la convergence et de la différence', *Genèses*, 71:2 (2008), 4–25.

van Daele, Jasmien and Müller, Christian, 'Peaks of internationalism in social engineering: a transnational history of international social reform associations and Belgian agency, 1860–1925', *Revue belge de Philologie et d'Histoire*, 90:4 (2012), 1297–319.

Vandendriessche, Joris, 'Arbiters of science: expertise in public health in nineteenth-century Belgian medical societies', in Joris Vandendriessche, Evert Peeters and Kaat Wils (eds), *Scientists' Expertise as Performance: Between State and Society, 1860–1960* (London: Pickering & Chatto, 2015), 31–48.

Velle, Karel, 'Arts, geneeskunde en samenleving: medicalisering in België in de 19de en de 20ste eeuw' (PhD thesis, Ghent University, 1988).

Zylberman, Patrick, 'Fewer parallels than antitheses: René Sand and Andrija Stampar on social medicine, 1919–1955', *Social History of Medicine*, 17:1 (2004), 77–92.

Part II

Institutions and beyond

5

Ways of knowing medicine

Renaud Bardez and Pieter Dhondt

An ideal physician should meet many different requirements. The person in question should have a vigorous mind, he or she should possess a large degree of common sense, be capable to act judiciously and decisively, have a well-balanced personality of high moral standing, combined with social consciousness and a practical knowledge of psychology, he or she should have a pleasant manner, a sympathetic appearance, a broad general culture, profound expert knowledge, and besides some non-negligible practical skills, if possible, it should be someone who can rely on the experience of a family tradition, and without doubt the person should also enjoy good health.[1]

Jean-Jacques Bouckaert, the dean of the medical faculty of Ghent University, gave this speech at the Royal Academy of Medicine in 1958, during a debate on the preparation of a reform of the medical curriculum. His words illustrate the high expectations that were put on physicians. Of course, the dean was aware that it is almost impossible to combine all these qualities in one and the same person. Nevertheless, his list aptly illustrates his view on what a medical education ideally should provide, at a time when he was urging for a thorough reform of the educational system at the end of the 1950s.

Bouckaert's characterisation of the ideal physician points to a continuous tension in medical education from the end of the eighteenth century onwards. Indeed, within the medieval and the early modern university, even the practically oriented field of medicine adopted a largely philosophical approach in line with the other disciplines – namely, not dealing directly with practical occupational skills and a study method consisting of the study of texts and empirical observation.[2] Medical degrees in the southern Netherlands – the region that became Belgium in 1830 – were primarily obtained at the University of Leuven, yet other types of medical education existed as well in a society built around corporations. This was especially the case for the professions of barber surgeons or midwives. Likewise, practical teaching in and close to hospitals remained a widespread practice.[3]

However, due to the obsession by the French revolutionaries with 'usefulness' (*utilité*), the focus in medical education briefly, yet radically, shifted towards vocational training. The Restoration of 1815 resulted in a partial return to practices of the *Ancien Régime*, but obviously the clock could not be turned back completely. Therefore, according to the 'Regulations on the Organisation of Higher Education in the Southern Provinces of the United Kingdom of the Netherlands', issued in 1816, the aim of the new medical faculties was to provide future physicians both with a broad general education and a profound practical training.[4]

During the second half of the nineteenth century, a third dimension was added: scientific schooling. Comprehensive medico-philosophical systems such as Brunonianism and Broussaisism, which explained the vital functions of their patients by indisputable physio-chemical processes in the humours and firm parts of the body, gradually gave way to treatment methods that were based on extensive medical research.[5] The treatment of symptoms and diseases by withdrawing excesses or bad humours from the body (through bloodletting and the use of laxatives and emetics) was increasingly replaced by the systematic detection of pathogens.[6] Moreover, students had to become familiar with this new approach through the introduction of practical courses in, for instance, microscopic pathological anatomy and in anatomy of the bronchial tubes. However, this modernisation process was clearly not welcomed by everyone. The scientification of medical education was not a straight-line development, but rather an evolutionary process with ups and downs. The increasingly dominant form of 'scientific' medical knowledge was sometimes highly contested as its opponents wished to return (at least partly) to the idea(l) of medicine as an art.

This chapter will focus on the shifts in the balance between general education, vocational training and scientific schooling at the medical schools and later the faculties of medicine in the southern Netherlands/Belgium from the end of the eighteenth century up until today. Bouckaert's opening quotation nicely illustrates how medical scientists also in his time were searching for a balance between these different dimensions. In their search for the perfect medical education, Belgian policymakers often took inspiration from German, French and English regulation, since their colleagues abroad were all struggling with the same issues. How, for instance, could the practical training at the bedside in increasingly specialised clinics be combined with the theoretical-scientific training offered in the laboratories? What kind of attitude did future physicians have to adopt in the discussion between, on the one hand, a specialised focus on the disease and its causes, and, on the other hand, the holistic approach of medicine, which paid attention to the individual patient with his or her entire medical and psychological background? And to what extent was there still room for 'medical uncertainty' within the 'objective' science of medicine? Generally speaking, the developments in medical education in Belgium largely resembled those in other European countries. And yet, specific choices and peculiar circumstances, both at the national and the local level, sometimes led to a unique outcome, as will become clear in this chapter.

Obviously, professors and university administrators played a major role in the discussions on medical education, but consistently they had to consider the preferences and interests of other parties concerned, such as the government, medical societies, professional associations and expert bodies like the Royal Academy of Medicine, which distinguished itself as a very active player from its foundation in 1841.[7] The opening quote is a good illustration of this situation. With regards to the nineteenth century, a literal transcription of most of these debates was included in the *Bulletin*, though during the twentieth century the continuous serial publications by the Academy also formed crucial primary sources for writing the history of medical education in Belgium, precisely because of the academy's highly influential role in educational matters. When it came to tackling the question of the training of specialists, for instance, it appears that the universities' manoeuvring strategy was rather limited due to the strong position of the academy in this case.

The rise of specialist education in medicine has received some specific historiographical attention,[8] but articles that focus on the transition from the nineteenth to the twentieth century are rather the exception to the rule with regard to the historiography on medical education in Belgium. First, apart from a few books that present a general overview of the issue and some typical jubilee publications, research that covers the entire last two hundred years is scarce. Second, the extensive list of studies discussing developments during the (long) nineteenth century is in great contrast to the extremely limited interest for the twentieth century. Among the most recent publications in the former category are undoubtedly our own doctoral dissertations, respectively on the history of the medical faculty of the Université libre de Bruxelles and on the debates around university education in Belgium (with a focus on the faculties of arts and medicine).[9] In 2019, Tinne Claes made an important contribution to the history of anatomical education with her extensive study on the history of anatomy in nineteenth-century Belgium.[10] Finally, two researchers wrote about the history of the medical faculty of the University of Leuven. Liesbet Nys's book retraces the history of the faculty since 1960, while Joris Vandendriessche's book focuses on the twentieth-century history of the academic hospital of the University of Leuven. The latter work gives a good insight in the organisation of practical education inside the hospitals.[11]

Learning to heal during the French occupation[12]

The transitional period around 1800 has been studied in detail.[13] On 1 October 1795, the French administration approved the annexation of the Belgian provinces and thereby extended all legal provisions and 'fundamental freedoms' to its territory. At that time, the University of Leuven was the only institution in the area that trained physicians. Its defiance of the republican command and its refusal of new political ideas led to its closure in October 1797. The training of surgeons offered during the *Ancien Régime* within the *collegia medica* subsequently disappeared a few years after the annexation due to the introduction of several new laws. The result was a period of wide-ranging freedom for the medical profession, although this came to an end in 1818 when the country was under the Dutch regime.[14]

Following the closure of the University of Leuven, the stage was set for several schools to open under private initiative in order to meet the demand for medical training in Brussels, Antwerp, Ghent,

Leuven and Bruges. These institutions were often modest, run from the physician's home and offering a rudimentary knowledge of medicine, surgery and obstetrics. Between 1804 and 1812, some (in Antwerp, Ghent, Brussels and Liège) were individually granted recognition by the French government. In these schools the body (sick or dead) became the centre of medical training, and it was essential to see, touch and transform it.[15]

These new concepts had started to circulate after the foundation by decree of *écoles de santé* ('health schools') in Paris, Strasbourg and Montpellier on 4 December 1794. The new way of learning embodied in these specialised schools was based on the acquisition of medical practice, and no longer mainly of philosophical-speculative medical knowledge.[16] The reorganisation was headed by Antoine Fourcroy, director of public instruction during the era of the French Consulate. His reform was based on a simple precept: 'read little, see and do much'.[17] This maxim illustrates the necessity to offer a vocational training that was useful to society. It stood in opposition to the purely theory-based teaching of the past, even though in practice the old ways often still dominated.

The officially recognised private medical schools in the provinces of the southern Netherlands were not granted permission to train physicians or surgeons but only 'medical officers', a military rank transferred to civil society by law in 1803. One could attend a practical medical school for three years or become an officer by assisting a private physician for six years, or for five years as a student in a civil or military hospital.[18] Even though they were considered second-class practitioners for a long time, these medical officers played an important role in bridging the gap between medicine and surgery because, for the first time, they were legally authorised to combine internal and external medicine. Medical officers formed the majority of the medical body up until the establishment of new universities in 1817 under the Dutch regime. Many physicians, surgeons and future professors practised medicine and surgery well before officially obtaining a university degree. Joseph Seutin, a powerful figure in the Belgian medical world during the first half of the nineteenth century, is a prime example of this practice.[19]

The fundamental change during the French occupation consisted of the institutionalisation of hospital-based schools, in line with the dominant practical orientation of (medical) education. Naturally, in-hospital training had existed before, but the full integration of schools into the hospital environment changed the way in which medical knowledge was taught. The first hospital-based schools were created in 1806 in Antwerp, Brussels and Ghent, developed from the previously existing private schools. In some cases, especially for those towns or cities without easy access to an *école de santé*, the hospital was the prime institution for the training of medical practitioners. The transformation of the hospital structure and the integration of teaching cemented the link between education and hospitals.

The hospital became the place where modern clinical observation techniques and the approaches used in anatomical pathology came together. The introduction of the new form of practical bedside teaching in the clinic as the base for medical training had an influence on the understanding and the treatment of healthy and diseased bodies, resulting in the very subtle and gradual transition from a focus on the diseased patient as a whole to a focus on the disease itself (see Chapter 7, p. 254). These conceptual changes took shape in the post-revolution years and quickly arrived in the provinces of modern-day Belgium. From the perspective of knowledge acquisition, however, the introduction of internships and externships (on-the-job training in the hospital) in 1808 was the biggest 'invention' in terms of medical education in the first half of the nineteenth century.[20]

Offering vocational training within a broad general education, 1815–76

Even though the Dutch administration copied the French system of internal and external students connected to the hospitals and increased the number of clinics, at the same time a much less practical approach once more returned to the medical faculties of the newly established state universities from 1817, in Ghent, Leuven and Liège. First, students in the clinics were no longer allowed to treat the patients themselves, but only to passively observe. Second, in most hospitals the number of patients was too small to offer enough variation of diseases (this was especially the case in the small city of Leuven, where it was a huge problem). And, third, in counter-reaction to the French practical orientation, the university system in general was characterised by a more scholarly-philosophical approach, inspired by some leading Prussian universities and realised through the appointment of many young professors from mainly smaller German-speaking institutions.

Yet, with regard to medical issues, most criticism was directed towards the reintroduction of the distinction between internal and external medicine in the law of 1818. The existing *écoles de médecine* remained open, but they acquired a new role. They now trained the future countryside *chirurgeons* by focusing on external medicine and the acquisition of practical knowledge. Only in cases of exceptional urgency were these *chirurgeons* authorised to treat internal diseases, but in principle internal medicine became an exclusive prerogative of the doctors of medicine educated at the universities. After obtaining a general degree in medicine, students could specialise in surgery, obstetrics or pharmacy, but they were never permitted to practise these different branches of medicine cumulatively. Also, when it came to the theoretical conception of medicine, the French approach was no longer continued, at least not everywhere. Whereas the medical school in Brussels and the faculty of medicine in Leuven still adored the ideas of the French physician François Broussais, it was quite the opposite in Ghent, where Jean-Charles van Rotterdam became one of his strongest opponents.

After Belgian independence and the complete reorganisation of the university system in 1835, the discussion concerning the division or unification of internal and external medicine continued. According to the law of 1835, students at the medical faculties still had to acquire a degree in medicine previous to their possible specialisation in surgery or obstetrics (pharmacy was thus no longer considered a university subject until its return at university level in the latter part of the 1840s). The hierarchisation underscored the predominance of (internal) medicine, but also hinted at a first step towards a future unification of degrees. Belgium was actually the first European state to create a common national university curriculum in 1849, culminating in the award of a single degree, the 'Doctorate of Medicine, Surgery and Obstetrics'. It was followed by Prussia in 1852, the Netherlands in 1865, and the United Kingdom in 1886. The formal unification of these programmes can be explained by the impact of the reforms introduced under the French and Dutch regimes, the innovative work of clinical study and the new role in medical training played by the hospitals.[21]

The doctoral degree in medicine consisted of a one-year preparatory degree in sciences, a one-year undergraduate degree in medicine and two years of study at the doctoral level, extended to three years from 1849. In addition to the preparatory degree in sciences, students had to pass a possible entrance examination and an additional literary test consisting of Greek, Latin, history of philosophy, logic, anthropology and moral philosophy, which was clearly a continuation of the broad general-philosophical education introduced by the Dutch government in 1816. However, in consequence of the continuous changes concerning the general entrance conditions, the preparatory education was gradually reduced to basic courses in chemistry, physics, botany, zoology and mineralogy (i.e. the curriculum of the preparatory degree in sciences, which barely changed between 1835 and 1876).

Similarly, the programme for the actual two-level medical degree also remained largely the same during this period. It consisted of classes in anatomy (and its various divisions), physiology, internal and external pathology, and also such related subjects as the theory of childbirth, hygiene and forensic medicine. In terms of the teaching of practical knowledge, the law of 1835 took a step backwards in comparison with the situation at the end of the Dutch period. The only obligatory attendance now was for anatomical demonstrations and for clinics in internal and external medicine and obstetrics. To sit the exams, one simply needed to present a certificate from the head of clinics which stipulated that the student had attended the clinics and acted diligently and successfully. However, this does not mean that clinical study was neglected by the universities, but the format of the given training changed into a more passive learning experience, despite the programme's general intention to offer a proper vocational training.

This curriculum was adopted by the state universities of Ghent and Liège, and largely copied by the free universities that had come into existence during the chaotic years between the independence of Belgium in 1830 and the introduction of a new law on higher education five years later. The establishment of the liberal Free University of Brussels and the Catholic University of Leuven (which replaced the state university in that city) presented the new Belgian government with a unique problem, which demanded a unique solution. How could universities under a different authority (the state, a group of freethinking liberals, or the church) and with a different curriculum grant the same degrees, especially when they had social implications, as was the case for degrees in law or medicine? The government did not have the right to inspect the free universities, but on the other hand, it did want to supervise professions, at least to some extent. After long-lasting debates, independent boards were created that would examine the students and grant the diplomas. Whereas the introduction of these boards enjoyed wide support, the composition of them and the question of who would appoint their members were heavily discussed in parliament between Catholics and liberals (see Chapter 2). The jury system was more than once overhauled and reconstituted, and became a constant stumbling block.

Nonetheless, by reserving the right to issue degrees and consequently control access to the profession, the state forced the otherwise free universities of Brussels and Leuven to conform to its logic and curricula. There were, however, some differences in the programmes and subjects on offer from one university to the other, due to the constitutional freedom of education. State recommendations were not always adhered to with regard to the subjects that were required. For example, the teaching of ophthalmology was speedily adopted by the state universities, while the free universities dragged their feet over whether to add it to the curriculum. In contrast, in 1855, professors in Leuven offered classes in mental illnesses, while at the same time, their colleagues in Brussels introduced a course on the 'illnesses of the elderly'. While the state controlled the granting of academic honours, the manoeuvring space for the free universities was limited.

The creation of an educational framework laid out by the state played a fundamental role in the definition of an orthodoxy of knowledge. This was determined through a debate among the different authorities concerned, namely the universities, the Royal Academy of Medicine, the provincial medical commissions, scientific societies and official medical journals issued by the state. Recent research by Vandendriessche has also emphasised the fundamental role played by the scientific societies as the most important space for sociability and for the regulation of science and scholarship.[22] The force of this orthodoxy became visible in controversies surrounding the teaching of disciplines that were considered minor (such as ophthalmology) or heterodox (such as homeopathy or animal magmatism). As a result, the alignment of doctrines became the cement between the medical profession and its social order. (The level and kind of) education thus undoubtedly occupied pride of place in the definition of a theoretical-professional order for the social group.[23]

From 1830 to 1870, medical orthodoxy was largely made up of general anatomy classes based on gross anatomy. Anatomical learning was both materialist and mechanical in nature, and was studied on a large scale, with scalpel, rather than with the aid of a microscope. Anatomy was heavily linked to physiology and pathology in this period and made the human body the focal point around which other branches revolved. The exam for the primary degree in medicine was heavily focused on anatomical branches such as general, descriptive and comparative anatomy and anatomical demonstrations and dissections.[24] Dissections became fundamental in the acquisition of anatomical knowledge. It contributed to the complete recognition of surgery, where teaching started to go beyond the skeleton, amputations and bleedings. Future surgeons were required to learn all the techniques and knowledge of what was known as 'modern' anatomy. In this context, anatomical specimens and cadavers were of educational importance for universities. The emphasis given to the collection of medical specimens was both the product of 'scientific prestige' and a competition between, and indeed within, universities. Each university sourced these 'raw materials' from their partner hospitals and the most interesting specimens were used as visual support in their theory classes (Figure 5.1). In this way, in the anatomical museum, theoretical and practical learning came together. Considered within the context of a history of medical learning, the first half of the nineteenth century is the era of anatomical museums and of the dissection amphitheatre, the latter becoming the place where a doctor in training could learn the basic gestures from his master or a fellow colleague.[25] The anatomical approach to medicine thus gradually transformed from being the core of 'scientific medicine' at the beginning of the nineteenth century, to being a typical characteristic of a rather practical orientation.

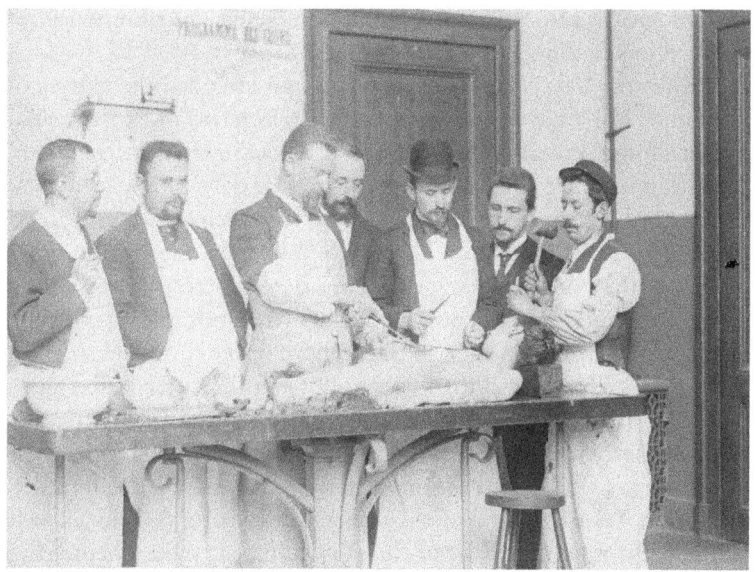

Figure 5.1 Anatomy lesson at St-Pierre Hospital, 1892.

Belgian universities, while having no problem with the teaching of practical anatomical knowledge, did struggle to combine it with scientific instruction. This was true across Belgian universities, where the majority of professors were also practitioners. Consequently, the university authorities were forced to recruit teachers from abroad, and especially from German-speaking areas, for courses in physiology and pathological anatomy in particular. German recruits included Karl Windischmann in Leuven, Vincent Fohmann and Antoine Frédéric Spring in Liège, Theodor Schwann who moved from Leuven to Liège and Gottlieb Gluge in Brussels. The influence of these German physicians, professors and researchers on the popularisation of pathological anatomy, as well as on new research in physiology, was immediately recognised by contemporaries. In his *Essay on the History of Contemporary Belgian Medicine* (1886), Léon Marcq, for instance, underscored their role from an educational point of view and their impact on the circulation of new knowledge in Belgium: 'The works of Fohmann on the lymphatic system, Schwann on cellular evolution, Spring on cardiac functions, ... Gluge on physiology, histology and particularly on pathological anatomy have spread and created an entire world of new understanding' (see Chapter 9, p. 321).[26]

Professors like Gluge and Schwann had attended the classes of Johannes Müller, the most notable figure in terms of experimental medicine in Germany in the first half of the nineteenth century.[27] The training that they received focused heavily on experimental laboratory research; thus realising the interconnection and interdependence of teaching and research.[28] In Belgium, on the other hand, at that time teaching was considered merely as the acquisition of practices and an entitlement to enter the profession. As a result, a course such as the 'Encyclopaedia and History of Medicine', which was introduced following the German example, never really took off, despite the support of a number of scientists such as Pierre van Meerbeeck. The course was intended to sensitise the students to the acquisition of a scientific and critical mindset. However, because many of them increasingly dropped out, it was subsequently abolished from the curriculum, first in Ghent, later in Liège and Leuven, and finally also in Brussels. The students, as was the recurring complaint, simply wished to obtain their diploma as soon as possible and did not have time for such 'useless' subjects. Repeatedly the debate on the utility of teaching history of medicine was taken up in the Belgian medical faculties. It was generally considered a way to combat a vision of medicine that was too positivist.[29]

So, up until the last quarter of the nineteenth century, most of the attempts of these German professors to introduce some kind of scientific schooling to the medical training remained largely in vain. The general ambition was rather to offer a vocational training within a broad general education. In order to realise the former part of this target, increasing emphasis was put on the clinics and on practical education in general. Clinical study became of critical importance in the relationship between the hospital and the university, and thus a permanent link was created between the towns (as the administrators of the hospitals) and their universities. The Free University of Brussels, enjoying a large number of patients in the hospitals of the capital, clearly was at the forefront in this regard, closely followed by Ghent University. Liège and particularly Leuven lagged behind due to the ongoing lack of patients. Nevertheless, in the early 1870s, in addition to the mandatory clinics, most of the universities had introduced clinics for mental illnesses, ophthalmology, syphilitic and cutaneous diseases and for the treatment of children and elderly people.

Practical, clinical education revolved around three complementary approaches. The first is intimately linked to the reorganisation of the hospital structure in the mid-nineteenth century and the launch of free consultations. This made a plethora of interesting cases available, giving the most advanced students the opportunity to make their first diagnoses. It should be noted though that the consultations were mostly done by 'privileged' students who had managed to obtain an intern- or externship in the hospital, rather than by 'normal' students. The second approach, which is part of collective memory, is that of crowds of twenty to thirty students charging through the wards together with the professor, making the diagnosis and discussing the treatment of six to eight patients within an hour. The third approach was located in the amphitheatre, away from the open clinical wards. In a private setting, particular cases were studied through physical examination, and a review of their medical history and applied treatments, by combining inputs from different medical disciplines. Ideally the three approaches were joined together to ensure an optimal result. The intensity and urgency of consultations called for rapid decision making, whereas the study of patients in bed allowed for wider considerations.[30] The role of the poor within this system should be highlighted. They were used as subjects for clinical teaching or, after their death, as cadavers for dissection.[31] Often, discussions arose between the hospital administration and the professors about the allocation of patients for clinical education, to such an extent that in 1874 the minister of public education intervened by deciding that all non-paying patients were allocated automatically to the university services.[32] However, as before, real practical experience could only be acquired by a selective group of internal and external students. Therefore, some professional medical associations made a plea for the introduction of obligatory apprenticeships for all medical students because 'medicine was based on observation and experience and was much more an art than a science', yet they could not stop the prevalent transition towards a more scientific (i.e. laboratory) approach of medical education.[33]

Searching for a new compromise between general education, vocational training and scientific schooling, 1876–1918

By the dawn of the 1860s, a physician's education was still widely seen as the acquisition of some practical knowledge and a professional right. And yet, a few professors from the universities of Ghent and Brussels began to develop another vision. Similar to their colleagues in Italy, the United Kingdom, Russia and the Netherlands, they turned their attention to German, particularly Prussian, universities. It was there that they found the spaces, the knowledge and the know-how that transformed their comprehension of sickness and medical practice. Concretely, the German influence was visible, for instance, in the introduction of the doctoral dissertation in medicine at the end of the 1850s, an evolution that signals a will to encourage medical students to participate in the production of knowledge. Very quickly, the debate focused on the issue of whether a more scientific approach had to be introduced through separate practical classes (in the laboratory) or rather within the existing theoretical lecture courses. For many professors in Liège, the transition was happening too fast and they therefore opted mainly for the second choice, largely because they feared an overload in the curriculum once new courses were added.

The first impulses for change clearly came from below, on the initiative of a handful of individuals, among whom were many of the German professors and a number of Belgian colleagues who had made a research trip to Germany. After completing their doctoral dissertation, they visited German and other European scientific institutes and attempted to introduce new technologies to their home universities, as well as the experience and knowledge that they had acquired during their trips. Gluge, for instance, became known for the introduction of the microscope at the University of Brussels because, as he put it himself, 'the microscope has become to the physician and the naturalist what the telescope is to the astronomer; one must learn to use it'.[34]

The 'German model'[35] of the scientific laboratory remained the ideal example for many of the professors at Belgian universities until the outbreak of the First World War. Gradually the laboratory developed into the perfect means to offer scientific schooling.

In order to realise this transition, a visit to German universities and/or research institutes became almost mandatory. It clearly demonstrates the link between centre and periphery in medical teaching. On the one hand, German universities embodied the archetypical scientific values pursued by Belgian institutions, but on the other hand, the system could only be implemented to a limited extent as it was subject to financial and national constraints; particularly the fact that the government only had an indirect impact on the curriculum at the free universities and that, concerning the state universities, huge differences of opinion between Catholics and liberals had to be overcome within parliament. The result was a typical Belgian compromise in 1876 consisting of a new law, which only introduced some elements of a scholarly training in science and medicine, such as an obligatory course in microscopic pathological anatomy.[36]

The importance of this change in the curriculum cannot be denied. However, just as its introduction had been the result of tough discussions and was certainly not welcomed by everyone, the implementation of the law of 1876 was not straightforward during the following decades. Its principal driving force was the development of laboratory science, but, first, academic expansion was not limited to the construction of laboratories and, second, the availability of laboratories was largely dependent on financial resources, which differed hugely from one university to the other. Jean Joseph Crocq, a professor at the medical faculty in Brussels, was one of the main proponents of a purely practical form of medical education. In his view, the German universities were anything but the model to copy because there, future physicians were offered a far too theoretical, specialised and unworldly scholarly training, as he explained during a debate at the Royal Academy of Medicine in the middle of the 1870s. Belgian students were already overwhelmed with theoretical courses, while the time spent in clinics with the patients was too limited to ensure a solid practical training.

In addition to cordial concerns about the necessity of an excellent vocational training for future physicians, Crocq's plea was at least partly inspired by the consideration that the university in Brussels was not able to carry the burden of the financial implications of organising proper scientific schooling. In consequence, he revealed himself as one of the major proponents of a division of education and research into two separate institutions. The choice to assign the vocational training to the university and the scientific schooling to a separate Institut central des hautes études was thus based on profound arguments as regards content, as well as on purely materialistic motivations. Because the funds to establish specialised laboratories and institutes were largely lacking, Crocq and some of his colleagues preferred to focus on the traditional strength of medical education in Brussels, namely the large number of hospitals and patients available for practical teaching. Instead of organising practical scientific exercises, they tried as much as possible to give a scholarly interpretation to the clinics.

Among differing reasons, the need also for a stronger philosophical embedding of the studies was once again increasing, resulting in more attention being paid to the general education of students. At the beginning of the 1870s, some professors repeated the plea for the introduction of a course on the history of medicine. In Germany, its importance to stimulate a scholarly attitude among the students had already been recognised for a long time, as was the case in Paris where a chair within this discipline had recently been founded. However, for most of the students the connection between history of medicine and the scientific study of this discipline was still too indirect. Nevertheless, Richard Boddaert, professor of surgery in Ghent, who was clearly one of the forerunners in a more scientific interpretation of medical education, defended the (re) introduction of some philosophical courses in the curriculum of natural sciences and medicine. His views were mainly determined by scientific concerns, and not so much by attempts to secure the general education of the students. According to Boddaert, just as in the famous medical school of Salerno in southern Italy, a course in logic and philosophy should be provided in order to enable the students to gain some insights into the human soul and to treat nervous and mental illnesses from a more theoretical background. The German *philosophische Fakultät*, in which human and natural sciences were combined, also functioned as one of his examples in this regard.

The rector in Leuven, Alexandre Namèche, supported the ideas of Boddaert, but primarily on moral grounds: 'If the study of natural sciences does not rest on the cultivation of human sciences, it easily leads to absolutism and materialism', he explained.[37] A colleague of Namèche, in his turn, justified the attention to human sciences in the education of physicians by appealing to 'an "exterior" reason: the conservation of their social rank'.[38] Anyhow the result was the same. The law of 1876 introduced obligatory courses in logic, moral philosophy and psychology in the preparatory degree in sciences. On its own initiative, the University of Leuven added obligatory courses in religion and general philosophy for those students who aimed for a legal degree; and anthropology, history of philosophy, Greek and Latin for the very small number of students who strived for a so-called scientific diploma.

The same law introduced obligatory practical scientific exercises, yet even though Namèche acknowledged the usefulness of these exercises, at the same time he warned against exaggerating their importance in the educational programme as a whole. It was his clear opinion that scientific interests should not exceed professional interests. A prerequisite for the well-being of the country and of society was, according to Namèche, that medical studies should not focus on the training of scholastics, but of smart practitioners who were educated in all aspects of the conscientious and complicated art of medicine. In a later speech of 1880, Namèche deliberately referred to the rectorial address of the by then deceased Antoine Frédéric Spring, who had been known for his tendency towards reform. Approximately a decade before, this famous pathologist of Liège had also argued in favour of paying more attention to the literary and moral education of future physicians. However, despite all of these attempts, by around 1880 vocational training was still at the forefront within the medical faculties, to the detriment of scientific schooling and, more particularly, of a general education.

In order to realise a more scientific interpretation of medical training, a significant extension of the curriculum was absolutely necessary. A large number of professors, along with a remarkable group of recently graduated doctors, offered optional subjects on their own initiative, often dealing with a very specific field of research. Furthermore, students should be offered the opportunity to specialise in subdisciplines such as ophthalmology or legal medicine.[39] Such a kind of specialisation, however, could only happen after having obtained the general doctoral medical degree.

Indeed, the struggle for the introduction of a common degree in medicine, surgery and obstetrics, which had taken place over many years, should not be in vain. It was the general opinion that because of the close connections between the different branches of medicine, all future physicians should receive a profound basic training in all three disciplines. Only afterwards could they then choose to focus on the treatment of a particular disease or a number of (more complicated) diseases. (On the access of women to medical education in Belgium, see Chapter 1, p. 37.)

And even then, the professional associations of physicians, which increasingly intervened in debates during the last quarter of the nineteenth century, pointed frequently to the danger of students losing their way in the case of a too early or a too extensive specialisation. In their opinion, specialisation was perhaps desirable from a scientific point of view, but certainly not from a professional angle. Along the same line of thought, they also warned of the danger of attaching too much importance to the scientific, practical exercises. These should not jeopardise the excellent vocational training as it existed up to that day. Possibly, obligatory internships should be included in the curriculum in order to secure practical training. The main concern of the associations of physicians in this period, however, was the assumed oversaturation of the market. The medical unions even accused the government of raising the number of physicians intentionally in order to weaken their competitive power and thus to undermine their material and social position.[40]

The realisation of all of these proposals, be it the introduction of philosophical courses to ensure the general education of the students, of practical scientific exercises or specialised subjects with a view on their scientific schooling, or of a more practical orientation to guarantee their vocational training, required more staff, more classrooms and more money, according to the physicians and professors Guillaume Rommelaere, Louis Deroubaix and Paul Heger in Brussels. Even though there were some important differences between the four universities with regard to the introduction of practical exercises, and even though each university emphasised different branches of specialisation, the diverging development of the medical faculties happened primarily in consequence of the huge differences concerning the availability of staff, classrooms, buildings and, crucially, money. The free universities suffered directly from the financial impact of the freedom of education and the lack of subsidies, this being the price to pay for the absence of government supervision. Nonetheless, according to the Brussels professors, it was of the utmost importance that they adopt the German model to some extent and avoid lagging behind in the scientification of medical education.

What could be seen, however, was the implementation of a system of common values between two entities. The peripheral position of Belgium in medical teaching in general can be observed from Abraham Flexner's 1925 report titled *Medical Education: A Comparative Study*.[41] At the European level, Belgian universities were slow to set up scientific institutions. In the early 1890s there were two sides from a university perspective. On the one hand, the state universities enjoyed a comfortable position in this regard. Between 1879 and 1893, the state earmarked almost ten million Belgian francs for the foundation of laboratories and institutes in Liège and Ghent. This funding enabled the creation of institutes of biology in Liège and Ghent and, more notably, an institute of physiology in Liège, headed by Léon Frédéricq.[42] On the other hand, there were privately founded institutes such as the Montefiore Institute in Liège (1883) and the Errera Institute (1892) and Solvay Institute (1895) in Brussels. The University of Leuven also jumped on the partnership with the industrial sector bandwagon, establishing its own medical and applied science laboratories. In 1890, for instance, the Jean-Baptiste Carnoy Institute was founded in this vein. The result was a shift away from theory-based training with little practice, towards a system based around practical classes, in-ward teaching and laboratory work. The educational paradigm shift also resulted in more autonomy given to the students, who were encouraged to reflect on case studies. So gradually a new generation came to the fore, being skilled in the use of the microscope and trained in laboratory studies. It also led to a wider appreciation of an independent 'scientific spirit'.[43] Obviously, the laboratory system did not limit itself to medicine, but was introduced elsewhere too.[44] The laboratory became an instrument of state building that went beyond questions of health and education and thus developed into a new political instrument (Figure 5.2).[45]

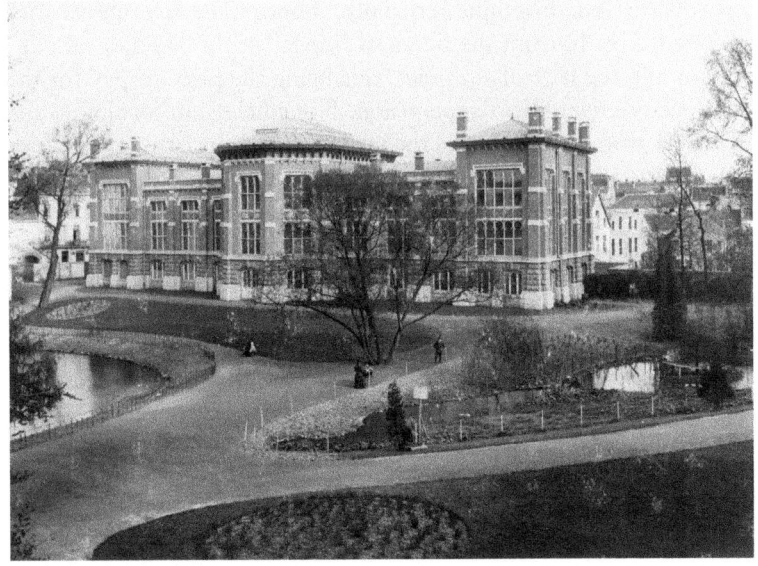

Figure 5.2 The Anatomical Institute of Brussels University, 1895.

Pure science during the interwar period

This trend, which typified the interwar period, began at the end of the nineteenth century when universities gained access to new ways to legally open their own laboratories. This was made possible in 1911, when they were granted the status of legal personality, enabling them to enter into contracts, own property, etc.[46] The First World War did not put an end to the importance of research in education. Wars in general lead to a rise in medical practices and research, and the First World War was no exception to this rule. During the war, research was done in several fields such as surgery and blood transfusion as well as in the design of prosthetics (on the post-war treatment of injured soldiers, see Chapter 8, p. 298). In Belgium, research essentially took place at the Ambulance de l'Océan in La Panne, which was founded by Antoine Depage. The institution's primary goal was to treat wounded soldiers close to the battlefield, but it additionally became a place for the procurement and circulation of knowledge during wartime and was conceived as a place of learning for students who were finishing up their education.

Ways of knowing medicine

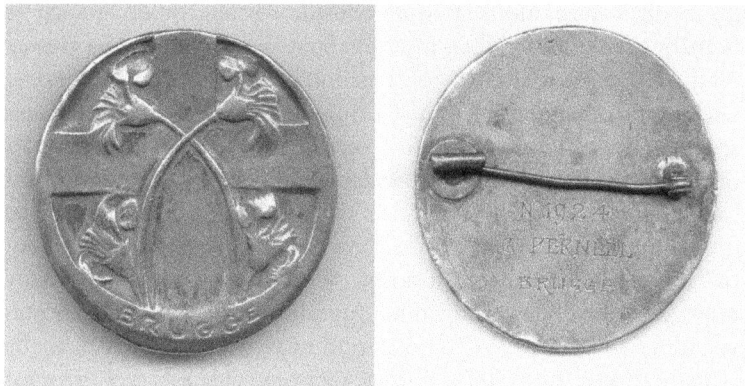

Figure 5.3 Pin of G[odelieve] Perneel, one of the nurses who graduated from the Catholic St Elizabeth School in Bruges, 1924.

The new hospital fitted Depage's idea of a modern hospital. The building, which contained several clinics, research laboratories and teaching and conference rooms, was managed by physicians and trained nurses.[47] The gradual replacement of nuns in hospitals by professionally trained nurses at the beginning of the twentieth century was an important factor in the competition between the secular and Catholic milieus (Figure 5.3; see also Chapter 2, p. 69). This change led to a revolution in the hospital sector: gradually the hospital itself was seen as a learning place both for physicians and nurses.[48] In the same way, the interwar period also marks a transition from hygienist policies to a global approach based on the education of public health in order to improve national health. Following a eugenic vision, the state, physicians, scientific societies and non-profit organisations worked together to promote medical educational policies and spread their knowledge on sickness and health to Belgian children and the working classes. The Red Cross, for instance, played a major role in this educational effort by publishing papers, leaflets and posters, organising conferences and even offering training courses for paramedics.[49]

At the end of the First World War, the Royal Academy of Medicine again took up its preponderant role in the debates around medical training. As mentioned previously, in its early decades the academy actively intervened, for instance, in the discussion on medical specialties that were considered 'unorthodox', such as homeopathy.[50] Its activities after the First World War can be viewed within the context of the reconstruction of Belgium and the funding allocated to the country by the Commission for Relief in Belgium specifically for higher education. Consequently, the medical academy distinguished itself again as a fundamental player in the reorganisation of teaching by the state. For the universities, this offered the unique opportunity to continue their efforts to introduce the scientific approach in medical education. With the influence of Germany now gone, the door was open for American, British and Dutch universities to be heard.[51] Over a period of two years, debates at the academy were led by Jules Bordet, recipient of the Nobel Prize for Medicine in 1919 and chief director of the Brussels Pasteur Institute. The central question was to determine the place given to pure science in medical teaching.[52] Yet one should not assume that clinical and laboratory medicine were in competition. The success of the former paved the way for the introduction of the latter, as a supplementary asset, while a student's deepening of practical understanding in turn improved the circulation of concrete knowledge.[53]

For Bordet and a number of fellow physicians, the future of medical education was in the hands of 'full-time' academics who were focusing on teaching and research instead of aiming for practical knowledge. This view was not immediately embraced by the majority. Some strong personalities were required to impose this idea on the medical landscape, among them Bordet himself, along with Joseph Denys, Pierre Nolf, Albert Brachet and Ernest Malvoz.[54] Thanks to their laboratories, Belgium was able to position itself among the elite of the European scientific nations, even though it still remained a secondary centre. Nevertheless, Bordet's Pasteur Institute became particularly attractive to foreign students despite the material poverty of Belgian laboratories in general, as described by some American students in their study reports.[55] This new vision on medical training remained marginal when compared to the dominant opinion that focused on the completion of mandatory theoretical learning by clinics, along with a number of optional courses for specialisation.

Around the same time, however, the various medical specialisations took on a more dominant position in the medical field and inevitably influenced medical training as well.[56] These specialisations questioned a unitary view of medicine. They prevailed in hospitals as well as at the universities, and at the same time specialist physicians created their own federations to hasten their official recognition inside the medical community. Both specialist societies and journals were created, their role being the legitimisation of the specific specialist discipline. Located at the crossroads between marketing and scientific strategy, these societies were the cornerstone for the defence and development of medical specialties.[57] Nevertheless, it was not yet possible to create separate, specialist study programmes, as the unitary perception of medicine and the weight of the general practitioners still prevailed in the debates. This led to years of long, yet ultimately unfruitful discussions, caused in part by friction with the Fédération Médicale Belge. The legal recognition and regulation of medical specialisations was eventually ordered by royal decree on 12 September 1957. Before this date, anyone could call himself a specialist.[58]

A cautious countermovement, hampered by neo-liberal developments

An increasing number of different specialist courses was continuously added to the programme, but without abandoning the unitary degree. Even though students were generally encouraged to specialise, this could only happen after having obtained the degree of doctor in medicine, surgery and obstetrics. This, according to a growing group of dissenting voices from the middle of the 1950s, resulted in an overloaded curriculum and an excessively long period of study. The training of surgeons, for instance, lasted for thirteen years: seven years for the general medical degree, followed by six years of specialisation. Might it not be possible to shorten the general programme specifically for those students who wanted to specialise afterwards, which was the case for almost 50 per cent among them? Moreover, the ever-progressing specialisation had also led to a focus on memorisation and the loss of an integrative or holistic approach, a challenge with which colleagues abroad were struggling as well. On the occasion of an international symposium on medical education at the Royal Academy of Medicine, William Hobson (education and training officer at the World Health Organization) complained that 'there is general dissatisfaction in many quarters with the present medical curriculum. It is felt that too much factual detail is being taught, particularly in such fields as anatomy and biochemistry, and that the training does not fit the future doctor for his role in society ... There is a strong need for more integration of the teaching of different subjects.'[59]

In this regard, the first attempts at change in Belgium already dated from shortly after the Second World War. In 1948, an internist at the University of Leuven, Jozuë Vandenbroucke, published a study about medical education (awarded by the Royal Academy), in which he argued for the shortening and simplification of basic medical education. In his view, two years of undergraduate study, followed by three years for graduation and a one-year internship had to be enough.[60] However, for more concrete proposals one had to wait for at least another decade. Many of these proposals were suggested on the common initiative of the French-speaking and Dutch-speaking sections of the Royal Academy. The academy had already split in 1938, and at the end of the 1960s the universities of Brussels and Leuven were also divided in two separate institutions. Despite this division along linguistic lines, the national curriculum in medicine was largely preserved, but more detailed research about possible local differences in the medical programme is missing.

During the long-lasting debate at the academy, the dean of the medical faculty in Ghent expressed the opinion of many of his colleagues: that medical knowledge had become so diverse and so extensive during previous decades that the educational programme could and should no longer strive for exhaustivity. It was also during this discussion that Bouckaert presented his views on the ideal physician, referred to at the beginning of this chapter. Most important was to sharpen the critical mind of the student, for instance by adding an obligatory course in philosophy. According to the final report of the mixed commission: 'Without neglecting the aspect of information that is necessary for the practitioner, the training should focus mainly on fundamental ideas of educational value.' Furthermore, 'future practitioners should no longer learn only "how" to act, but also understand the "why" of their actions. They can no longer limit themselves to applying standard procedures, "recipes" so to say, when coming into contact with different situations.' Or, as the German physician Hans

Schulten explained: students had to be taught to make a distinction between what they know and what they believe.[61] Through integrative lessons in which different specialists presented their own view on the same subject, a more holistic approach of medicine was promoted once again.

A large part of the reform proposals aimed for a revaluation of the profession of general practitioner, which had lost a degree of popularity due to the ongoing pressure to specialise. As faculty dean, Vandenbroucke not only scheduled the year of internship one year earlier (so that the last year of training could function as a kind of pre-specialisation), but he also allowed students to take their internship at a local family doctor's surgery instead of exclusively at the hospital, in order to experience a normal doctor's practice. Concerning the hospitals, an increasing number of regional hospital centres were integrated into the educational system.[62] Associate professors in family medicine were finally appointed, which happened exceptionally early in an international perspective. When Leuven took the lead in 1968, only Edinburgh and Utrecht had preceded it. Antwerp followed in 1972, Ghent in 1980 and Brussels in 1987, as the last Dutch-speaking university in this regard.[63]

In several European countries, a similar cautious countermovement against the dominant scientific and specialist approach in medicine could be seen. The new medical faculty in Maastricht, for instance, experimented in the middle of the 1970s with a model of so-called problem-oriented education with 'self-activity', 'permanent evaluation' and 'attitude-development' as its key words. The transfer of knowledge stood no longer at the centre, but actively acquiring it.[64] In Finland, the orientation to society was strengthened in the same period by introducing more social and preventive medicine and work with patients outside of hospitals. Practical, clinical studies were given a higher priority, whereas theoretical parts of the curriculum were reduced. Medical students strongly promoted these developments all along the way.[65]

In Belgium also, the majority of students supported the changes, but at the same time many of them were quite disappointed that often the reform proposals remained dead letters. Student societies had, for a long time, called for a shift in attention within the medical curriculum to the social role of the physician and the psycho-social dimension of medicine, but somatic medicine nevertheless clearly remained at the centre. Despite the pioneering work of the University of Leuven in comparison to the other Belgian universities in reducing the heavy theoretical elements of the programme, the ever-growing number of students largely prevented a more personal approach. Also, the ongoing discussion within the European Economic Community about the mutual recognition of diplomas at the end of the 1980s delayed some of the actual changes.[66] It clearly shows how the local, national and international level were closely connected to each other.

Another reason why many suggestions to shift the focus away from the theoretical, scientific part of the programme were never realised, was the succession of major breakthroughs in medical science during this period; breakthroughs that the students needed to be aware of, according to their professors. On the one hand, the still ongoing specialisation was 'solved' to some extent by moving specific disciplines to separate medical faculties of, for instance, pharmaceutical sciences or movement and rehabilitation sciences. Yet, on the other hand, in order to become good practitioners, students had to be at the same time excellent researchers, not only familiar with recent findings in virology (e.g. human immunodeficiency virus (HIV)), genetics (e.g. the human genome project) or oncology, but also be able to critically access the increasingly complicated kind of research practices in these fields.

This last skill is essential within the concept of evidence-based learning, which became popular from the 1980s. However, it proved to be almost impossible in the Belgian context to replace the tradition of so-called authority-based learning. Professors themselves complained about the lack of a proper research attitude among the students, but did not manage sufficiently to encourage them to assess or develop new knowledge critically.[67] The ambition of a psycho-social and more holistic approach was replaced by continuing specialisation and discipline formation, processes that could not be countered by existing attempts of interdisciplinarity, which moreover too often only had a rhetorical character. In order to be able to develop critical thinking (being included in the idea that future physicians should not only be trained, but also be educated), a certain degree of interdisciplinarity was needed, particularly the ability to escape from prevailing theories in one's own discipline. To what extent were future physicians still made aware of the uncertainty of medicine, which itself raises doubts about the infallibility of evidence-based medicine?[68] Medical students sometimes had the impression that they were taught to consider their textbooks the 'medical bible'.[69]

The neo-liberal policies from the last quarter of the twentieth century changed the way knowledge is produced, exchanged and taught. The new market economy, new ways to fund research, the development of new technologies, sciences and organisational politics have profoundly modified the way we produce and acquire knowledge. A good example of this trend is the recently gained strategical importance of research and development departments within the health industries. These departments are in direct competition with the university laboratories for both fundamental and applied research. However, the pharmaceutical industries and the Belgian universities quickly developed durable links that are visible in the production and financing of research at the universities. A significant part of fundamental research is thus 'subcontracted' to university laboratories for directed research.

Besides doing fundamental research, university hospitals are present at other levels in the production of new products and knowledge. A good example of this practice is the collaboration between hospitals, laboratories and physicians in the field of clinical research. Here, the doctors and universities play a primordial role in approving products or practices that come forth out of a knowledge-based economy. This shift in research conditions was accompanied by a rise in the number of people who produce knowledge and invent new practices. Chemists, biologists, statisticians and computer scientists have joined the doctors in the field of research, as 'experts' of all kinds have gained a central role in the process. Applied research thus takes more and more space in the production of medical knowledge, both inside and outside the universities.[70] As the academic and industrial fields have grown closer since the Second World War and the era of neo-liberalism, so too has the production of knowledge taken on a more 'businesslike' approach. Researchers not only publish and protect their results and discoveries, but they also develop distribution and commercial strategies in close relation with the health industries, an approach that is characteristic of the first decades of the twenty-first century.[71]

The specificity of medical education in Belgium

However, one should be careful when making broad statements about medical education in Belgium during this period as research assessing these recent developments is largely missing. In fact, this applies almost to the twentieth century as a whole. Indeed, publications focusing on a particular institution during a specific (often short) period of time do exist, but they enable us to have a view on changes in medical education only to a limited extent. Particularly, possible variations between different universities or between Dutch- and French-speaking Belgium remain somewhat underexposed. In consequence, we can only hint at the tension between the local, regional, national and European level, yet unfortunately we are not able to develop this interesting and promising approach extensively. Nevertheless, it has become clear how the attitude towards medicine as an art or a science in medical education has been continuously reciprocating, in relationship with changing political, social and cultural circumstances.

On the one hand, medical education in general followed a similar line of development in Belgium as in most other European countries, yet on the other hand, many specific circumstances also created a unique situation. Most important in this regard was, first, the early introduction and the exceptionally long preservation of the unified degree of doctor in medicine, surgery and obstetrics. Second, the competition between state and private universities often resulted in small differences in the curriculum, yet sometimes the policy of the latter was decided not so much by choice, but rather out of necessity due to their long-lasting difficult financial position. Finally, the traditional conflict between Catholics and liberals led to specific conditions, such as the somewhat more holistic approach at the Catholic University of Leuven (also shown by its pioneering role in the countermovement of the 1960s and 1970s). Classroom history and other methods and concepts from the discipline of the history of education could be helpful in expanding this kind of more detailed research further.[72]

Notes

1 J.-J. Bouckaert, 'Geneeskundige opleiding', *Verhandelingen van de Koninklijke Academie voor Geneeskunde van België*, 20 (1958), 11–12.
2 R. Walter, 'Themes', in *A History of the University in Europe. Volume I: Universities in the Middle Ages*, ed. H. de Ridder-Symoens (Cambridge, UK: University Press, 1992), 25–30.
3 C. Bruneel and P. Servais (eds), *La formation du médecin: des lumières au laboratoire. Actes du colloque du 9 décembre 1988* (Louvain-la-Neuve: UCL, 1989), 5–43.
4 P. Dhondt, *Un double compromis. Enjeux et débats relatifs à l'enseignement universitaire en Belgique au XIXe siècle* (Ghent: Academia Press, 2011), 65–8.
5 E. Lacroix, 'Negentiende eeuw: van speculatieve naar wetenschappelijke geneeskunde', in *Wetenschappelijke ontwikkeling van de geneeskunde in de negentiende eeuw. Bijdrage van enkele Belgische artsen* (Brussels: Académie royale de Médecine de Belgique, 2002), 9–33.
6 K. Velle, *De nieuwe biechtvaders. De sociale geschiedenis van de arts in België* (Leuven: Kritak, 1991), 87. A selection of literature is available on the transformation towards a fundamentally different view on disease in which the symptoms are no longer the centre of attention, but rather the causes. Some examples include: C. Huerkamp, *Der Aufstieg der Ärzte im 19. Jahrhundert. Vom gelehrten Stand zum professionellen Experten: Das Beispiel Preussens* (Göttingen: Vandenhoeck & Ruprecht, 1985); W. F. Bynum, *Science and the Practice of Medicine in the Nineteenth Century* (Cambridge: Cambridge University Press, 1994); and C. Bonah, *Instruire, guérir, servir. Formation et pratique médicales en France et en Allemagne pendant la deuxième moitié du XIXe siècle* (Strasbourg: Presses universitaires, 2000).
7 G. Willems, 'De maatschappelijke rol van de Academie Royal de Médecine de Belgique (1841–1914)' (unpublished master's diss., KU Leuven, 2003).
8 R. Schepers, 'Om de eenheid van het medisch beroep. Het debat over de specialisatie in België (1900–1940)', *Gewina*, 16:3 (1993), 155–70; and I. Meul and R. Schepers, 'De opkomst en consolidering van medische specialisten in België (1857–1957)', *Belgisch Tijdschrift Voor Nieuwste Geschiedenis*, 43:2 (2013), 10–45.
9 R. Bardez, 'La Faculté de Médecine de l'Université Libre de Bruxelles: Entre Création, Circulation et Enseignement ses Savoirs (1795–1914)' (PhD diss., Université libre de Bruxelles, 2015); and Dhondt, *Un double compromis*. See their bibliographies for key works on the topics of research in this field.

10 T. Claes, *Corpses in Belgian Anatomy, 1860–1914: Nobody's Dead* (New York: Palgrave Macmillan, 2019).
11 L. Nys, *Van mensen en muizen. Vijftig jaar Nederlandstalige faculteit geneeskunde aan de Leuvense universiteit* (Leuven: Leuven University Press, 2016); and J. Vandendriessche, *Zorg en wetenschap. Een geschiedenis van de Leuvense academische ziekenhuizen in de twintigste eeuw* (Leuven: Leuven University Press, 2019).
12 This and the following two sections of this chapter are largely based on Bardez, 'La Faculté de Médecine de l'Université Libre de Bruxelles' and Dhondt, *Un double compromis* – specific references to original sources and additional literature can be found there.
13 See, for instance, P. Dhondt, 'La situation précaire de l'enseignement supérieur dans les départements belges entre 1797 et 1815', *Revue belge de philologie et d'histoire*, 82:4 (2004), 935–67, and the large number of references included in the article.
14 J. Vandendriessche, *Medical Societies and Scientific Culture in Nineteenth-Century Belgium* (Manchester: Manchester University Press, 2018), 15–28; R. Schepers, *Artsen in Gebreke. Zelfregulering door het medisch beroep* (Leuven: Lannoo Campus, 2008), 121–6.
15 E. T. Hurren, *Dying for Victorian Medicine: English Anatomy and Its Trade in the Dead Poor, 1834–1929* (New York: Palgrave Macmillan, 2012), 303–11.
16 R. Schepers, 'Towards unity and autonomy: the Belgian medical profession in the nineteenth century', *Medical History*, 38 (1994), 237–54; J. Vandendriessche, 'Wetenschapsbeoefening en belangenbehartiging: naar een nieuwe geschiedschrijving van negentiende-eeuwse medische genootschappen in de Lage Landen', *Studium. Revue d'Histoire des Sciences et des Universités*, 7:1 (2014), 36–49.
17 L. Brockliss and R. Rogers, 'L'enseignement médical et la Révolution. Essai de réévaluation', *Histoire de l'éducation*, 42 (1989), 84.
18 C. Dickstein-Bernard, 'Panorama de l'enseignement supérieur en Belgique au XIXe siècle (1795–1876)', in Bruneel and Servais, *La formation du médecin*, 63.
19 M. Crosland, 'The *officiers de santé* of the French Revolution: a case study in the changing language of medicine', *Medical History*, 48 (2004), 229–32; R. Heller, '*Officiers de santé*: the second-class doctors of nineteenth-century France', *Medical History*, 22 (1978), 27–9; E. Ackerknecht, *Medicine at the Paris Hospital, 1794–1848* (Baltimore, MD: Johns Hopkins Press, 1967), 56.
20 T. N. Bonner, *Becoming a Physician: Medical Education in Britain, France, Germany, and the United States, 1750–1945* (New York: Oxford

University Press, 1997), 105; J. V. Pickstone, *The Ways of Knowing: A New History of Science, Technology and Medicine* (Manchester: Manchester University Press, 2001), 18.

21 W. F. Bynum and R. Porter (eds), *Companion Encyclopedia of the History of Medicine* (London: Routledge, 1993), 1151.

22 Vandendriessche, *Medical Societies and Scientific Culture*; J. Vandendriessche, 'Anatomy and sociability in nineteenth-century Belgium', in *Bodies Beyond Borders: Moving Anatomies, 1750–1950*, ed. K. Wils, A. Sokhieng and R. De Bont (Leuven: University Press, 2017), 51–72.

23 P. Bourdieu, *Homo Academicus* (Paris: Les éditions de Minuit, 1984), 87; N. Gevitz, 'Unorthodox medical theories', in Bynum and Porter, *Companion Encyclopedia of the History of Medicine*, 603; W. F. Bynum, *Medical Fringe and Medical Orthodoxy, 1750–1850* (London: Croom Helm, 1987).

24 W. F. Bynum (ed.), *The Western Medical Tradition: 1800 to 2000* (New York: Cambridge University Press, 2006), 155; A. Dalcq, 'L'enseignement et les recherches des anatomistes belges de 1830 à 1930', *Le Scalpel* (June 1931), 7.

25 M. Sappol, *A Traffic of Dead Bodies: Anatomy and Embodied Social Identity in Nineteenth Century America* (Princeton, NJ: University Press, 2002), 51; J. Reinarz, 'The age of museum medicine: the rise and fall of the medical museum at Birmingham's School of Medicine', *Social History of Medicine*, 18 (2005), 437; Claes, *Corpses in Belgian Anatomy*, 161–84.

26 L. Marcq, *Essai sur l'histoire de la médecine belge contemporaine* (Brussels: Académie royale de médecine de Belgique, 1866), 134.

27 D. Knight, *The Making of Modern Science: Science, Technology, Medicine and Modernity: 1789–1914* (Cambridge, UK: Cambridge University Press, 2009), 123–4.

28 R. Anderson, *European Universities from the Enlightenment to 1914* (London: Oxford University Press, 2004), 51–6.

29 Vandendriessche, *Medical Societies and Scientific Culture*, 217–23.

30 L. Deroubaix, 'Clinique chirurgicale de l'Hôpital Saint-Jean. Observations et leçons cliniques recueillies par M. Lebrun, aide de clinique, depuis le 1er octobre 1877 jusqu'au 1er juillet 1879', *Annales de l'Université de Bruxelles. Faculté de médecine*, 1 (1880), 1–3; A. Uytterhoeven, *Notice sur l'Hôpital Saint-Jean de Bruxelles, ou étude sur la meilleure manière de construire et d'organiser un hôpital de malades* (Brussels: Tircher, 1852), 74–5.

31 A. Cunningham, O. P. Grell and R. Jütte (eds), *Health Care and Poor Relief in 18th- and 19th-Century Northern Europe* (London: Ashgate, 2012); R. Fuchs, *Gender and Poverty in Nineteenth-Century Europe* (Cambridge, UK: Cambridge University Press, 2005).
32 L. Elaut, *Een epos. Het Gentse akademisch ziekenhuis* (Kapellen: De Nederlandsche Boekhandel, 1977), 23–7.
33 *Rapport sur quelques questions relatives à l'enseignement supérieur adopté par le cercle médical liégeois en Assemblée générale du 29 novembre 1872* (Liège: Denoel, 1872), 4, 7–8.
34 G. Gluge, 'Séance solennelle de réouverture des cours de l'Université de Bruxelles. Discours de M. Gluge, pro-recteur pour l'année 1870–1871', *La Presse médicale belge*, 22:45 (1870), 360.
35 G. Vanpaemel, 'The German model of laboratory science and the European periphery (1860–1914)', in *Sciences in the Universities of Europe, Nineteenth and Twentieth Centuries, Academic Landscapes*, ed. A. Simoes, M. P. Diogo and K. Gavroglu (Dordrecht: Springer, 2015), 216–17.
36 Vanpaemel, 'The German model of laboratory science', 211–15.
37 A. Namèche, 'Discours prononcé le 6 octobre 1875, jour de l'ouverture des cours académiques', *Annuaire de l'Université catholique de Louvain*, 40 (1876), 411.
38 G. Verriest, 'Sixième congrès international de médecine à Amsterdam, 1879. Conférence de M. le prof. Virchow sur l'éducation médicale', *Journal des sciences médicales de Louvain*, 4 (1879), 535.
39 The best introduction to the increasing specialisation in medical education is G. Weisz, *Divide and Conquer: A Comparative History of Medical Specialization* (Oxford: Oxford University Press, 2006).
40 J. de Maeyer, L. Dhaene, G. Hertecant and K. Velle (eds), *Er is leven voor de dood. Tweehonderd jaar gezondheidszorg in Vlaanderen* (Kapellen: Pelckmans 1998), 173–4. Especially the supposedly too easy recognition of diplomas obtained abroad, was heavily criticised.
41 A. Flexner, *Medical Education: A Comparative Study* (New York: Macmillan, 1925).
42 G. Vanpaemel, M. Derez, and J. Tollebeek (eds), *Album van een wetenschappelijke wereld. De Leuvense universiteit omstreeks 1900* (Leuven: Lipsius Leuven, 2012), 35; P. Héger, *Réponse à Mr. Léon Frédéricq* (Brussels: Hayez, 1891), 2–3; L. Frédéricq, *Paul Héger et les Instituts Universitaires de Gand et Liège* (Liège: Vaillant-Carmanne, 1891); A. Firket, 'Les nouveaux éléments de l'éducation médicale en Allemagne', *Bulletin de l'Académie royale de médecine* (1907), 283–35.
43 Bonner, *Becoming a Physician*, 221.

44 L. Diser, *Wetenschap op de proef. Laboratoria in het Belgisch overheidsbeleid, 1870–1940* (Leuven: Universitaire Pers, 2016), 439.
45 Vanpaemel, 'The German model of laboratory science', 218; R. Fox and A. Guagnini, *Laboratories, Workshops and Sites: Concepts and Practices of Research in Industrial Europe, 1800–1914* (Berkeley: University of California, 1999), 191; S. Dierig, 'Engines for experiment: laboratory revolution and industrial labor in the nineteenth-century city', *Osiris*, 18 (2003), 118–19.
46 E. Lamberts and J. Roegiers, *De universiteit te Leuven, 1425–1985* (Leuven: Universitaire Pers, 1986), 212–13.
47 A. Depage, *Pages écrites à la Panne en 1917* (Brussels: Bothy, 1918).
48 P. Dhondt, 'Social education or medical care? Divergent views on visiting nurses in Belgium in the interwar years', *History of Education and Children's Literature*, 7:1 (2012), 505–22; C. Jacques, 'Les infirmières dans l'entre-deux-guerres et l'action des dames d'oeuvres', *Sextant*, 3 (1994), 107–26; Vandendriessche, *Zorg en wetenschap*, 71–95.
49 S. G. Solomon, L. Murard and P. Zylberman (eds), *Shifting Boundaries of Public Health: Europe in the Twentieth Century* (New York: Rochester Press, 2008), 63–86.
50 A. H. Baal, *In Search of a Cure: The Patients of the Ghent Homeopathic Physician Gustave A. van den Berghe (1837–1902)* (Rotterdam: Erasmus, 2008); K. Velle, 'De homeopathie in België in de 19de eeuw', *Geschiedenis der Geneeskunde*, 2 (1994), 18–27.
51 E. Malvoz, 'Le doctorat en médecine: diplôme scientifique et diplôme professionnel', *Bulletin de l'Académie royale de médecine* (1920), 1353–7.
52 'Discussion sur la réforme des études médicales', *Bulletin de l'Académie royale de médecine* (1920), 396–418, 826–34, 872–7, 890–7; (1921), 40–59, 116–35, 160–82, 217–27, 261–80, 399–413, 469–91, 526–49; (1922), 53–71, 105–19, 415–23, 445–67; (1923), 43–62, 89–108, 137–63, 207–26.
53 R. Sternberg and J. Horvath, *Tacit Knowledge in Professional Practice: Researcher and Practitioner Perspectives* (London: Lawrence Erlbaum Associates, 1999), 75–6; A. Cunningham and P. Williams, *The Laboratory Revolution in Medicine* (New York: Cambridge University Press, 1992), 5–7.
54 Rockefeller Archive Center, RFA, 1.1., 707.1: Report of Dr R. M. Pearce about Medical Education in Belgium 1920–1926. Thanks to Kenneth Bertrams for sharing this information.
55 Archives of the Belgian American Educational Foundation, Box 5.1: Final and Preliminary Reports of American Fellows in Belgium, 1920–1924, Report of Miss C. Bernice Rhodes, 12 December 1923.

56 Meul and Schepers, 'De opkomst en consolidering van medische specialisten in België', 10–45; Vandendriessche, *Zorg and wetenschap*, 47–70.
57 Vandendriessche, *Medical Societies and Scientific Culture*, 250–78.
58 Meul and Schepers, 'De opkomst en consolidering van medische specialisten in België', 42–3.
59 'Bespreking', *Verhandelingen van de Koninklijke Academie voor Geneeskunde van België*, 21 (1959), 185.
60 Nys, *Van mensen en muizen*, 36–7; Vandendriessche, *Zorg en wetenschap*, 127–50.
61 'Verslag van de Gemeenschappelijke Commissie belast met de studie van het vraagstuk omtrent de hervorming der geneeskundige studiën', *Jaarboek en verslagen. Koninklijke Academie voor Geneeskunde van België* (1963), 184–5; Bouckaert, 'Geneeskundige opleiding', 9.
62 J. Vandendriessche and L. Nys, 'Expansion through separation: the linguistic conflicts at the University of Leuven in the 1960s from a medical history perspective', *BMGN: Low Countries Historical Review*, 132:1 (2017), 38–61, at 46.
63 Nys, *Van mensen en muizen*, 39; J. C. van Es, *Een halve eeuw huisartsgeneeskunde. Van ambacht naar professie* (Houten: Bohn Stafleu van Loghum, 2007); L. François and J. de Maeseneer (eds), *Omzien naar de toekomst. Huisartsgeneeskunde op de drempel van de 21e eeuw* (Ghent: RUG, 2000).
64 P. J. Knegtmans, *De Medische Faculteit Maastricht. En nieuwe universiteit in een herstructureringsgebied, 1969–1984* (Assen: Koninklijke van Gorcum, 1992).
65 S. Aalto, *Medisiinarit, ammattiin kasvaminen ja hiljainen tieto. Suomalaisen lääkärikoulutuksen murroksen vuodet 1933–1969* (Helsinki: University Press, 2016), 10.
66 Nys, *Van mensen en muizen*, 84, 129.
67 Ibid., 209.
68 T. C. Bolt, *A Doctor's Order: The Dutch Case of Evidence-Based Medicine (1970–2015)* (Apeldoorn: Maklu, 2015).
69 P. Dhondt and N. Vansieleghem, 'The idea of a university: a universal institution in a globalised world', *History of Education and Children's Literature*, 9:1 (2014), 193.
70 'Université et recherche', *Les Dossiers du Crisp*, 27 (1987), 1–27; A. Vincent, 'L'industrie pharmaceutique en Belgique', *Courrier hebdomadaire du CRISP*, 12:598–9 (1973), 1–48.
71 A. M. Brett, D. V. Powers, M. F. Betz and C. Alsanian, *Higher Education in Partnership with Industry: Opportunities and Strategies*

for *Training, Research, and Economic Development* (San Francisco, CA: Jossey-Bass, 1988); S. Muller (ed.), *Universities in the Twenty-First Century* (Providence: Berghahn Books, 1996).

72 P. Dhondt, 'University history as part of the history of education', in *University Jubilees and University History Writing: A Challenging Relationship*, ed. P. Dhondt (Leiden: Brill, 2015), 233–49.

Selected bibliography

Bardez, R., 'La Faculté de médecine de l'Université Libre de Bruxelles: entre création, circulation et enseignement des savoirs (1795–1914)' (Unpublished PhD diss., Brussels Free University, 2015).

Dhondt, P., 'Social education or medical care? Divergent views on visiting nurses in Belgium in the interwar years', *History of Education and Children's Literature*, 7:1 (2012), 505–22.

Dhondt, P., *Un double compromis. Enjeux et débats relatifs à l'enseignement universitaire en Belgique au XIXe siècle* (Ghent: Academia Press, 2011).

Meul, I. and Schepers, R., 'De opkomst en consolidering van medische specialisten in België (1857–1957)', *Belgisch Tijdschrift voor Nieuwste Geschiedenis*, 43:2 (2013), 10–45.

Nys, L., *Van mensen en muizen. Vijftig jaar Nederlandstalige Faculteit Geneeskunde aan de Leuvense universiteit* (Leuven: Universitaire Pers Leuven, 2016).

Vandendriessche, J., *Zorg en wetenschap. Een geschiedenis van de Leuvense academische ziekenhuizen in de twintigste eeuw* (Leuven: Universitaire Pers Leuven, 2019).

Vandendriessche, J. and Nys, L., 'Expansion through separation: the linguistic conflicts at the University of Leuven in the 1960s from a medical history perspective', *BMGN: Low Countries Historical Review*, 132:1 (2017), 38–61.

6

Medicine, money and mutual aid

Dirk Luyten and David Guilardian

In 2015, average out-of-pocket patient payments would amount to some 18 per cent of healthcare expenditures, almost 80 per cent being paid for by the national compulsory health insurance scheme, while revenues from voluntary insurances fund less than 5 per cent of the total amount.[1] Two hundred years ago, a patient would have to pay the total bill by themselves or turn to local public welfare. In the last two centuries, the financing of healthcare obviously went through major changes. This chapter will highlight the shift of both healthcare and hospital financing, from local welfare to state intervention through the creation of private schemes and institutions, especially mutual aid societies.

Economic and financial issues in medical history have not received as much attention in Belgium as compared to the Netherlands, Great Britain or France.[2] And most of the time they have been touched upon indirectly. In the 1990s sociopolitical literature on the history of social security, for instance, the financial aspects of medicine in Belgium have been analysed at macro level, but always in the context of a larger political and social history. Publications on the history of the mutual aid sector are another place to look for indirect examinations of the Belgian healthcare economy. The history of public healthcare institutions constitutes a third field of research that has allowed historians to peek at the financial realities of medicine in the past.

The economy of the private healthcare sector and the study of social groups financing medical care through their own means remain a blind spot in current research. And although the development of private health insurance companies has been less significant in Belgium than in a neighbouring country such as the Netherlands, the specificities of the Belgian private health insurance sector are still to be studied in detail.³ Drawing from the existing historiography, this chapter will thus mainly explore the public or semi-public spheres of healthcare.⁴

Healthcare and hospitals before 1795

If we divide the population roughly between the wealthy, the poor and the middle class, there are three different possibilities as to healthcare consumption. To the higher classes, private home care was the norm. The wealthiest paid in full the remedies of their pharmacist, the visits of their physician or the rare operations that the surgeon would perform in their living room. For the poor, public and private welfare would intervene, especially in cities where the local authorities paid for a doctor and surgeon whose task was to care for the poor, and where a hospital would offer them nursing care.⁵ As for the craftsmen and workers who were neither rich nor poor, membership to a craft guild or a brotherhood often offered the benefit of some form of mutual assistance. The most thriving among these organisations set up 'sick funds' or even built their own almshouses to spare their members the humiliation of having to resort to charity in time of sickness.⁶ An alternative would be to turn to home care congregations such as the Black Sisters or Alexians.⁷

Institutional healthcare, provided by hospitals, was limited to nursing care provided essentially by religious congregations, with very little physician involvement. Financially, they relied almost entirely on the income of their estate and gifts from wealthy patrons.⁸ All who could afford it avoided these establishments for they bore the mark of poverty and death. Local public authorities in main cities only intervened when they feared for public health and security; they, for instance, funded the construction of '*pesthuyskens*' (plague houses) or institutions for the mentally ill.⁹ What percentage of the population would turn to a doctor in the *Ancien Régime*? Considering most people in the countryside would resort mainly to religious or superstitious relief (e.g. quacks), a doctor would only be called for by the bedside when death already approached. In cities, doctors were more frequently consulted. In Brussels, extrapolations on the basis of a series of practitioner records around 1780 would indicate that some 16 per cent of the population would ask for a doctor.[10]

The French reorganisation and the dual society (1794–1850)

The French *Régime* would fundamentally change the financing of healthcare by introducing two new ideas. The first idea contended that the well-being of citizens could no longer be left to the goodwill of philanthropists and charitable organisations but needed to be a major concern to the nation as a whole. The French Revolutionary Constitution of 1793 asserted: 'Public relief is a sacred debt. Society owes subsistence to its less fortunate citizens.'[11] Although the French *Assemblée* quickly realised that free universal healthcare was financially unviable, it ordered the nationalisation of all private care institutions, foundations and almshouses (*décret du 23 messidor II*).[12] Institutional healthcare would be automatically public, and directed by a newly created local board called civil hospitals (*hospices civils*). At the same time, poor relief and healthcare were entrusted to the new local welfare bureaus (*bureaux de bienfaisance*), who appointed the 'poor doctors' (Figure 6.1). Placed under the control of local authorities, welfare did not rest directly on the purse of the central state; only the care of certain categories of destitute people (blind people, profoundly deaf people, or prostitutes arrested by the police, for instance) remained state-financed.[13] The reform did cause welfare institutions to lose parts of their traditional incomes (tithes, feudal rights, annuities from guilds, etc.).[14] In Leuven, the annual income of the city hospital and hospices dropped by 38 per cent (from almost 120,000 F before the French annexation to less than 75,000 F in 1800), a deficit that municipalities would have to compensate.[15]

The second idea had to do with the new role of the revolutionary state: it was believed that the state should be the main recourse of its citizens in time of need and that private intermediary organisations should be done away with. Craft guilds, brotherhoods and their mutual aid systems were abolished. Those who could not afford the

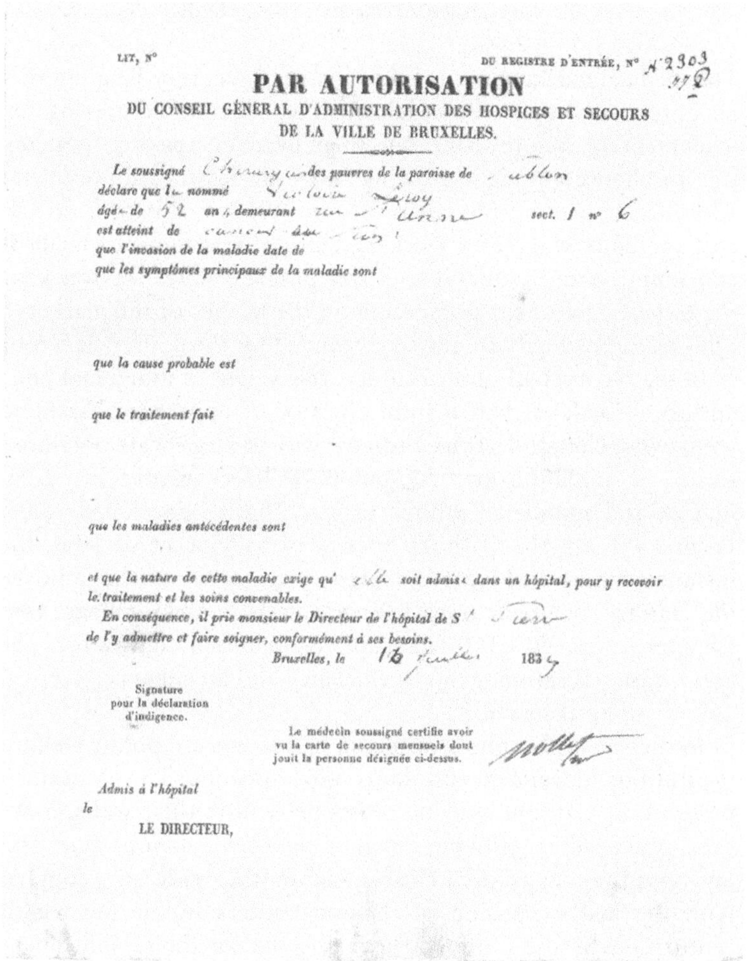

LIT, N° DU REGISTRE D'ENTRÉE, N°

PAR AUTORISATION

DU CONSEIL GÉNÉRAL D'ADMINISTRATION DES HOSPICES ET SECOURS
DE LA VILLE DE BRUXELLES.

Le soussigné *des pauvres de la paroisse de*
déclare que l *nommé*
âgé de 52 *an, demeurant* *sect.* 1 *n°* 6
est atteint de
que l'invasion de la maladie date de
que les symptômes principaux de la maladie sont

que la cause probable est

que le traitement fait

que les maladies antécédentes sont

et que la nature de cette maladie exige qu' *soit admis dans un hôpital, pour y recevoir le traitement et les soins convenables.*

En conséquence, il prie monsieur le Directeur de l'hôpital de S
de l'y admettre et faire soigner, conformément à ses besoins.

Bruxelles, le 183

Signature
pour la déclaration
d'indigence.

Le médecin soussigné certifie avoir
vu la carte de secours mensuels dont
jouit la personne désignée ci-dessus.

Admis à l'hôpital
le

LE DIRECTEUR,

Figure 6.1 Poor doctor's certificate, issued for the director of St-Pierre Hospital in Brussels, indispensable for admission, 1837.

cost of private care would now have to turn automatically to public welfare, which acquired some kind of monopoly. The 'French system' would be maintained but challenged, especially after 1850, both by the return of Catholic charities, and by the need for new mutual aid societies.

Private charity returns (1850–1900)

The medical marketplace in mid-nineteenth-century Belgium was an unregulated space in which qualified doctors competing for 'clients' were free to determine their fees and (paying) patients free to choose among a growing range of healthcare providers. Although expensive physician fees (in 1850 a visit to a doctor cost the daily wage of a worker), cultural resistance to medical consumption and availability of free public medical services kept the largest part of the population on the fringes of the market,[16] options for medical care slowly expanded for the poorer class too.

In the second half of the century, the weight of individual philanthropy, such as that of local elites or of upper-class Catholic women's societies, decreased to give way to large-scale organised forms of philanthropy. As public welfare institutions grew in size and number, Catholic private charity developed too.[17] From 1841 on, the Catholic Society of St Vincent de Paul, for instance, established local 'conferences' in many parishes all over the country and built outpatient hospitals in small villages (see Chapter 2, pp. 70–1).[18] This shift to organised charity brought about rationalisation, gains in efficiency and an enhanced control over the poor it served.[19]

In theory, all hospitals were and had to remain public welfare institutions dependent on local governments. The continued presence of Catholic nursing personnel within their walls, however, often led to growing tensions between religious staff and lay boards of directors. This is one of the reasons – coupled with the fast expansion of religious orders in the nineteenth century – why the Catholics kept pushing for the establishment and financing of their own private institutions. New private hospital foundations with independent boards had, in fact, been authorised under French ruling (*Arrêtés* from the years X, XII and 1806), provided that they were placed under the supervision of public welfare.[20] Unlike the situation in France, religious charity in Belgium was allowed to keep a crucial place in the national landscape of healthcare. It would also take part in the mutual aid system.

Workers' health insurance: social control and a first step towards collective responsibility, 1850–94

In the first half of the nineteenth century, most workers lived at a subsistence level. After 1850, a modest rise in salary rates allowed the better paid among them to start saving modestly. Most then elected to invest in small-scale initiatives of the labour movement such as mutual societies or cooperatives.[21] Mutual societies grew out of the principles of reciprocity and resource pooling. They allowed workers with too low an income to mutualise limited savings to no longer rely on public assistance in time of sickness.[22] Outside of the paternalistic, charitable, partisan sphere of liberal and Catholic organisations, some mutual societies had been set up by workers themselves with a different set of rules and aspirations. Workers belonging to one specific occupational group, especially craftsmen, would pool a fraction of their income together to cover the risk of sickness of their peers, thus somehow picking up the thread that had been cut by the French reorganisation.[23]

In the mid nineteenth century, most mutual aid societies only paid their members a daily sickness allowance when illness, old age or an accident prevented them from working. They also partially compensated the cost of the funerals of deceased members. Considering the limited efficacy of orthodox therapeutics at the time, the rarity of practitioners in the countryside and the high cost of medical treatment, monetising was, in working-class culture, often more oriented towards the dead than the living. Proper funerals, with the social and religious obligations they entailed,[24] were prioritised over the receiving of standard medical care.[25]

Despite mutual aid alleviating some of the pressure put on Welfare funds, the 1851 law on mutual societies ratified by a wary Liberal government in the wake of the social protest of 1848, hints at the authorities' distrust and prudent ways of dealing with these new types of organisations. For the latter, legal recognition and fiscal advantages came at the price of direct control by the municipality and sanctions in case of non-compliance with the law.[26] While philanthropic (liberal or Catholic) mutual funds, or societies set up by employers and factory owners, were tolerated, the authorities did not hesitate to enforce the 1791 coalition ban against organisations of factory workers, arguing that they sometimes functioned as secret trade unions. The mid-nineteenth-century textile sector in Ghent counted 12 factory-based mutual societies, with a total membership of 2,200.[27] In 1886, mutual aid funds in Belgium served 65,000 affiliated members (of a national population of about 6 million in 1890); this was less than in 1850 (70,000 members for a total population of 4.3 million in 1846). For the government, the moralisation of workers needed to be the primary goal of these organisations; prizes were awarded to those, particularly of bourgeois origination, most successful in educating the poorer classes.[28]

Moralisation was central to the mission of Catholic mutual societies created in the 1850s and 1860s too, just as was the preservation of the Catholic faith in the face of the secularisation policies adopted by a succession of Liberal governments. Organised at parish level and often embedded in charity structures, Catholic mutual societies were managed and partly funded by members of the elite, or so-called honorary members who contributed high membership fees without being entitled to any benefits. Both liberal and Catholic developments in the field of mutual aid sought to prevent the emergence of socialism and workers' organisations.[29]

But the social unrest of the late nineteenth century forced new issues into the conversation. Spurred by a severe economic recession in the industrial regions of Wallonia, the violent strikes of 1886 brought the appalling working and living conditions of Belgian workers to national attention. As a political response to the strike, the Parliamentary Inquiry Commission tasked with investigating this state of affairs advocated in favour of mutual aid funds as tools of social pacification. Even further, it encouraged class cooperation and worker involvement in the management of these organisations.

The issue of mutual aid came at the forefront of public attention again in 1895 during the debates on the reform of public assistance. Socialists from the newly founded Labour Party (the Parti Ouvrier Belge, or Belgische Werkliedenpartij) favoured a system of compulsory social insurances as an alternative to public assistance. They were of the opinion that obligation should stem from solidarity: such a system would entail the redistribution of the national income and contribute to the advancement of society as a whole rather than providing insurance solutions for isolated individuals.[30] The Catholics had already raised the idea of a compulsory health insurance during their annual Catholic Congresses in the late 1880s, but only for low-paid industrial workers and financed by the industry itself.[31] At that time, concern of the governing class for the moralisation of working-class citizens and for their learning of simple principles of financial caution trumped technical issues of funding and sparse medical considerations. In addition, a curtailing of the free market still seemed an undesirable prospect for most.[32] For the first time, however, the idea of a nationwide system of shared responsibility for healthcare costs had been put forth.

Subsidised liberty (1894–1944)

All in all, the last quarter of the nineteenth century was a period of growth in healthcare thinking and strategising. Economic crises and social unrest demanded that the state face up to the situation of the working class and spurred a national public reflection on the issue of healthcare for all. As a growing number of people and political organisations looked to forms of organised solidarity to remedy the costly plague of ill health, the state sought to unburden the load of public assistance by acting as a distant unifying force in a sector still mostly livened up by Catholic initiatives. At the same time, the growing influence of the socialist movement forced most political families to adopt one or other aspect of the socialist agenda, lest they lose a portion of their constituency. This set off a century-long search for more democratic and universal solutions to the problem of healthcare financing.

In public debates about the health of the Belgian population, the focus moved away from moral concerns towards the cost of care in and of itself: the possible ways to calculate it, to contain it, to share or allocate it. New techno-financial tools and arguments were introduced into healthcare planning and mutual aid thinking. All the while, the idea of a national system of compulsory insurance kept resurfacing time and again, but political and ideological discords prevented it from materialising into more than words.

With the new 1894 law on mutual aid societies, direct control and threats of sanction gave way to a new regime of 'subsidised liberty'. The central state preferred to restrict its role to the subsidising from afar of independent organisations. From 1898 on, mutual societies with an official accreditation could qualify to receive state subventions. Municipal control abated. This new system, in combination with the rise of workers' living standards and renewed efforts – particularly from the Catholics – to set up more organisations, led to an increase in mutual aid membership. In 1890, Belgian state-accredited mutual funds counted 54,347 members. In 1900, this figure reached 185,201.[33]

In the two last decades of the nineteenth century, habits of medical consumption changed due to the democratisation of the medical market,[34] the development of antiseptic surgery and the increase of purchasing power. Mutual aid offers transformed as workers became more willing to invest part of their income in medical services that they could not afford or were not interested in before. In the late 1880s in the province of Namur, mutual societies started to trade the system of daily sickness allowance for a system of reimbursement of medical expenses.[35] A series of factors – state subsidies, centralising and rationalising incentives, industrial accident risk coverage transferred to private insurance companies (1903) and disability insurance passed on to the more generously state-funded federations of mutual organisations – enabled local mutual aid funds throughout the country to propose an expanding range of options, starting with a basic 'medical-pharmaceutical' coverage (reimbursement of doctor fees and pharmacist bills). Some promoted preventive healthcare or offered additional coverage for specialised treatments like surgical operations.[36]

Inevitably, the growing involvement of mutual societies in medical care led to conflicts with a fast-organising medical profession still bent on defending a patient's free choice of practitioner and a physician's right to freely set his fees. To contain the cost of medical care, mutual societies offered physicians contracts with fixed fees to take up the care of all their members.[37] Medical practitioners resented this type of agreement. Some accepted, however, to ask less for the treatment of workers but not for that of the craftsmen who made up a large part of mutual aid membership. In their dealings with pharmacists, mutual societies used as leverage the threat of opening their own 'people's pharmacies'.[38] In 1912 in Antwerp, disgruntled physicians organised a strike against the (liberal) society

Help Uzelve (Help yourself). The latter offered free basic, and later specialised, medical care to a growing membership, steadily eroding the independent practitioners' share of the medical market.[39]

But the better organised the medical profession became, the greater weight it was able to hold in its negotiations with mutual aid funds. The firmer demands of physicians constituted a new unpredictable variable in the system of healthcare financing. By comparison, the costs of daily sickness allowance paid to a society's members were easy to control: the fee lowered the longer the sickness lasted, always had a time limit (often six months) and decreased on a sliding scale the older a member got. Often membership was denied to applicants over forty-five or fifty years old.[40] But since payment for medical care had a more open-ended character, mutual aid organisations had to establish new strategies of cost limitation. To solidify their position, Brussels mutual societies organised in 1863 into a federation; the pooling of local mutual aid resources and cooperation between contracted physicians helped pushing the development of healthcare provision further.[41] In Ghent, the local mutual aid society took on the payment of sickness allowances, while the coverage for medical care was organised at the federation level and funded by a separate contribution from members.[42] The most radical solution to skyrocketing and unpredictable costs consisted simply in no longer offering members the 'medical-pharmaceutical' coverage and to increase the amount of the daily sickness allowance instead, which could then be used to pay a doctor. An alternative was to put an upper limit – per year and per member – to the coverage of medical expenses, which would then allow mutual funds to extrapolate their maximal budgets for each year.[43] In the countryside, physicians and mutual aid societies often opted for an alternate subscription system: the organisation paid a fixed fee per member to a number of local physicians between whom healthcare-seeking members were free to choose. This was an interesting solution that provided practitioners with a stable income in areas with low medical demand.[44]

The development of mutual funds must also be studied in the political context of what is termed today the 'pillarisation' of Belgian society; a process of fragmentation and reorganisation of the country's social life around the three main dominant political families competing for national dominance. Most organisations and institutions belonged to one of the three political 'pillars' – whether socialist, Catholic or liberal – and each of these pillars controlled a large part of the social and cultural infrastructures of the country. Because it privileged organisations over the state, pillarisation impeded direct state intervention and state institution-building. Unsurprisingly, it agreed with the idea of subsidiarity, the cornerstone of Catholic social ideology and of the social policy of the Catholic governments in office between 1884 and 1914. The expansion of mutual aid societies was one of the numerous expressions of this pillarisation process, a process that would deeply inform the shape of care provision and preventive medicine in the twentieth century. While Catholic congregations and organisations used this situation to expand their institutional and medical reach,[45] socialist mutual societies started building small surgical facilities – they were not able yet to support the building of a comprehensive infrastructure – to offer healthcare to workers potentially interested or already invested in socialism and challenge the Catholic dominance in this field.[46]

Although the system of subsidised liberty improved health coverage at the turn of the twentieth century, it left three population groups vulnerable. First, in rural regions, mutual societies predominantly organised the wage earners and had difficulties attracting the self-employed, particularly farmers. Similarly, rural elites, unlike their urban counterparts, were little inclined to support the development of mutual aid. Local authorities, too, felt no urgency to bolster mutual funds because they did not have to cope like cities had with fluctuating poverty resulting from the business cycle. The usually lenient positions adopted by public assistance institutions towards the needy in sparsely populated rural communities further tempered the perceived need for such solidarity mechanisms.[47] In the rural province of Namur, the farmers' lack of interest in mutual aid was attributable to the influence of local priests who favoured traditional charity too, and did nothing to stimulate the foundation of Catholic mutual funds.[48]

The second underrepresented group among mutual aid members were women and children. As a general rule, mutual societies only covered (male) breadwinners. Insuring every member of a family was far too expensive and women were considered to be at higher risks than men. In 1900, women made up only 5.5 per cent of the total number of members in mutual societies.[49] The creation of women and children's, or so-called familial, mutual societies provided a first solution to this problem.[50]

Low-paid workers constituted the third group, among which mutual society membership was rare, a group whose situation the proponents of a compulsory system of health insurance particularly wanted to see improve.[51]

The political debate about the possibility of implementing such a compulsory system provided various occasions to discuss the financial coverage mechanisms of medical care for the lower social classes. The 1912 project of the Catholic government, inspired by the British system (Lloyd George), defended the continuation of subsidised liberty. In that system, workers who could not pay or were refused membership to a mutual aid fund were to be insured, with lower benefits, via state mutual funds organised at regional level. Those outside the labour market would remain dependent on public assistance.[52] Liberals and socialists criticised the Catholic scheme by using new arguments based on financial methods such as risk assessment: these 'regional councils', they asserted, could not be financially viable since their members combined a high-risk profile with limited financial means to pay their contribution. According to them, this type of risk should be covered by repartition, and thus solidarity.

The 1913 project of socialist politician Camille Huysmans hints at a growing consciousness of the cost of care as well; it contended that a compulsory sickness insurance scheme could be financed simultaneously by employers, their employees and the state. But employers, resisting the idea of state intervention and of their own responsibility towards their workers, opposed actuarial risk principles to that socialist notion of solidarity: young wage earners should not contribute the same amount as their older counterparts, since they were less likely to get sick; the risk of illness was purely personal and premiums should be calculated on an individual basis, using mortality and sickness tables. Additionally, the cost of ill health should be borne by the workers alone.[53]

The First World War brought a new awareness of the vulnerability of the population and of the need to preserve the productive forces of the country. Belgium had always relied on international imports for a significant portion of its food needs. Suddenly plunged into deep economic disarray and weakened by trade embargoes, the country under German rule faced massive unemployment rates, a general impoverishment of the population and a risk of famine on an unprecedented scale. Many people could no longer afford medicine or the visit of a physician. In September 1914, to prevent the worst, several members of the Belgian economic elites founded, with the support of the exiled Belgian government, the National Relief and Food Committee, a 'parallel social state' that gathered and distributed national and international aid within the country. The committee coordinated social policies in cooperation with organised labour. In addition to food, it provided free medical care to the unemployed and redistributed funds to mutual aid societies, but this time on the condition that they offered coverage not only to individual male breadwinners, but also to every member of their family, for the lives of women and children needed protection too. The committee organised care for babies and children, and supplied meals to expectant mothers. Preventive care (against tuberculosis among others), too, became central to the committee's efforts and continued well after the war.[54]

After 1918, despite the achievements of the innovative National Relief and Food Committee, the Belgian government resumed its policy of subsidised liberty. Catholic opposition to state intervention in an area that had historically been the prerogative of religious organisations was partly responsible for the status quo. Catholic pushbacks also ensured that the creation of a standalone Ministry of Health would not come to be until after the Second World War.[55] State financial support to mutual aid organisations increased after 1918, however, and became a permanent feature of interwar governmental policies. The National Committee's efforts towards the coverage of the working-class and families were carried on by the various coalition governments that followed the end of the war (and often included the Socialist Party). The largest part of this support went to the financing of medical-pharmaceutical services.[56] Specialised structures for women within mutual aid organisations took over the role of independent women's mutual societies.[57] Large sums were invested in tuberculosis prevention. Other categories of preventive care had to do with pregnant women, babies and children: open-air holiday camps, for instance, were offered as part of tuberculosis preventive efforts. Since the receipt of subsidies was subject to compliance to certain conditions, the system of state subsidies led to more uniform practices in healthcare provision.[58] The financing of mutual aid and the development of healthcare infrastructures also resumed at province and local level, primarily through subsidies or cooperation with private actors.[59]

More and more people gained access to health coverage, which became relatively less expensive. In 1934 a visit to a general practitioner costed 8 BF, while an unskilled worker in the building industry in Brussels earned 4,10 BF per hour.[60] In 1926, 75 per cent of the rural *Kempen* population already enjoyed membership to a local mutual aid fund.[61] In the 1920s, generous state subsidies initiated by the socialist minister of labour Joseph Wauters, as well as a slow reorganisation and centralisation of mutual aid, allowed for the pooling of resources at regional level.[62] This process contributed to the general expansion of the medical offer,[63] including to the construction of brick-and-mortar facilities, to the multiplication of prevention initiatives and of specialised services.

The introduction of universal male suffrage in 1919 and the country's post-war swing to the left positively impacted the development of the socialist flank of the mutual aid sector. To keep abreast of the growing specialisation of medical care, socialist mutual organisations built their own polyclinics, offering specialised care and the benefit of up-to-date technological equipment to the working class at a fixed affordable fee.[64] Socialists also built clinics, such as the People's Clinic in Ghent, one of the strongholds of socialist organised labour. In that specific clinic, cost control was achieved by applying the principles of division of labour: each patient was examined by a general practitioner before being sent to a specialist and each patient had a personal file. Maintaining a healthy financial balance, however, proved to be difficult; the price of medical care had to be raised and patients were expected to pay an entrance fee in addition to the cost of their treatment.[65] In the 1920s, as a countermove to the flourishing of socialist structures, industrial employers created at company level a parallel network of mutual aid organisations that similarly contributed to the general expansion of health coverage: in 1931, however, about a million workers still remained uninsured.[66]

As for the Catholic labour movement, it first lagged behind but soon caught up, broadening and diversifying its medical infrastructure, building clinics and sanatoria like their political rivals. In this context of growth, cost control and the regulation of the health market became crucial. Individual mutual aid organisations each implemented their own system of cost containment, usually involving the hiring of physicians with fixed-fee contracts. In 1920, attempts to conclude a national agreement between the medical profession and the mutual aid sector pushing for the standardisation and capping of medical fees, failed. Conventions at regional and provincial levels, however, were successfully negotiated.[67] While socialists like the leader of the national federation of socialist mutual funds, Arthur Jauniaux, argued again for the existence of one single mutual society with a unified fee policy, Catholics advocating organisational pluralism still stood in the way of a compulsory health insurance scheme.[68] Nevertheless, healthcare financing and the mutual aid sector, now enjoying the full and permanent support of the state, were moving towards centralisation and standardisation.[69]

Hospitals no longer only for the poor (1890–1944)

By the end of the nineteenth century, the private healthcare institutions would not only be organised by a Catholic congregation or a mutual aid society, but sometimes founded by surgeons or specialist physicians, for a middle- and upper-class population eager to benefit from new technologies originally developed in hospitals. Operating outside of what had been thus far the charitable logic of institutional medicine, these establishments initiated a new financing model resting entirely on patient-paid revenues. Although the admission of occasional wealthier paying patients had been customary in Belgian public hospitals in the nineteenth century, it had always been with the understanding that the better-off did not really belong there.

In contrast to the development of private medical services and mutual aid clinics, municipalities experienced great difficulties in sustaining and growing their network of public hospitals. The cost of hospital construction – especially of new specialised facilities – and of everyday hospital management was as prohibitive as ever. In the Brussels area, a few hospitals built after 1883 (Laeken, Forest,

Molenbeek) closed after the First World War. Few municipalities banded together to create inter-municipal institutions; most kept sending their poorer residents to the better-equipped city hospitals.[70] The search for private – sometimes foreign – funds was one of the ways municipalities got around their lack of capital. To rebuild the city's historic St-Pierre Hospital according to the new scientific and technological standards of the time, for instance, the Brussels Public Welfare and the Brussels University successfully sought the support of the American philanthropic Rockefeller Foundation directly after the First World War.[71]

The provision of affordable healthcare through mutual aid clinics and polyclinics negatively impacted the rate of public hospital use since mutualists no longer depended on public assistance physicians and institutions. One of the solutions available to municipal hospitals experiencing a decline in their user population was to open their doors to paying patients. While not doing so explicitly, the 1925 Law on the Reform of Public Assistance (which merged each municipality's welfare bureaus and hospitals into one single Commission d'Assistance Publique (CAP)/Commissie van Openbare Onderstand) and the ensuing debates admitted the necessity of attracting and accommodating a wider array of patients, mutual aid members and insured individuals included.[72] Hospitals could become an affordable option for lower-middle-class and middle-class patients seeking specialised and technological treatments; in return, patient-paid revenues would constitute a significant input to the finances of public institutional medicine. Now CAPs were free to open clinics for paying customers with comfortable private rooms.[73]

Paying public hospital users were charged the basic legal daily rate, plus a series of additional charges for blood transfusion, medicine, nursing material, radiography, laboratory analysis, radiumtherapy, transportation, etc. They also paid their physician's or surgeon's fees separately, especially if the latter did not belong to the hospital staff.[74] Between 1926 and 1934, the proportion of paying patients treated in the two main CAP hospitals of Antwerp (St-Elisabeth and Stuivenberg) would range yearly from 8 per cent to almost 25 per cent. In 1934, private CAP clinics opened in both hospitals.[75] In Brussels, CAP welcomed a proportion of paying patients of nearly 16 per cent and 12 per cent in its two

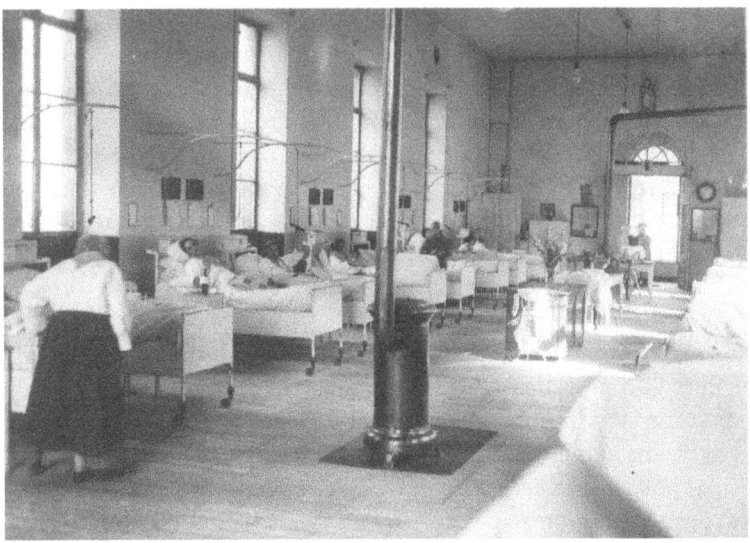

Figure 6.2 Two possibilities in the 1930s: either the common sick ward, free (as in this picture), or the single room with private bathroom, for paying patients. Ward 14, St-Jean Hospital in Brussels, around 1935.

major hospitals during the year 1926.[76] However, the income from paying admissions only amounted to 8 per cent and 5 per cent of the hospitals' global expenses (Figure 6.2 and Table 6.1).[77]

In 1935, a wing of the freshly rebuilt St-Pierre Hospital, named Clinique Héger, was exclusively dedicated to paying patients while the main building itself remained allocated to the poor. Four years later, the new specialised Cancer Institute Jules Bordet combined four floors for the poor with three floors for paying patients (who occupied one-third of the beds).[78] Despite these changes the public healthcare system kept losing money. By 1933, the CAP hospitals of the capital suffered a deficit of 9.5 million F.[79]

Notwithstanding the hardships of public healthcare financing, the development of medical institutions carried on, galvanised by the mushrooming of mutual aid clinics and private health institutions, the general public's interest in safe surgery, technological innovations and the antibiotic revolution of the 1930s. The

Table 6.1 Paying patients in the two main Brussels hospitals (1926)

Hospital	Number of beds	Total number of patients admitted during the year	Number of paying patients admitted during the year	%	Income from paying patients	Total hospital expenditure	%
Brugmann	760	5,657	891	15.8	546,671 F	6,735,902 F	8.1
St-Jean	570	5,410	642	11.9	256,255 F	5,166,126 F	5.0

Source: Rapport Annuel de 1926 (Brussels: Assistance Publique, [1927]), 24–5.

number of hospital beds (psychiatry included) grew from 40,000 in 1933 to nearly 52,000 in 1940, showing a growth rate of about 1,700 beds a year.[80]

Regulation and control: the Belgian welfare state since 1944

During the Second World War, German occupiers considered implementing a compulsory health insurance in Belgium resembling that of the German healthcare system. This vision was frustrated by Catholic civil servants from the Ministry of Labour and Social Affairs who feared that marginalising the role of mutual organisations would undermine Catholic efforts in healthcare and weaken Catholic presence in the life of the Belgian people.[81] It is, instead, a clandestine pact of social solidarity concluded just before the end of the war between some Belgian union and employer representatives assembled under the name *Comité patronal-ouvrier* that brought about change. A blueprint for a national social security policy, the pact served as a draft for the Social Security Act for salaried workers of December 1944. The decree law that followed instructed that all Belgian employees, regardless of their wage level, be protected by a compulsory health insurance that would be funded by the state, employer contributions and deductions from employees' salaries. For the first time in the history of the country, all employers had no choice but to support the general provision of medical care for the men and women they employed.[82] Despite the fears of the Catholics, mutual societies were to remain central to the functioning of the system: insurance payments would be channelled through them. For the self-employed, an obligation to contract a basic insurance – to cover 'major' medical 'risks' at least – followed in 1964. A year later, the same requirement applied to civil servants, and in 1969, to the whole population.[83]

The new compulsory insurance scheme of 1944 transformed the role of the state. The financing of healthcare became part of public service and authority in the matter was progressively delegated to a new administrative body: the National Institute for Health and Disability Insurance, or INAMI/RIZIV. But if the system was based on the principle of national solidarity between wage earners, risks were unevenly spread among mutual organisations since they catered to social groups with different risk profiles. Because blue-collar workers made up most of their membership, socialist mutual aid funds, for instance, had to deal with higher risks than their Catholic counterparts while also taking in far less income since member contributions were wage based. This resulted in early financial problems for the new system: in 1948, it registered a deficit for the first time, which rapidly acquired a permanent character. Rising expenses were caused by demographic expansion, the development of medical sciences and expensive technologies, as well as by the inclusion into insurance services of social groups entitled to health benefits despite not being able to pay their share. Deficits varied across the mutual aid market: in 1949, for instance, most mutual societies were losing money, except for the Catholic organisations united within a federation of Christian mutual funds (De Landsbond der Christelijke Mutualiteiten/La Mutuelle Chrétienne).[84]

Belgian historian Guy Vanthemsche has offered a sophisticated analysis of the compromise reached in 1949 to bridge the Catholics' and socialists' opposing views on solidarity. For socialists, who still wished for the creation of a single mutual society, national solidarity should prevail over all other concerns (i.e. the state should close the gap between incomes and expenses by granting more subsidies to mutual organisations in deficit). To the Catholics, solidarity should be organised only among the members of each individual mutual society. The 1949 compromise specified, on the one hand, that contributions to health insurance funds should be distributed among all mutual societies, taking into account the risk profile of each society's membership (organisations with members more in need of care received a bigger part of these contributions); on the other hand, mutual societies had a financial responsibility and – this was a demand coming from the Catholic side of the sector – in case of deficit, should ask an extra contribution from their members or lower the benefits that they offered. In the 1950s, a period of great political polarisation, the unstable compromise was called into question; it is only in 1963 with the implementation of the Leburton law on sickness and invalidity insurance that a long-lasting reform could be achieved (Figure 6.3). The latter pushed the separation of benefits compensating the loss of wage and reimbursements of healthcare expenses, and it secured higher financial support from

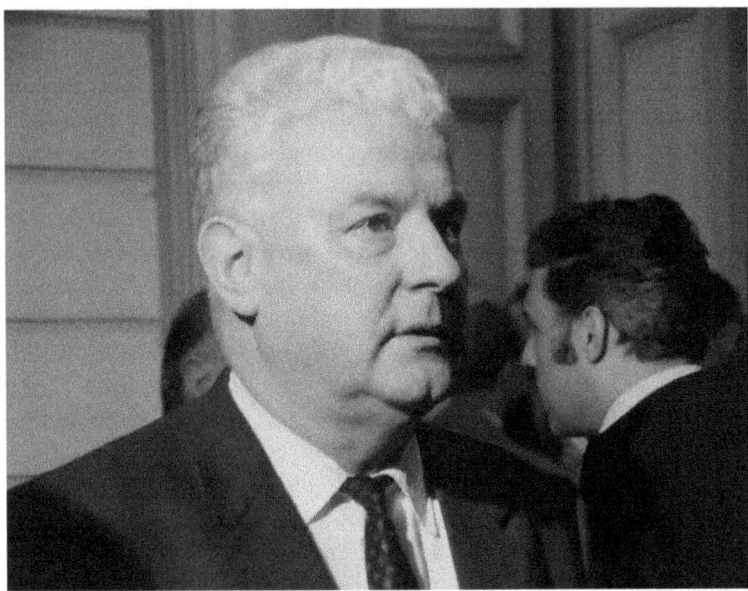

Figure 6.3 Edmond Leburton (1915–97), the minister who gave his name to a law on financing of the sickness insurance in 1963. Screencap from video 'Conseil des Ministres sur la grève des mineurs du Limbourg', 1970.

the state. All the while, the mutual aid sector agreed to assume a greater level of financial responsibility.

The transformation of healthcare after 1944 impacted the medical profession too. To maintain the financial viability of the system, medical fees, for general practitioners as well as for specialists, had to be regulated, with a central role for the state. This restricted the freedom of doctors to determine their fee: as a consequence of the compulsory character of sickness insurance for wage earners, regulated fees covered more patients: a medical journal estimated the expansion of people covered by a sickness insurance after the introduction of social security from 3.5 to 5 or 6 million.[85] Regulation attempts met with resistance as conflicts between the state, the medical profession and mutual funds – acting, in the name of their members, as a pressure group – multiplied. In 1961 an agreement about official fee rates was concluded between the mutual aid sector and associations of medical professionals, but was opposed by the

League of Belgian Physicians. Another organisation, the Syndikale Kamers der Geneesheren, reacted by staging a doctors' strike against the provision of the 1963 law that encouraged fee regulation through the signing of conventions between mutual funds and physicians' organisations and provided penalties for doctors who did not respect the agreed fees.[86] It took nearly twenty years to bring about stabilisation in the financing mechanism of the new public healthcare insurance system.

The post-1944 transformations had consequences for mutual societies as well. Competition between them changed in nature. Since all the wage earners were now insured and entitled to equal benefits,[87] expansion was only possible at the expense of a competitor. As a result, mutual organisations redirected their competitive energy to the so-called free insurance market (i.e. the selling of additional health coverages not included in the compulsory social security package, such as the reimbursement of funeral costs or home nursing). Often, they shaped their 'free' offer to attract a particular profile of wage earners. Some Catholic insurance funds, for instance, organised pilgrimages to attract the most pious among the Belgian workers. Up to 1964, free insurances were also key to the health coverage of the self-employed, farmers and civil servants, whose medical expenses were not covered by social security. Because it lined up with Catholic ideas of subsidiarity, precaution and solidarity, Catholic mutual aid organisations prioritised the development of that particular market and soon became the biggest player in this field. During the *Trente Glorieuses*, the breadth of health coverage expanded in all sense of the term: the number of insured individuals grew, just as did the variety of risks covered.

The economic crisis of the 1970s put a halt to further expansion of the post-war system. In the following decade, major budget cuts in state support increased the share of healthcare costs payable by users, driving up the prices of medical services and stirring up calls for privatisation. In that impoverished context, the situation of healthcare workers degraded. In 1988, a law proposal from Flemish minister Jan Lenssens triggered an unprecedented wave of protest throughout the whole healthcare sector. Nurses, social and hospital workers, youth and disability care workers took to the streets, mostly of Flanders, in a movement of 'White Fury' ('*Witte Woede*', as it was referred to at the time) to denounce low and

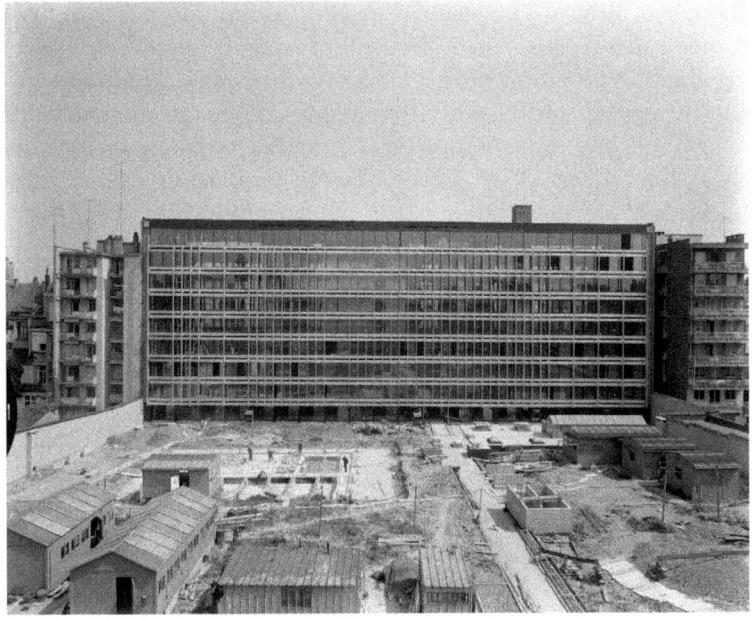

Figure 6.4 Construction of a new building for the INAMI inaugurated in 1974, when the economic crisis of the 1970s started.

unpaid salaries, high work pressure due to short-staffing and a general lack of recognition for their work (Figure 6.4).[88]

In the same period, private insurance companies that had entered the market of complementary insurances in the late 1960s established themselves as serious competitors for mutual funds. They offered hospital insurance (an insurance that was progressively coming to be seen as a necessary component of any salary-related benefit package) or insurance for those who sought the security of an additional sickness allowance in case of ill health. Mutual societies reacted by turning the non-compulsory hospital coverage into a complementary insurance product themselves, taking it out of their basic coverage and thus pushing it outside of the solidarity mechanism binding together their membership. On the other hand, the growing share of patient financial participation in healthcare costs, the reduction in social security reimbursements and the freedom physicians still enjoyed in some areas in the fixation of their own fees, created conditions in which the healthcare market could resume an easier expansion. In the late 1980s, the mutual aid sector broke into the market of international health coverage, which had been dominated up to then by private companies.[89]

In the past decades, the system has become more selective. Even though special supplementary benefits are directed at lower-income groups,[90] individuals and families with insufficient means of subsistence have found themselves pushed progressively to the margins of healthcare. Despite efforts from the mutual aid sector to develop an offer aimed at the poorest, remedying the gaps in medical care has fallen more and more to non-governmental organisations (NGOs) such as Médecins du Monde/Dokters van de Wereld (Doctors of the World), a non-profit organisation that provides direct medical support to drug addicts, the homeless, undocumented and other people who have fallen off the healthcare radar.[91] In other areas of public health today, NGOs will focus on specific diseases, like cancer for instance; by means of large-scale public campaigns, often with support from the media, they raise money to finance research and provide financial support to cancer patients.[92]

Hospitals increasingly under state control after 1944

The compulsory health insurance scheme had an immediate effect on public hospital finances. In the years following the 1925 reform of public assistance and the opening of public health facilities to paying patients, the patient population of the St-Elisabeth Hospital in Antwerp, for instance, was still made up of 60 to 80 per cent of indigent patients whose treatment had to be supported by municipalities. In 1945, that figure dropped to 10 per cent and stayed between 8 and 12 per cent the following years.[93] This meant that roughly 90 per cent of the St-Elisabeth Hospital users now belonged to the 'paying patient category'; they could pay for their treatment themselves or, more likely, had insurance. The new compulsory system of health insurance generated a financial windfall, flowing directly from the state and the mutual aid sector to public hospital accounts. Hospitals were not used to receiving such large amounts of capital for the services they provided. In Brussels and in Antwerp, the local CAPs split the sums that they received from the INAMI in two, one half going to their hospitals, the other half to the salaries of public assistance physicians. A pool system was set up to redistribute the latter half between the CAPs' various departments; part of it was also reserved for medical equipment. However, this development did not solve the depth of the global public assistance deficit: in 1948, the shortfall of the ordinary accounts of all the CAPs was still estimated at 1 billion BF. As a result, the state created a new 'Fonds communal d'Assistance publique' (Vermeylen Law of 24 December 1948)[94] – later referred to as the 'Fonds spécial d'Assistance publique' (law of 27 June 1956) – to help municipal CAPs reduce their debts. By 1962 the cumulated yearly deficit of the CAP hospitals was cut down to 755 million F.[95]

The salaries of public assistance – and, in particular, hospital – physicians were another point of contention in the financing mechanism of the new healthcare system. In the first half of the twentieth century, hospital work was still considered charity work and the function of 'hospital doctor' was attractive mostly for the research possibilities it offered, the prestige it afforded and as a springboard for a career in private medicine. Hospital physicians were granted a temporary mandate, earned nothing more than a small symbolic compensation for their services and had to rely financially on their private practice to earn their living. That is the reason why most doctors in this period would only spend two hours a day at the hospital, generally in the morning, and few hospital medical activities took place in the afternoon.[96] After the Second World War, the system of temporary mandates with limited compensation no longer seemed acceptable. Doctors aspired to become full-time employees and to fully take part in the daily life of their hospital. It took twenty years for this goal to be achieved, as is exemplified by the cases of Brussels (1967) and Antwerp (1971), both resulting in the creation of a professional union of hospital physicians. In Brussels the reorganisation of public assistance physician contracts and salaries was influenced by the new Centres Hospitaliers Universitaires (CHU) (university hospital centres) reform in France (1960), which pushed for financial support from universities and sought to define a better balance between on-site curing, teaching and research activities.[97] In the aftermath of the physician strike of 1964 and a successful compromise on state-regulated medical fees, a national Joint Commission was tasked in 1967 to create a statute for hospital physicians but failed to reach a definitive solution. Minister Jean-Luc Dehaene settled the issue twenty years later, in 1986.[98] In the meantime, the total number of physicians in all branches of medical services multiplied by three, going from 8,000 in 1950 to 24,000 in 1980.[99]

With the introduction of social security, the hospital sector became subject to more state regulation. Hospital accreditation appeared in 1945, funding the (re)construction of hospitals in 1950 (public) and 1953 (private).[100] The Custer's law on hospitals of 1963 was the final step in the reorganisation of the Belgian health insurance system. Its purpose was, among others, to keep hospital admission free of charge for those who met the conditions of the compulsory health insurance policy. It was also to subsidise hospitals by contributing to the payment of daily hospitalisation fees (now calculated on a national basis), and to help abate the budget gaps burdening local CAPs and the municipalities that they were tied to. In that same movement, hospitals all came under state supervision.[101] To be part of the system, each institution had to apply for accreditation, keep up with quality requirements, as well as adopt nationally standardised bookkeeping methods that would allow a comparison of hospital rates and statistics for the whole country. The standardisation of hospital administrative practices such as accounting was both a consequence of, and a condition to, the implementation of a national public healthcare system. In Belgium, the art and science of hospital management emerged as an issue before the Second World War and became a specialised field around the major post-war healthcare reforms. In the academic institutes of the St Raphael Hospital in Leuven, for instance, professionalisation began in 1940 and led to the creation of the first Centre for Hospital Sciences of the country in 1961.[102]

In the 1970s, the Ministry of Public Health was also compelled to reduce hospital funding, and initiated programmes supporting merger operations or aiming at reducing the number of hospital beds in Belgium. In 1976, the CAPs in charge of welfare and public healthcare in each municipality were renamed Centre Public d'Aide Sociale (CPAS) or Openbaar Centrum voor Maatschappelijk Welzijn (OCMW), but this did nothing to improve the indebted situation of public healthcare institutions. To allow more flexible governance practices and alternative financing sources and methods, hospital administrations were offered the possibility of a transfer into new administrative structures. In Brussels, all CPAS hospitals were integrated into the new Interhospitalière Régionale des Infrastructures de Soins (IRIS) hospital network in 1996. Antwerp followed in 2004, gathering its public hospitals together into its own Ziekenhuis Netwerk Antwerpen (ZNA) network.[103] After years of debating the issue, CPAS themselves are now gradually being incited (Wallonia) or forced (Flanders) to merge with their municipalities. Tendencies towards cost control are hardening after the sixth state reform and the announcement of a necessary cut of 1 billion euros in healthcare expenditures. Among the actions taken recently is the grouping of all existing Belgian hospitals within a maximum of 25 different 'local-regional networks', each with their own legal personality and management body. One of the many objectives of this ongoing reform is to foster more effective coordination and collaboration between facilities, and allow the elimination of duplicate departments within the same network.

To replace the old subsidy system based on hospital daily rates, the law of 7 August 1987 created a new administrative body – the Budget of Financial Means or Budget des Moyens Financiers (BMF) – tasked with determining the subsidy amount to be allocated yearly to each accredited hospital. The new calculations were based on each facility's number of 'certified' beds and on the total number of hospitalisation days recorded each year. That calculation scheme changed again with the law of 14 January 2002. Concurrently, a complex new system of financing was implemented: state subsidies would no longer be drawn from the budget of the Health Ministry, but instead would come from 'alternative financing', in this case VAT revenues (2004).[104] In 2018, the main sources of hospital income can be summarised as follows: BMF subsidies from the health ministry (40 per cent), INAMI funding for healthcare and medical drugs (60 per cent).[105]

Concluding remarks

The sources for financing individual care multiplied as industrialisation made its way and social protection became a political issue. In the early nineteenth century, public authorities, charity and personal financial means financed care. Mutual societies were a means to pool small savings for investment in health, initially on a professional and segmented basis. The development of mutual societies and the financial support of public authorities included more and more people in the healthcare system. It was only after 1944 that employers had to contribute in a structural way to finance the health insurance of the wage earners. Even if since the late nineteenth century, it was argued that healthcare was a matter of national solidarity, it took some time for this idea to make its way. The two world wars were factors of acceleration in this process: after the First World War, the national state intervened more systematically in healthcare, while with the Second World War came the idea of social security.

Medical care can be thought of as a product to be consumed in the marketplace. This is the dominant point of view adopted by most researchers working on the history of social protection today. According to that perspective, social protection is a service offered by a series of market actors (mutual societies of various kinds, commercial insurance companies, etc.).[106] In Belgium, the mutual aid sector, working within the three political pillars (Catholic, socialist and liberal) that structure Belgian social life, became the biggest provider of health coverage, for wage earners in particular. This dominant position is partly due to the system of subsidised liberty and the ever-increasing financial support of the state throughout the twentieth century. The implementation of the Belgian social security system after the Second World War changed very little in that regard because mutual aid funds retained their position as intermediary between the new public healthcare financing scheme and consumers.

Moreover, the fact that all the wage earners and not only those with a modest salary as in the Netherlands were covered limited the market for private companies. Those who were integrated later in the social security system such as the self-employed and civil servants could be served by the so-called free insurances offered by the mutual societies. This might explain the limited role of commercial insurances, as compared for instance to the Netherlands.[107] The situation changed when after the crisis of the 1970s the coverage of the financial cost of care via the public system diminished: there was a market for additional insurances, covering hospital care. This market is a secondary market, not replacing basic care, and mutual societies are active on this market as well.

The provision of medical care in Belgium today is carried out by a mixture of public institutions and private non-profit initiatives springing from the mutual aid and Catholic sectors. This is the result of a long historical evolution. In the nineteenth century, local public relief institutions organised according to principles dating back from the French Revolution constituted the core of healthcare infrastructures. To counter the development of public intervention in the healthcare sector, Belgian Catholics expanded their own network of medical institutions. At that time, the central state had very little involvement in the provision of medical care. From the end of the nineteenth century on, it used the system of 'subsidised liberty' as a policy instrument and favoured private initiatives from mutual aid societies and Catholic organisations. Although state involvement grew significantly after the First World War, this tendency toward supporting and leaning on private initiatives was never fully reversed. As a result, Catholic institutions obtained a dominant position in the national field of healthcare.

Though it is very difficult to encompass the cost of care, nowadays it is assumed that both health and social care represent some 10 per cent of the GDP.[108] The 'unbearable' burden of this cost is constantly being stressed in the media, which justifies the cuts in state subsidies.[109] For half a century, the state has been struggling with the challenging equation between maintaining the solidarity principle of the post-Second World War social security and applying business logic to all aspects of society, especially healthcare.[110] Is it possible to monetise the body?

Notes

1 https://ec.europa.eu/eurostat/statistics-explained/index.php?title=File:Healthcare_expenditure_by_financing_scheme,_2015_(%25_of_current_healthcare_expenditure)_FP18a.png (accessed 27 May 2021).

2 Martin Gorsky and Sally Sheard (eds), *Financing Medicine: The British Experience since 1750*, Routledge Studies in the Social History of Medicine, 24 (London: Routledge, 2006); H. F. van der Velden, *Financiële toegankelijkheid tot de gezondheidszorg in Nederland*.

1850–1941. *Medische armenzorg, ziekenfondsen en verenigingen voor ziekenhuisverpleging op nationaal en lokaal niveau (Schiedam, Roordaziekenhuis en Amsterdam)* (Amsterdam: Amsterdam Unviersity Press, 1993); *Un siècle de protection sociale en Europe. Colloque tenu au Sénat octobre 1996* (Paris: Association pour l'étude de l'histoire de la sécurité sociale, 2001).

3 Catharina Lis and Guy Vanthemsche, 'Sociale zekerheid in historisch perspectief', in *De sociale zekerheid verzekerd? Referaten van het 22ste Vlaams Wetenschappelijk Congres*, ed. Marc Despontin and Marc Jegers (Brussels: VUB Press, 1995), 23–79, at 64; Robert Vonk, *Recht of schade, 1900–2006. Een geschiedenis van particuliere ziektekostenverzekeraars en hun positie in het Nederlandse zorgverzekeringbestel* (Amsterdam: Amsterdam University Press, 2013).

4 A good introduction and overview is Jan De Maeyer, Lieve Dhaene, Gilbert Hertecant and Karel Velle (eds), *Er is leven voor de dood: tweehonderd jaar gezondheidszorg in Vlaanderen* (Kapellen: Pelckmans, 1998).

5 Claude Bruneel, 'L'aurore de la médicalisation dans les Pays-Bas autrichiens', *Annales de la Société belge d'histoire des hôpitaux*, 28 (1993), 3–33.

6 See, for example, Sandra Bos, 'A tradition of giving and receiving: mutual aid within the guild system', in *Craft Guilds in the Early Modern Low Countries: Work, Power, and Representation*, ed. Maarten Prak (London/New York: Routledge, 2006), 174–93.

7 Pierre-Jean Niebes, *Les frères cellites ou alexiens en Belgique. Monasticon* (Brussels: Archives générales du Royaume, 2002).

8 Detailed information for the Antwerp hospital in several chapters in Jacques De Haes et al. (ed.), *750 jaar gasthuis op 't Elzenveld 1238–1988* (Brussels: Gemeentekrediet, 1988).

9 An overview of local interventions is in several chapters of *L'initiative publique des communes en Belgique. Fondements historiques (Ancien Régime). 11ᵉ colloque international Spa 1982*, Collection Histoire, série in-8°, n° 65 (Brussels: Crédit Communal, 1984).

10 Claude Bruneel, 'L'aurore de la médicalisation'; Claude Bruneel, 'Ziekte en sociale geneeskunde: de erfenis van de verlichting', in De Maeyer et al., *Er is leven voor de dood*, 18–19, 25–6.

11 In the text: 'Les secours publics sont une dette sacrée. La société doit la subsistance aux citoyens malheureux'.

12 See, for instance, Dora Weiner, *The Citizen-Patient in Revolutionary and Imperial Paris* (Baltimore, MD: Johns Hopkins University Press, 1993), 6–14.

13 Jean Imbert, 'La centralisation administrative des hôpitaux et de la bienfaisance dans les communes du département de la Dyle', *Revue d'histoire du droit*, 19 (1951), 58–104, 296–335; Jean Imbert, 'L'influence de la législation hospitalière dans les département belges et luxembourgeois (1795–1814)', *Annales Universitatis Saraviensis*, 2:4 (1953), 286–99. In 1856, on 2,531 municipalities, 2,514 had a welfare bureau, and 174 a civil hospitals commission. See P. Lentz, *Des institutions de bienfaisance et de prévoyance en Belgique. 1850 à 1860. Résumé statistique* (Brussels: Ministère de la Justice, 1866), 4 [Extrait de l'exposé de la situation du Royaume].

14 Claire Dickstein-Bernard, 'L'histoire des hôpitaux bruxellois au XIXe siècle: un domaine encore inexploré', *Annales de la Société belge d'histoire des hôpitaux*, 15 (1977), 68.

15 Ibid., 69–70. For the finances of the hospices of Louvain, see G.-J. Servranckx, *Mémoire historique et statistique sur les Hospices civils et autres établissements de bienfaisance de la ville de Louvain* (Louvain, 1843; reprint AGR no. 2, Brussels, 1995), 45–53.

16 Karel Velle, 'De overheid en de zorg voor de volksgezondheid', in De Maeyer et al., *Er is leven voor de dood*, 130–50, at 139; Karel Velle, 'De belangenverdediging van de geneesheren', in De Maeyer et al., *Er is leven voor de dood*, 167–78, at 177; Paule Verbruggen, 'De volkskliniek: een socialistische polikliniek in Gent', in De Maeyer et al., *Er is leven voor de dood*, 233–41, at 233; Geert Souvereyns, *Solidair in gezondheid. 100 jaar christelijk mutualisme in de Kempen* (Leuven: CM/KADOC, 2001), 22; Karel Velle, *De nieuwe biechtvaders. De sociale geschiedenis van de arts in België* (Leuven: Kritak, 1991), 98.

17 Marie-Sylvie Dupont-Bouchat, 'Entre charité privée et bienfaisance publique: la philanthropie en Belgique au XIXe siècle', in *Philanthropies et politiques sociales en Europe (XVIIIe–XXe siècles). Association de recherche sur les philanthropies et les politiques sociales. Actes du colloque Paris 1992*, ed. Colette Bec, Catherine Duprat, Jean-Noël Luc and Jacques-Guy Petit (Paris: Anthropos, 1994), 29–44, at 40.

18 Jacques Lory and Jean Luc Soete, 'Implantation et affirmation (1845–1914)', in Jan De Maeyer and Paul Wynants (eds), *De Vincentianen in België. Les Vincentiens en Belgique 1842–1992*, Kadoc Studies 14 (Leuven: Universitaire Pers, 1992), 45–80, at 69; Rudolf Rezsohazy, *Histoire du mouvement mutualiste chrétien en Belgique* (Paris: Erasme, 1957), 57; Souvereyns, *Solidair in gezondheid*, 22–3; Wilfried Wouters, 'De bewogen start van het Sint Vincentius a Paolo genootschap in België (1841–1848)', in De Maeyer and Wynants, *De Vincentianen in België*, 27–43.

19 Lis and Vanthemsche, 'Sociale zekerheid in historisch perspectief', 47, 52–3; Patricia Quaghebuer, *Welzijn door vooruitzicht. Een kijk op de christelijke mutualiteitsbeweging in het arrondissement Gent tijdens de 19de en 20ste eeuw* (Ghent: Verbond der Christelijke Mutualiteiten van het arrondissement Gent, 1986), 38.
20 Lentz, *Des institutions de bienfaisance*, 5–7. See also Chapter 2, pp. 68–9.
21 Jos De Belder, 'Het arbeiderssparen 1850–1890', in *De Belgische spaarbanken. Geschiedenis, recht, economische funktie en instellingen* (Tielt: Lannoo, 1986), 91–120.
22 Souvereyns, *Solidair in gezondheid*, 40; Dominque Boucher, 'Les catholiques et le mouvement mutualiste dans la province de Namur de 1886 à 1914', in *Le Monde Catholique et la Question Sociale (1891–1920)*, ed. Françoise Rosart and Guy Zelis (Brussels: EVO, 1992), 89–112, at 92.
23 Karel Veraghtert and Brigitte Widdershoven, *Twee eeuwen solidariteit. De Nederlandse, Belgische en Duitse ziekenfondsen tijdens de negentiende en twintigste eeuw* (Amsterdam: Aksant/HiZ, 2002), 42.
24 Velle, *De nieuwe biechtvaders*, 98.
25 Rezsohazy, *Histoire du mouvement mutualiste chrétien*, 74; Jolien Gybels, 'Reassessing the pauper burial: the disposal of corpses in nineteenth-century Brussels', *Mortality*, 23 (2018), 184–98; Tinne Claes, '"By what right is the scalpel put in the pauper's corpse?" Dissections and consent in late nineteenth-century Belgium', *Social History of Medicine*, 31 (2018), 258–77.
26 Paule Verbruggen, 'The mutualist movement in Belgium', in *Social Security Mutualism. The Comparative History of Mutual Societies*, ed. Marcel van der Linden (Bern: Peter Lang, 1996), 419–20; Boucher, 'Les catholiques', 91; Souvereyns, *Solidair in gezondheid*, 32.
27 Veraghtert and Widdershoven, *Twee eeuwen solidariteit*, 44.
28 Griet van Meulder, 'Mutualiteiten en ziekteverzekering in België, 1886–1914', *Belgisch Tijdschrift voor Nieuwste Geschiedenis*, 27 (1997), 83–134, at 86; Veraghtert and Widdershoven, *Twee eeuwen solidariteit*, 44.
29 Boucher, 'Les catholiques', 92; Verbruggen, 'The mutualist movement, 421; Rezsohazy, *Histoire du mouvement mutualiste chrétien*, 61.
30 Van Meulder, 'Mutualiteiten', 86; E. Gerard, 'De christelijke mutualiteiten', in *De christelijke arbeidersbeweging in België 1891–1991*, ed. E. Gerard, Kadoc Studies 11 (Leuven: Universitaire Pers, 1991), vol. 2, 66–145, at 73; Rezsohazy, *Histoire du mouvement mutualiste chrétien*, 337, 361.

31 Jan De Maeyer and Lieve Dhaene, 'Sociale emancipatie en democratisering: de gezondheidszorg verzuild', in De Maeyer et al., *Er is leven voor de dood*, 151–66, at 152; Van Meulder, 'Mutualiteiten', 94–7, 103.
32 Jo Deferme, *Uit de ketens van de vrijheid. Het debat over de sociale politiek in België, 1886–1914*, KADOC-Studies 32 (Leuven: Universitaire Pers, 2007), 337, 414.
33 Van Meulder, 'Mutualiteiten', 103–5.
34 As can been witnessed through the evolution of pharmaceutics and medical services advertising. See Velle, *De nieuwe biechtvaders*, 99.
35 Boucher, 'Les catholiques', 95.
36 Verbruggen, 'The mutualist movement', 424–5; De Maeyer and Dhaene, 'Sociale emancipatie', 156; Verbruggen, 'De Volkskliniek', 235; Souvereyns, *Solidair in gezondheid*, 119; Deferme, *Uit de ketens*, 340; Rezsohazy, *Histoire du mouvement mutualiste chrétien*, 136.
37 Karel Velle, 'De belangenverdediging van de geneesheren', in De Maeyer et al., *Er is leven voor de dood*, 167–78, at 173.
38 Souvereyns, *Solidair in gezondheid*, 127.
39 Daniel Vanacker, *Een averechtse liberaal. Leo Augusteyns en de liberale arbeidersbeweging* (Ghent: Academia Press/Liberaal Archief, 2008), 365–78.
40 Rezsohazy, *Histoire du mouvement mutualiste chrétien*, 109.
41 Michel Vermote, *Gezondheid. 75 Jaar Nationaal Verbond van socialistische mutualiteiten* (Ghent: AMSAB, 1988), 22.
42 Quaghebeur, *Welzijn door vooruitzicht*, 61.
43 Souvereyns, *Solidair in gezondheid*, 68–72, 127–8; Rezsohazy, *Histoire du mouvement mutualiste chrétien*, 139.
44 Souvereyns, *Solidair in gezondheid*, 127.
45 Els Witte, Alain Meynen and Dirk Luyten, *Histoire politique de la Belgique de 1830 à nos jours* (Brussels: Edition Samsa, 2017), 117–56; De Maeyer and Dhaene, 'Sociale emancipatie en democratisering', 151–66.
46 Verbruggen, 'De Volkskliniek', 236.
47 Souvereyns, *Solidair in gezondheid*, 119.
48 Boucher, 'Les Catholiques', 101.
49 Van Meulder, 'Mutualiteiten', 118; Griet van Meulder, 'Vrouwenmutualiteiten of familiemutualiteiten? De betekenis van het mutualisme voor vrouwen rond de eeuwwisseling (1885–1914)', *Brood en Rozen*, 3 (1997), 38–349, at 40.
50 Souvereyns, *Solidair in gezondheid*, 125; Van Meulder, 'Vrouwenmutualiteiten', 40.
51 De Maeyer and Dhaene, 'Sociale emancipatie', 156.

52 Van Meulder, 'Mutualiteiten', 119–20.
53 Ibid., 112, 120–5.
54 Claudine Marissal, *Protéger le jeune enfant: Enjeux sociaux, politiques et sexués (Belgique, 1890–1940)*, (Brussels: Editions de l'Université de Bruxelles, 2014), 109–28; Godelieve Masuy-Stroobant, 'Le choc de la guerre de 14–18: une avancée pour les oeuvres de l'enfance', in *Mères et nourrissons: de la bienfaisance à la protection médico-sociale (1830–1945)*, ed. Godelieve Masuy-Stroobant and Perrine C. Humblet (Brussels: Labor, 2004), 159–75; Gerard, 'De christelijke mutualiteiten', 90; Vermote, *Gezondheid*, 35; De Maeyer and Dhaene, 'Sociale emancipatie', 156–8; Luc De Munck, *Altijd troosten. Belgische verpleegsters tijdens de Eerste Wereldoorlog* (Amsterdam: Amsterdam University Press, 2018).
55 The First Ministry of Health created in 1936 was short-lived. See Velle, 'De overheid', 136–8.
56 Verbruggen, 'De Volkskliniek', 236.
57 Ibid.; De Maeyer and Dhaene, 'Sociale emancipatie', 158–63.
58 Gerard, 'De Christelijke mutualiteiten', 100.
59 Velle, 'De overheid', 139; Piet Clement, *Government Consumption and Investment in Belgium, 1830–1940: 1940: The Reconstruction of a Database* (Leuven: Leuven University Press/Koninklijke Vlaamse Academie van België voor Wetenschappen en Kunsten, 2000), 114.
60 Ineke Meul, 'De professionalisering van het medisch-specialistisch beroep in het kader van de verplichte Ziekte-en invaliditeitsverzekering in België (1944–2014)' (PhD thesis, University of Antwerp, 2016), 89; Peter Scholliers, 'Loonontwikkeling, conjunctuur en arbeidsverhoudingen in het bouwvak in Brussel en Parijs, 1855–1940', *Belgisch Tijdschrift voor Nieuwste Geschiedenis*, 21 (1990), 1–47, at 42.
61 Souvereyns, *Solidariteit in gezondheid*, 167.
62 Lis and Vanthemsche, 'Sociale zekerheid in historisch perspectief', 68.
63 Verbruggen, 'The mutualist movement', 426.
64 Vermote, *Gezondheid*, 35.
65 Verbruggen, 'De Volkskliniek', 238.
66 De Maeyer and Dhaene, 'Sociale emancipatie', 156–8; E. Geerkens, 'Les mutualités professionnelles, un axe majeur de la politique sociale patronale pendant l'entre-deux-guerres en Belgique?', *Revue Belge de Philologie et d'Histoire*, 80 (2002), 1275–349.
67 Quaghebeur, *Welzijn door vooruitzicht*, 176.
68 Vermote, *Gezondheid*, 67.
69 Verbruggen, 'The mutualist movement', 425; Souvereyns, *Solidair in gezondheid*, 205.

70 Claire Dickstein-Bernard, 'L'initiative communale en matière hospitalière entre 1795 et 1940, et plus particulièrement à Bruxelles et dans les faubourgs de la capitale', in *L'initiative publique des communes en Belgique, 1795–1940, Actes du 12e colloque international, Spa 1984*, Collection histoire, série in-8°, 71 (Brussels: Crédit communal, 1986), 395–6, 400–4.

71 David Guilardian, 'Saint-Pierre et Bordet: De l'Art Deco au Modernisme', in *Du monumental au fonctionnel: l'architecture des hôpitaux publics bruxellois (XIXe–XXe siècles)*, ed. Claire Dickstein-Bernard, David Guilardian, Astrid Lelarge and Judith Le Maire (Brussels: CIVA, 2005), 75–7.

72 'Hospitals which, yesterday still, were considered asylums for the poor, have become healthcare establishments offering all the required guarantees, frequented not only by the poor but by a large clientele made out for the most part of individuals who, thanks to social security, are now paying or semi-paying patients.' J. Glineur and P. Rochet, *Guide pratique de l'administration des CAP* (Brussels, 1955), 11 (see also p. 194); Dickstein-Bernard, 'L'initiative communale', 393–4.

73 Glineur and Rochet, *Guide pratique*, 194–5; Dickstein-Bernard, 'L'initiative communale', 393–4.

74 Jacques De Haes et al., 'De overlevingsstrijd van een ziekenhuis', in De Haes et al., *750 jaar gasthuis*, 256–7.

75 Note that the number of patients was not calculated on the same basis throughout the period. De Haes et al., 'De overlevingsstrijd', 255.

76 *Rapport Annuel de 1926* (Brussels: Assistance publique, [1927]), 24–5.

77 Ibid., 12 and 32–3.

78 Guilardian, 'Saint-Pierre et Bordet', 91, 94, 105, 109.

79 Dickstein-Bernard, 'L'initiative communale', 389.

80 Beds in military hospitals are not included in these figures. See Bernard Delvaux, 'Les hôpitaux en Belgique. Évolution de l'infrastructure et de la politique hospitalière', *Courrier Hebdomadaire du CRISP*, 1140–1 (1986), 6.

81 Karel Vanacker, *Kroniek van een overleving: de Belgische ziekenfondsen tijdens de Tweede Wereldoorlog* (Ghent: AMSAB, 2010); Gerard, 'De christelijke mutualiteiten', 103.

82 Guy Vanthemsche, *De beginjaren van de sociale zekerheid in België, 1944–1963* (Brussels: VUB Press, 1994), 56–77.

83 Peter Heyrman, Joris Colla and Noortje Lambrichts, *De sociale zekerheid van zelfstandigen in België 1937–2017. Solidariteit en verantwoordelijkheid* (Herent: KADOC/Zenito, 2017), 147–8.

84 Vanthemsche, *De beginjaren*, 127.

85 Meul, *De professionalisering*, 126.
86 Vanthemsche, *De beginjaren*, 127–157; Klaartje Schrijvers, 'De artsenstaking van 1964. Of hoe de artsen een machtig eenheidsfront wisten te vormen in hun strijd tegen de overheid', *Bijdragen tot de Eigentijdse Geschiedenis*, 16 (2005), 57–89; Guy Vanthemsche, 'Les mutualités et la protection sociale en Belgique (milieu du XIXe–fin du XXe siècle)', *Histoire et Sociétés. Revue européenne d'histoire sociale*, 16 (2005), 20–31; Meul, *De professionalisering*, 163–4.
87 Except for the young men and women entering the labour market but who often remained loyal to their parents and family's insurance fund anyway.
88 For the 'Witte Woede' movement, see Erik Henderickx et al., *Ze vragen zoveel mijnheer. De kwalitatieve kant van de witte woede* (Antwerpen: Ruca Rijksuniversitair Centrum, 1993); and Marianne De Troyer, 'Blouses blanches en colère. Quelles sont les résultantes des mouvements de grèves et des négociations des dernières années (1989–1992)?', *L'année sociale* (1992), 110–19.
89 Etienne Arcq and Pierre Blaise, 'Politieke geschiedenis van de sociale zekerheid in België', *Belgisch Tijdschrift voor Sociale Zekerheid*, 40 (1998), 491–746, at 673–6; Herman Deleeck, *De architectuur van de welvaartsstaat opnieuw bekeken* (Leuven: Acco, 2000), 421.
90 Bea Cantillon and Linde Buysse, *De staat van de welvaartsstaat* (Leuven: Acco, 2016), 51.
91 Arcq and Blaise, 'Politieke geschiedenis', 677.
92 www.komoptegenkanker.be (accessed 27 May 2021).
93 It would rise again after 1957 in this hospital, but not in Stuivenberg. See De Haes et al., 'De overlevingsstrijd', 257–60.
94 Anne Moureaux-van Neck, 'Assistance publique 1856–1956', *Acta Historica Bruxellensia. Travaux de l'Institut d'Histoire de l'Université Libre de Bruxelles*, 1 (1967), 62–71.
95 'Le problème hospitalier en Belgique', *Courrier hebdomadaire du CRISP*, 395 (1968), 6.
96 De Haes et al., 'De overlevingsstrijd', 286; Marcel Franckson, 'Plan Badon', in *Du côté de Brugmann. Un hôpital dans son siècle*, ed. Daniel Désir (Brussels: Éditions Ercée, 2006), 83–4.
97 Madeleine Moulin, *La genèse de l'hôpital Erasme. Un essai de sociologie compréhensive* (Brussels: Editions de l'ULB, 1987), 94–6.
98 De Haes et al., 'De overlevingsstrijd', 281–2.
99 Samuel Halter, 'Les hôpitaux belges de 1830 à 1980', *L'Hôpital Belge*, 148 (1980), 20.
100 Arrêté du Régent 21 March 1945, art. 56; Arrêté du Régent 2 June 1949; Halter, 'Les hôpitaux belges de 1830 à 1980', 20.

101 *30 jaar ziekenhuiswet in België* (Brussels: Ministry of Health, 1993); 'Le problème hospitalier en Belgique'.
102 Joris Vandendriessche, 'Reforming on paper: Accounting practices in the Leuven academic hospitals, 1920-60', in Axel C. Hüntelmann and Oliver Falk (eds), *Accounting for health: Calculation, paperwork and medicine, 1500–2000* (Manchester: Manchester University Press, 2021).
103 On the financial background in Brussels, see *Centre public d'aide sociale de Bruxelles. 18 ans au service des Bruxellois. 1977–1995* (Brussels: CPAS, 1995), 110–15; '40 ans de chantiers hospitaliers bruxellois. Entretien avec Arnold Czerwonogora', in Christine Dupont ed., *Hôpitaux bruxellois. De la charité à la santé publique*, Cahiers de la Fonderie, 52 (Brussels: La Fonderie, 2017), 39–46.
104 See, for example, the report by the Cour des Comptes, *Nouvelles règles de financement des hôpitaux*, Brussels, February 2006, 8, 11–12.
105 See the latest statistics summarised by the Health Ministry in www.health.belgium.be/sites/default/files/uploads/fields/fpshealth_theme_file/vue_densemble_donnees_generales_hopitaux_2019_3.pdf (accessed 7 June 2021).
106 Jacques van Gerwen and Marco van Leeuwen (eds), *Studies over zekerheidsarrangementen. Risico's, risicobestrijding en verzekeringen in Nederland vanaf de Middeleeuwen* (Amsterdam: Den Haag, 1998).
107 Vonk, *Recht of schade?*
108 Federal statistics, see the Introduction to this volume.
109 See also the problems with the increase of life expectancy and ageing population in Iris Loffeier, Benoît Majerus and Thibauld Moulaert (eds), *Framing Age: Contested Knowledge in Science and Politics* (London: Routledge, 2017).
110 For example, Jean Hermesse, 'Soins de santé: logique commerciale et/ou solidariste?', *La Lettre des Académies*, 8 (2007), 4–5.

Selected bibliography

De Maeyer, Jan, Dhaene, Lieve, Hertecant Gilbert and Velle, Karel (eds), *Er is leven voor de dood: tweehonderd jaar gezondheidszorg in Vlaanderen* (Kapellen: Pelckmans, 1998).

Dickstein-Bernard, Claire, 'L'initiative communale en matière hospitalière entre 1795 et 1940, et plus particulièrement à Bruxelles et dans les faubourgs de la capitale', in *L'initiative publique des communes en Belgique, 1795–1940, Actes du 12e colloque international, Spa 1984*, Collection histoire, série in-8°, vol. 71 (Brussels: Crédit Communal, 1986), 375–404.

Lis, Catharina and Vanthemsche, Guy, 'Sociale zekerheid in historisch perspectief', in Marc Despontin and Marc Jegers (eds), *De sociale zekerheid verzekerd? Referaten van het 22ste Vlaams Wetenschappelijk Economisch Congres* (Brussels: VUB Press, 1995), 23–79.

Van Meulder, Griet, 'Mutualiteiten en ziekteverzekering in België, 1886–1914', *Belgisch Tijdschrift voor Nieuwste Geschiedenis*, 27 (1997), 83–134.

Vanthemsche, Guy, *De beginjaren van de sociale zekerheid in België, 1944–1963* (Brussels: VUB Press, 1994) [in French: *La sécurité sociale: les origines du système belge, le présent face à son passé*, Politique et Histoire, 15 (Brussels: De Boeck, 1994)].

Velle, Karel, *De nieuwe biechtvaders. De sociale geschiedenis van de arts in België* (Leuven: Kritak, 1991).

Veraghtert, Karel and Widdershoven, Brigitte, *Twee eeuwen solidariteit. De Nederlandse, Belgische en Duitse ziekenfondsen tijdens de negentiende en twintigste eeuw* (Amsterdam: Aksant/HiZ, 2002).

Verbruggen, Paule, 'The mutualist movement in Belgium', in Marcel van der Linden (ed.), *Social Security Mutualism: The Comparative History of Mutual Societies* (Bern: Peter Lang, 1996), 419–29.

7

The material culture of caring and curing

Valérie Leclercq and Veronique Deblon

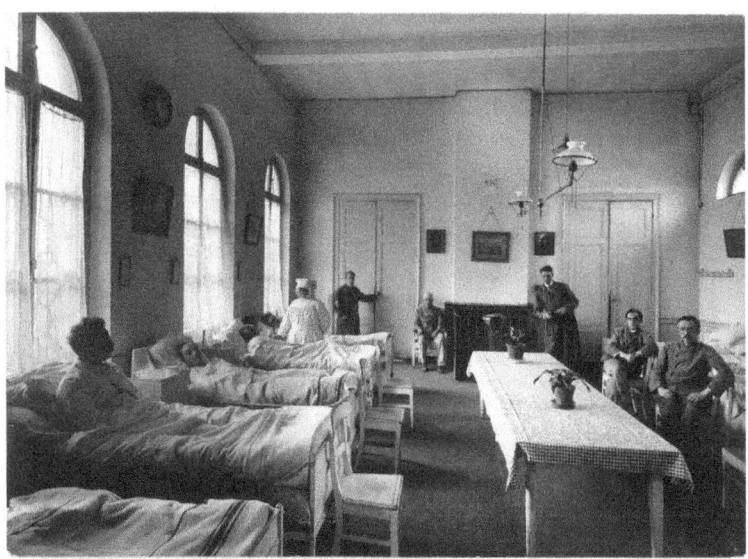

Figure 7.1 Photograph of a sick ward of the psychiatric facilities of the St-Jean Hospital in Brussels (1930).

Brussels, 1930. Bedridden patients, nurse and physician of the Hôpital St-Jean pose for a photograph (Figure 7.1). The picture presents a clean, well-ordered sick ward with frames hanging on the walls, beds, chairs and bedside tables. A piece of furniture as seemingly inconsequential as a bedside table can tell us a lot about the historic reality of such institutions. Bedside tables, just as their adjoining beds or chairs, were elements of comfort. They delineated an intimate, individual space that, even in its humble narrowness, not everyone could afford on the outside. In the drawers or on the tabletop, patients kept the few precious possessions that made them feel themselves: purses, administrative documents, but also small objects and images of sentimental value. Pieces of food (to be eaten, sold or slyly handed over to visiting family members) or pleasurable items such as cigarettes, pipes and alcohol also frequently found their way into the table drawers, in defiance of hospital rules. But if bedside tables allowed patients to retain some degree of joy and privacy in everyday ward life, they were also vulnerable to institutional intrusion. To curtail food trafficking, for instance, nuns and hospital wardens were often free to check the content of the tables whenever they pleased and to punish patients found at fault.[1] This invasion was all the more brutal because often the items stored in their bedside tables were all that patients had, the only material extension of themselves authorised in the spacious wards. Patients had no wardrobes or lockers. They wore uniform. Their civilian clothes had been disinfected and stored away in hospital cloakrooms.

As shown here, the tension between individual dynamics and institutional control that characterised the situation of public hospital patients in interwar Belgium is all there, contained in this object sitting at the side of patient beds. Looking at it closer gives us a glimpse of what it meant to be treated in a hospital; and it tells us what was believed – by hospital administrators and the larger society – to be a poor patient's rights, needs and duties in the early twentieth century.

Narratives of teleological progress and of social control have for a long time dominated the analytical discourse of medical historians. Since the 2000s, these narratives have been challenged through the consideration of the material aspects of medical culture and the ways that these aspects tie to the complex ideological, social and economic organisation of society. This 'material turn' in the history of medicine – and in history in general – set out to reconstruct what anthropologist Arjun Appadurai termed 'the social lives' of objects.[2] It surmises that artefacts (objects made or modified by humans) are 'historical events' that, like other historical events, do not 'just happen' but have a social history and are the product of multiple causes.[3] In addition to their intended function, artefacts reflect 'directly or indirectly, the beliefs of the individuals who commissioned, fabricated, purchased, or used them and, by extension, the beliefs of the larger society'.[4] The case of the bedside tables exemplifies how material culture can add layers and nuance to the history of medical institutions. The ways pieces of furniture, domestic objects, scientific instruments and architectural environments are built, used and adapted give us insight on everyday practices detached from the text of the rules and laws that regulated them. They also often engage a rich array of historical actors – patients, nurses, servants or other medical professionals – who have often been overlooked by traditional historical narratives. Complicating the history of institutional social control, recent material studies have, for instance, highlighted the 'domestic ideology' prevalent in nineteenth-century hospitals, pushing the idea that institutions (and society as a whole) should be modelled after middle-class home life and mirror family hierarchy.[5] To study material culture also means to learn, as historians, to interpret the absence of objects as well as their presence.[6]

In Belgian medical historiography, material culture has only recently turned up on historians' radar. Previously, studies of the material aspects of medicine in Belgium have mostly focused on two areas: hospital architecture and museum collections (on anatomical museums and health exhibits, see Chapter 9, pp. 326–31).[7] Hospitals in particular have received considerable attention, especially after the creation of the Société Belge d'histoire des hôpitaux/ Belgische Vereniging voor de Geschiedenis van de Hospitalen in 1963, but the resulting studies mostly focused on the history of individual institutions.[8] Benoît Majerus and Sophie Richelle were among the first to explicitly approach their subject through the lens of material culture. Both looked at spaces and artefacts to recreate a poignant history of twentieth-century psychiatric hospitals and nineteenth-century nursing homes.[9]

Building from the existing historiography, this chapter will stay mostly in the institutional space of hospitals and asylums but will attempt to move beyond the study of architectural design. It will shed light on the ways the different materiality levels of the hospital – built environment, spatial organisation, artefacts – reflected ideas of cure and care, and can offer glimpses of past healthcare practices. Hospital design evolved in conjunction with scientific development, although it has continuously been subjected to other influences too, be they social, economic, religious or other. Historian Annmarie Adams showed that medical spaces, in addition to materialising medical theories, were also 'produced' by all social groups partaking in the everyday life of the institution (from patients, to caregivers and visitors).[10]

The material and architectural history of hospitals in Belgium has been heavily shaped by wider trends in hospital design and international architectural theories that were themselves informed by scientific progress and socio-economic changes in the Western world. Throughout the nineteenth and twentieth centuries, Belgian architects and physicians travelled out of the country to study the features of foreign institutions and imported new design models from abroad. What specificities, then, could be ascribed to Belgian healthcare institutions? Local context is key here, as prevailing theories on design could rarely be adopted without adjustments to *in situ* conditions. The persistent and imposing presence of religious congregations in the Belgian healthcare system, for instance, had a huge impact on hospital organisation in the country. Belgian hospital material culture points to the interconnectedness of care and cure, the tensions between freedom and control, and makes obvious the different meanings medical professionals and Catholic caregivers assigned to these concepts.[11] This chapter will raise further questions about domesticity, privacy and hygiene in connection to institutional medicine, and explore the local, practical solutions found to address these issues.

The first section of this chapter will focus on the topic and practices of good ventilation, a central concern in the management of nineteenth-century medical institutions. Next, the ideology of domesticity told through the materiality of hospitals and asylums will be discussed. We will then go on to observe how the domestic ideal came to be supplanted by a new imperative of cleanliness that impacted hospital architecture, environment and furniture. However, the crusade against germs and the development of new scientific technologies did not alone shape nineteenth-century medicine. Hospital design and organisation also depended on moral and social norms, materialised through physical segregation and religious symbols. Finally, the emergence of the block hospital marked a turn in modern medicine; hospitals evolved to answer the social transformations of the twentieth century and new healthcare needs.

The last section of the chapter will explore the businesslike management style of these new institutions and the impact it had on their design.

Hospital organisation

Up until the nineteenth century, care for the ill and destitute in the southern Netherlands was in the hands of Catholic congregations. Daily life in the hospital partly replicated the strict daily structures of convent life and hospital architecture mimicked religious buildings. For example, the medieval Bijloke Hospital in Ghent was modelled after its adjacent Gothic convent. After the French Revolution and the annexation of the southern Netherlands to France, healthcare was radically reformed and charitable establishments were placed under the supervision of local governments. In municipalities with a hospital, a local board on civil hospitals was in charge of public medical care (see Chapter 6, pp. 208–9).[12] In the years following the French reorganisation, members of Catholic congregations returned to the hospitals and hospices, where they stayed active as nursing personnel until the mid twentieth century. As such, the hospital functioned as more than just a place of cure. Hospital work was part of the charitable and spiritual mission of religious congregations (see Chapter 2, pp. 68–75), while the interest of the state in taking over healthcare lay partly in the safeguard of public health and social order.[13]

In the early nineteenth century, old hospitals proved insufficient to provide medical therapy and failed to prevent contagion.[14] One of their substantial drawbacks was their odour. Bad hospital smells not only determined visitors' negative view of the institution – which at the time was exclusively dedicated to the care of the poor[15] – but these scents were also seen as an active threat to patients' health. The medical community identified foul odours, or miasma, as a cause of infection; putrid odours were associated with the dangers of contagious disease and epidemics.[16] The fear of miasmic infection instigated medical professionals to reorganise hospitals and eliminate as much as possible the contagious odours of disease.

The search for a design that allowed air circulation, space and light led to the introduction of the pavilion plan. The use of pavilions (or long 'blocks' isolated from each other) resulted in the installation of unconnected sick wards, with enough space to separate patients from each other. High windows flooded the ward with natural light and enabled good ventilation. In both psychiatry and general healthcare, the idea that architecture itself was curative gained traction. Nineteenth-century physicians became actively invested in hospital planning. The Ghent psychiatrist *avant la lettre* Joseph Guislain advocated for medical professionals to serve as 'the architect's guide'.[17] A well-organised hospital or hospice was not only designed to facilitate air circulation, but also to make possible the classification and segregation of patients according to their type of disease, gender or social status. Discipline, order and the discrimination of diseases, were thought to prevent the perpetuation of ill health and contribute to the healing process.

In Brussels, the St-Jean Hospital (1843) was known as Belgium's first pavilion construction. Its architect, Henri-François Partoes, was influenced by the latest standards in hospital design and had researched the organisation of several foreign facilities during study trips to Paris, Lyon and Plymouth.[18] Although the very first English and French pavilion hospitals dated back from the late eighteenth century,[19] pavilion construction only gained popularity in the nineteenth century. The St-Jean Hospital consisted of nine pavilions, connected by a two-storey covered gallery, where some patients took their walks. The design included separate floors for men and women and allowed segregation between contagious patients, patients with fevers and injured patients.[20]

Hospital style and appearance also came under increasing discussion. More and more voices turned against overly aesthetic hospital architecture. The surgeon André Uytterhoeven defended St-Jean's sober neoclassical style, stating that 'splendid ornamentation only adds to the cost [of the hospital], and does nothing to achieve its sanitary goal'.[21] In the second half of the nineteenth century, functional buildings should be prioritised. This was also the opinion of the Superior Health Council (Conseil supérieur de la santé), a commission of non-medical administrators founded in 1849 to supervise city planning and the construction of public buildings (see Chapter 4, pp. 144–5). Compelled by the poor hygienic circumstances of Belgian institutions, the council created national guidelines concerning the location and spatial organisation of hospitals.[22] They recommended the use of open galleries for the connection of hospital wards (instead of covered courtyards) and encouraged the use of pavilions. Although strict regulations for architects were imposed, once the council approved the plans of a hospital, there was no leverage to ensure the rules were actually followed.[23] Architects and administrators therefore retained some autonomy, even enjoying some room for experimentation.

Frans Baeckelmans, the architect of the Antwerp hospital Stuyvenberg (1884), for instance, designed circular patient wards.[24] The absence of corners was thought to prevent the accumulation of pathogens in typically dirty room areas. The sick ward radial plan also facilitated nursing supervision: caregivers could keep every patient in sight from their post at the centre of the cylindrical space.[25] Although Stuyvenberg's plan met both the hygienic and surveillance concerns of the time, the Superior Health Council was reluctant to approve its experimental design. The council favoured instead the layout of the Mons civil hospital (1869), made of four semi-detached pavilions connected through a pedestrian bridge.[26] The need to distract patients from their surroundings also preoccupied hospital administrators. The austere architectural style of the St-Jean Hospital was enlivened with flowerbeds and courtyard plants.[27]

Despite their modernity, nineteenth-century hospitals had an image problem. The indigent class perceived them as places where 'they [w]ere used for experiment, and after death ... for instruction'.[28] Indeed, public hospitals allowed clinical research in their wards and the dissection of its non-paying population in their anatomical theatres (see Chapter 5, pp. 180–3).[29] Due to their limited recovery rate, hospitals were often seen as places of last resort. However, some medical professionals believed that this perception could be improved by opting for the luxurious architecture some of their colleagues decried. Physician Constant Crommelinck, for instance, claimed that, although hospitals 'evoke repugnance among the poor', beautiful facilities would encourage the destitute not to postpone medical care.[30] Inspired by foreign hospital architecture, physicians saw beautiful hospital architecture as a way to legitimise institutional healthcare in the eyes of the reluctant poor.

Hospitals' (luxurious) appearance manifested the benevolence of their patrons and founders. The choice of a particular architectural

The material culture of caring and curing 251

style could also express an institution's ideological ties. Architect Adolphe Pauli, in charge of Ghent's new Bijloke Hospital (1863–78),[31] matched part of his eclectic design to the Gothic architecture of the medieval Bijloke convent[32] and in doing so, highlighted the Catholic identity of the hospital; other neo-Roman elements echoed Ghent's nineteenth-century urban landscape and pointed to the hospital's link to the (liberal) city council.

The domestic ideal: between home and institution

When the new asylum in Ghent opened in 1857, the press praised it as a 'Byzantine palace' and stressed its material comfort.[33] Its rich, eclectic architectural style answered to the bourgeois taste of the nineteenth century. As in most hospitals, the furniture and spatial organisation of sick wards were guided by the domestic ideals of the middle and upper class. For example, every patient had their own bed. Having one's own bed was a self-evident fact for the upper class, yet remained unusual in the homes of the destitute. Extreme deprivation was not uncommon in nineteenth-century Belgium.[34] Crowded unsanitary housing, dampness and coldness were the unfortunate lot of many families, who usually lived in one- or two-room dwellings where all family members shared the same bed. The degree of material comfort and privacy enjoyed by institutional patients can only be judged in relation to this broader material context. In 1845, a visitor to the newly opened St-Jean Hospital particularly lauded the unexpected cosiness of the heating system in the galleries: 'by way of precaution, which resembles tenderness, they have conducted the hot air under the benches so the sick can sit without catching a cold'.[35] The domestic ideal was further translated to the style of hospital furniture. Beds and bedside tables were painted to imitate wooden oak furniture.[36] Many hospital beds had closable curtains that separated patients from the rest of the ward (Figure 7.2). Curtains around the bed were meant to turn the space of the bed into a 'personal refuge' for patients and shielded their agonies and (painful) treatments from other patients.[37]

Medical professionals further embraced the domestic ideal in the organisation of institutional care, as is evidenced by two competing

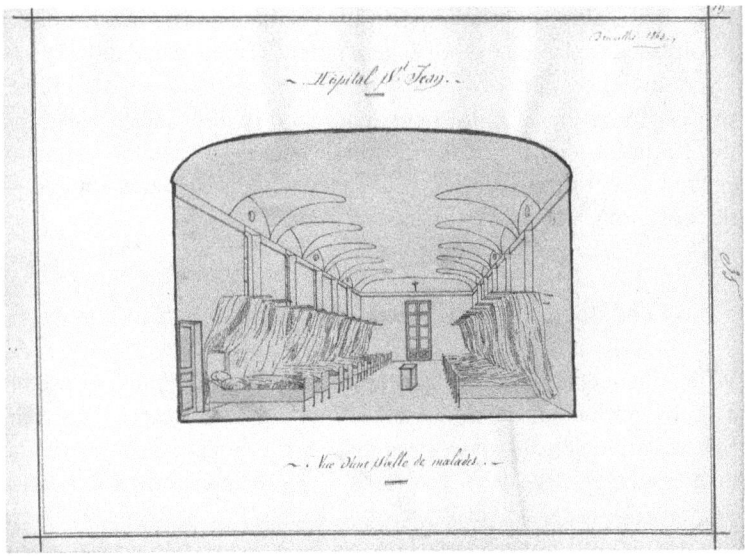

Figure 7.2 Vue d'une salle de malade (patient ward of the St-Jean Hospital in Brussels), painting on paper (1863).

regimes that structured Belgian psychiatric care: asylum care and community care. In Gheel, a village in the rural Campine region, the mentally ill were placed with local foster families. There, they enjoyed a relative amount of freedom and were allowed to move around freely in the village. In exchange for their care, lodgers helped out with household chores or performed agricultural labour.[38] In general, family care in Gheel was lauded for its philanthropic spirit, yet some medical professionals dismissed it and proclaimed asylums the only suitable place for psychiatric treatment (see Chapter 8, pp. 294–8).

The nineteenth century saw the rise of 'moral treatment', the first institutional therapeutic approach to madness. Moral treatment was based on the idea that the mentally ill could be cured if they were talked to, reasoned with and if a strict set of moral beliefs and a routine of order and labour were imposed on them. Chains and other forms of restraint were avoided as much as possible. Architecture was crucial in the reform of the nineteenth-century psychiatric landscape and proved an important tool to the propagation of moral treatment. Joseph Guislain, one of Belgium's first advocates of moral treatment, campaigned for new, purpose-built pavilion asylums and translated his medical ideas into elaborate architectural plans. The ideal asylum was situated in a rural area – far away from the pathogenic influence of the industrial city. Guislain called the new institution Maison d'hommes aliénés, a 'home' for alienated men. Mechanisms of confinement were concealed as much as possible from patients and the public. Windows were enhanced with 'decorative bars', which were aesthetically pleasing but still prevented escape. The wall around the domain was designed to recall the convent wall rather than the prison wall and it was camouflaged with a hedge.[39] All these manoeuvres were intended to distract patients from their confinement. Nineteenth-century asylum architecture in general aimed to create a feeling of domesticity,[40] while in Belgium the institutional orientation towards domesticity also allowed it to compete with community care.[41]

Despite the fierce medical critique, the public opinion remained favourable towards community care or family treatment. To the government, it was much cheaper to lodge the (insane) destitute with families than to provide (often lifelong) institutional care. Yet, physicians and government administrators agreed on the necessity of reforming Gheel's community care and ordered the installation of an 'infirmary' or sick bay. Guislain's influence on the reform of the colony was accordingly brought to bear through the construction of this infirmary.

Controlling mechanisms similar to those of the Ghent asylum were employed. For example, patients were classified in different categories (from 'tranquil' to 'agitated') and accordingly housed in different parts of the village; similar windows with decorative bars were installed. The infirmary served as a disciplinary space where patients were observed, isolated and received therapy. The colony's director, Jean Bulckens, explained to his peers: 'the patients are not free, but at least they have the illusion of freedom'.[42] After the reform, the enthusiasm grew for family care and the organisational model of the Gheel colony was exported to several foreign countries such as France, Germany and even Japan.[43]

Medicine after the Pastorian revolution and its impact on hospital architecture

Up to the 1930s, the pavilion plan remained the norm for hospital design in Belgium. It was still strongly favoured by the Superior Health Council in its 1928 instructional leaflet.[44] The history of Belgian hospitals in the wake of the 'Pastorian revolution' is thus not that of a radical transformation of architectural spaces. What we observe instead is the constant upgrading and readjustment of structures still firmly rooted in nineteenth-century hygienist principles. While elements such as ventilation and light remained central to the reasoning of hospital building experts, the new leitmotiv of 'decentralisation' encouraged the gradual division and isolation of hospital units. Furthermore, the application of new scientific knowledge and inclusion of new medical technologies gave shape to a material environment more and more unique to the hospital. To understand the slow permutation of the pavilion system, we must distinguish between various interconnected areas of medical development. Each had an impact on hospital design and organisation.

First, the evolution of medical knowledge itself was decisive. The work of Pasteur, Lister and Koch in the second half of the nineteenth century redefined our understanding of disease. No longer caused by an undetermined miasmic manifestation, it was now revealed to be the product of a variety of microorganisms. The germ theory led to new hygienic practices. Dust, rather than elusive miasmas, came to be seen as the new pathogenic force to oppose.[45] From then on, hospital cleanliness would rely on the creation of easily washable and disinfectable environments. Architects still wanted their hospitals flooded with natural light too, for sunlight not only allowed hospital cleaners to better spot dusty areas but also 'exert[ed] a sterilising influence on bacteria'.[46]

For the most part, the pavilion model seemed to satisfactorily accommodate the hygienic ideas and practices derived from the bacterial theory. It also allowed the containment of different germ types (i.e. groups of patients) in separate pavilions. The principle of 'decentralisation' adopted by most hospital administrations at the time encouraged, for sanitary reasons, the strict separation of departments, each forming their own independent unit.[47] In Brussels and its surrounding municipalities, the Military Hospital (1888), the Brugmann Hospital (1923), including its Psychiatric Institute (1931), or the Reine Élisabeth Hospital (1930) were all comprised of a large set of ground-floor pavilions.[48]

Between 1880 and 1930, the traditional two-department structure of the earlier healthcare institutions (medicine and surgery) was also confronted with the gradual emergence of new medical specialties such as ophthalmology, otorhinolaryngology, gynaecology, psychiatry, urology, etc. As medical knowledge and teaching grew more specialised, physicians demanded that distinctive spaces be created within the hospital to accommodate the new specialties. In existing hospitals, this often led to the reorganisation of the internal layout of the buildings. But administrators and physicians often struggled to maintain the coherence and practicability of their hospital's original design and to provide clear separations between the various departments.[49] The construction of new buildings was far easier.

Luckily, the pavilion system allowed for a convenient expansion of an institution's housing capacity. The last decades of the nineteenth century and the early decades of the twentieth thus saw an impressive multiplication of pavilions on hospital grounds. As a late example of pavilion construction, the Brugmann Hospital perfectly illustrates the expansive logic of a system that became increasingly more costly over time: designed by art nouveau architect Victor Horta, it consisted of no fewer than sixteen different departments, each comprising of one to five individual pavilions. Its myriad of buildings sprawled out across a twenty-hectare park located in one of the peripheral neighbourhoods of the capital.[50] The ever-growing number of individual pavilions not only demanded the purchase of bigger and bigger hospital lots, but also meant the pricey duplication, for each edifice, of a series of utilitarian spaces (entrance hall, kitchen, consultation areas) and building features (roof, cellars, walls). This phenomenon, of course, was affecting hospital construction everywhere. In Lyon, France, the colossal Edouard-Herriot Hospital had twenty-three departments located in twenty different pavilions. By the time the hospital was ready to open its doors to the public in 1933, it had cost 206 million francs instead of the budgeted 13 million.[51]

The development of the medical profession and the exponential number of medical students also increased the need for teaching spaces within public or university hospitals. Clinical lessons moved from the patient wards to makeshift classrooms, to auditoria. Technological innovation demanded the further moulding of hospital space to accommodate new tools, therapeutic procedures and – often cumbersome – equipment (i.e. X-rays, blood and urine testing laboratories, hydro- or electrotherapy, etc.), sometimes even necessitating the creation of whole new departments.

Germs and easily washable surfaces: a new cleanliness

The material environment of hospital and asylum patients changed drastically after the 'bacterial revolution'. It soon came to be defined by three distinct characteristics: smoothness, imperviousness and sparseness. Because Belgian physicians imported antisepsis methods and theories at least a decade later than their French or British counterparts,[52] that transformation mostly began in the 1890s and early 1900s. The discovery of germs demanded a redefinition of what constituted a salubrious environment.

First, the walls and floors of the patient wards could no longer be made out of absorbent, dust-catching or friable material. Walls, often the object of crude whitewashing in the past,[53] were now stripped of their wooden panelling or mouldings, covered with cement, enamel, stucco or earthenware tiles and received multiple layers of light-coloured paint and varnish.[54] The cheap and soft pinewood floors of older hospitals, which were dry scrubbed with coffee grounds or moist sand,[55] were also discouraged. Preference was given to watertight and seamless materials.[56] The Superior Health Council and the Brussels Hospital Administration favoured oak or 'bituminous wood' floors coated with specific waxes.[57] In the early 1900s, the new public hospital in Charleroi opted for *torgament* imported from Leipzig: a compressed mixture of magnesium chloride, sawdust, resin and cement.[58] Floors had to withstand repeated washing with disinfectant solutions. In 1928, the Superior Health Council specifically recommended that pieces of furniture be 'constructed so that they may be washed and disinfected without deteriorating', preferably in iron or (treated) wood.[59] In a report to the city authorities dating from 1903, physicians from the Brussels public hospitals explained the measures they were about to take

The material culture of caring and curing   257

to ensure a safer ward environment: 'Furniture will be reduced to what is strictly necessary (beds, chairs, benches, night tables, fireplaces, large tables, spittoons, washbasins, mirrors) ... Most cabinets can be placed in separate rooms. The carpets, curtains, and table-cloths which you can still find in some [places] will be done away with.'[60] Indeed, heavy fabrics caught dust and germs easily. So did non-human organisms, which also had to be removed from the patients' direct environment. New regulations forbade keeping 'plants or live animals which at the present time ... are reintegrated into the rooms [after disinfection], thus rendering incomplete and illusory the results of the operation'.[61] In another section, the report continued: 'whenever possible, wooden objects will be gradually replaced by other metal and glass objects'.[62]

Without the immediacy demanded by the management of surgical environments, with lesser financial means and a huge patient population to provide for, psychiatric institutions seemed to have been slower to meet the new standards of Pastorian hygiene. In the interwar period, some of the patient beds of the Beau-Vallon asylum, near the city of Namur, were still made of wood.[63]

All these changes partly prompted the 'modern' look and feel of the twentieth-century hospitals and, to a lesser extent, institutions for the insane. There were legitimate scientific imperatives behind the use of materials favoured by modernist architects, like glass, metal, stone, enamel or bricks.[64] With the addition of new therapeutic, surgical and diagnostic equipment too, hospital environment acquired a new scientific character, setting it more distinctively apart from everyday domestic settings than ever.

Wards and individual rooms

Despite undergoing a triple process of medicalisation, technologisation and specialisation, which earned them a growing legitimacy as places of medical and surgical treatment, turn-of-the-century hospitals remained firmly anchored in the realm of moral and charitable care. Confinement and discipline still characterised a large part of their therapeutic approach and heavily defined their materiality. The judgement of poor hospital patients, just like that of asylum patients at the time, was often perceived as irrational and unlikely to lead to good decision making and better health. In many situations, it was thought that patients had to be protected from themselves.

Large wards remained central to the experience of a majority of hospital and asylum patients well into the twentieth century. They marked healthcare institutions as collective spaces and made discipline a managerial necessity. But the kind of discipline demanded by the open wards also had a moralising – and thus therapeutic – effect. It commanded that patients behave appropriately towards each other and respect social hierarchy, that they assimilate the habits of good collective hygiene and contribute to the community by taking care of the communal space.

The size of that communal space decreased progressively. Whereas wards of twenty to twenty-five beds were still the norm in 1853, this ideal number decreased to 'no more than 20 beds' in 1911.[65] By the late 1920s, the Superior Health Council had decided that six or seven was the maximum number of patients a decent hospital ward should accommodate. In the small private Hôpital Français, located in Berchem Ste-Agathe, rooms had no more than nine beds.[66] Opened a few years before, in 1923, the gigantic Brugmann Hospital favoured three different ward formats: eight, twelve or sixteen beds.[67] When the Brugmann Psychiatric Institute opened in 1931, however, most of its wards still contained twenty-two beds.[68] Indeed, psychiatric patients had to endure the reality of large dormitories for a longer time.

This does not mean that there were no individual rooms in nineteenth- and early twentieth-century Belgian hospitals. There were in fact many of them. They, however, served two very specific functions. Their first purpose was that of medical isolation. Some small individual rooms, usually located next to the wards, were set up to receive patients who had to be separated from the ward population for medical reasons: contagious, dying, delirious or malodorous patients, for instance.[69] Another type of individual room provided for its part a means of social isolation. Usually built far from the wards, private rooms for 'paying patients' were a rare luxury reserved for a class of people that would not have tolerated being associated with the general population (see Chapter 6, pp. 220–4).

Since the law on public charity did not explicitly forbid it, the presence of middle-class patients in publicly funded hospitals had been accepted as customary.[70] Few mid-nineteenth-century bourgeois, however, would have dreamt of setting foot in a hospital. But

The material culture of caring and curing 259

things slowly started to change at the turn of the twentieth century for two reasons. First, the development of hospital surgery, medical technology and scientific knowledge about diseases brought a new effectiveness and attractiveness to hospital medicine. Second, these same developments drove up the costs of private healthcare and made it more difficult for even the better-off to afford certain expensive treatments. From the 1880s on, Belgian public hospitals experienced an ever-growing demand from middle-class patients looking for more specialised and cheaper treatment options.[71] This prompted most hospital administrations to seek ways to better integrate this 'new' lucrative population into their managerial outlook. In 1903, administrators of the small Turnhout Hospital decided to set up two three-bed rooms to accommodate its middle-class patients.[72] In the municipal hospitals of Tournai and Charleroi, private patients got their own quarters in, respectively, 1891 and 1910.[73]

Social order and material segregation

Cohabitation between the various social groups forced into the same restricted space was impacted by a fear not only of medical, but also of social contamination. Indeed, the therapeutic mission of hospitals called for the upholding of an environment that was not only medically but also socially and morally salubrious. Health could not be achieved without social and moral orderliness. The physical layout of hospitals and asylums sheds light on the views that physicians and administrators held on this sanitary-social order.

First of all, it was understood that patients had to be kept separated from the outside world. This required that both hospitals and asylums remained, to a certain degree, secluded spaces. It is no coincidence that, in official hospital and asylum jargon, patients leaving the premises without warning were said to have 'broken out'. Social segregation within the institutional space was also deemed essential to a healthy institutional order. Bourgeois and poor workers were kept separated in different buildings or parts of the buildings. In the Beau-Vallon asylum, better-off patients were welcomed from the mid 1920s on in the pavilions 'Charles' and 'Marie-José', where they enjoyed the privilege of individual rooms and a bourgeois interior that was set up with a reading room and paintings on the walls.[74] To avoid social mixing, the Brussels public hospitals went as far as allowing patients to occupy private rooms based on their social status even when they could not pay for their hospital stay.[75] Hospital and asylum architecture in the first half of the twentieth century continued to prevent interaction between female and male patients.

The prevention of moral contamination led, in addition, to complex marginalising processes of both spaces and patient groups within the hospital walls. The management of venereal patients perfectly illustrates this assertion. In earlier healthcare institutions, men and women with venereal diseases were often treated in the general wards. This was the case in the old public hospital in Liège, where syphilitic patients shared the same space as other patients. But in 1876, physicians of that hospital argued in favour of creating an isolated unit of six to eight beds dedicated to the exclusive treatment of female venereal patients.[76] If this request could be ascribed to an early process of specialisation, it was also clearly motivated by the perceived necessity to seclude patients thought to be a corrupting influence on others 'because in the presence of young ladies, they [were] rude and [made] inappropriate comments'.[77] It was commonly assumed at the time that female syphilitic patients were dissolute women. In the St-Pierre Hospital in Brussels, women and men with venereal afflictions had been treated in a specialised department since the mid nineteenth century. But additional 'moral' and material divisions were perpetuated within the department itself. 'Venereal women' who were registered as prostitutes by the police were not allowed in the proximity of other venereal patients and could only receive treatment in closed quarters from which they were forbidden to leave. It was often months before the head physician decided they were cured and agreed to their release.[78] The 'prostitute quarters' were comprised of eighteen beds (then four, after 1904) and had bars on the windows.[79] They also served as a disciplinary space for badly behaving women from the open syphilitic wards. In 1895, for instance, two female patients were demoted to the closed quarters after having been caught kissing each other in the yard.[80] But even further segregation was implementable; the quarters also had '*cachots*' (cells) to isolate disobeying prostitutes.[81] From the general ward, to the venereal ward, to the prostitute quarters, to

The material culture of caring and curing 261

the cell: this trajectory was that of a gradual social regression built into the hospital architecture itself. The closed quarters remained a feature of St-Pierre until the hospital's destruction in 1929.

Chapels, statues and cross pendants: religious discipline, religious healing

Members of hospital and asylum religious personnel helped enforce the many moral and social segregations of the institutional space and were particularly attentive in preventing illicit contacts between men and women.[82] But their religion, too, reinforced the institutional order with its own form of moral discipline.

In Catholic hospitals, hospices and asylums, the centrality and sometimes striking luxury[83] of the chapel was a constant reminder of the desirability of spiritual life and of a believer's obligations towards God, his brethren and himself. The call to mass marked the rhythm of institutional life. In the old Onze-Lieve-Vrouw Hospital in Oudenaarde, an abundant number of statues of Christ, of the Virgin Mary and of the saints adorned the walls of each ward (Figure 7.3); they were supplemented with a ceiling-high

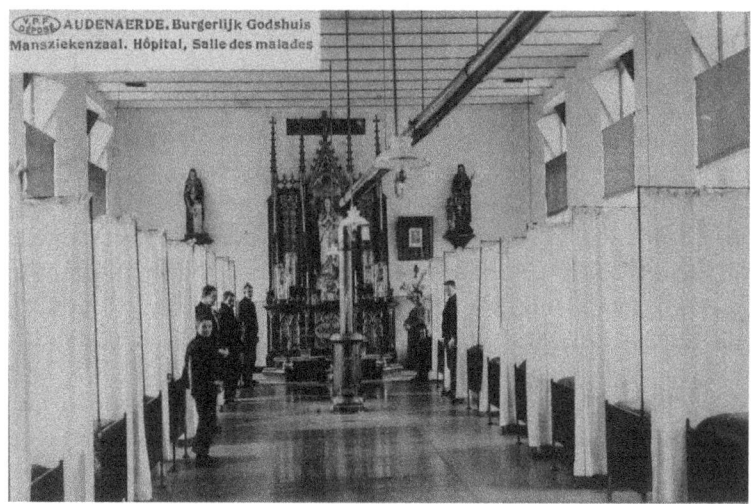

Figure 7.3 Postcard of a sick ward of a hospital in Oudenaarde (1915).

wooden altar at one end of the room.[84] Catholic statuary invited the patients to emulate the examples of the holy figures offered to their view and, in their time of suffering, to trustfully submit to divine authority, like they trustfully submitted to their physician's orders. In the Sisters of Charity-run Beau-Vallon asylum, the chapel and cemetery ensured the religious autonomy of the institution and provided a religious framework for the life of its residents, up to their death.[85]

At the turn of the twentieth century, a substantial proportion of hospitals, and almost all psychiatric institutions, remained in the hands of Catholic congregations.[86] For this reason, the secularisation process of the Belgian healthcare system had nowhere near the virulence and impact it had, in the same period, in a neighbouring Catholic country like France. Public hospitals, especially in liberal or socialist municipalities, did, however, experience tensions between their Catholic staff and lay administrations. But the prolonged need for 'cheap' religious nursing personnel and the extremely high percentage of public hospital patients still identifying as Catholic ensured the continued presence of religion in the everyday life of non-confessional institutions too.[87] That presence materialised around patients in many ways, although, much more than in private Catholic institutions, it had the distinct characteristic of being pushed from the bottom up. The installation of a centrally located chapel and of sparse Christian and Marian statues was usually conceded and engineered by lay hospital administrations themselves.[88] But the religious marking of public hospitals was as manifest in the candles carried by Catholic sisters, in the clothes they wore and in the holy water they threw on dying patients, sometimes in violation of hospital regulations. In the St-Jean Hospital, rosaries, prayer books and leaflets distributed by the hospital chaplains, similarly, encouraged religious contemplation and discipline.[89] As for patients, a portion of them – mostly non- (or non-practising) Catholics – were reluctant to pray, to go to mass and confession or to receive the Last Rites. But many others were eager to take part in spiritual life. In 1886, female patients from the public St-Pierre Hospital in Brussels petitioned to get a Christ on the cross for one of the open venereal wards: 'You must understand, Sir, that it is sad for us to be without Christ because, in the room we left, we had one', they wrote to the Superintendent, who quickly sought to satisfy their wish.[90] In public nursing homes in Brussels, residents often hung their own crucifixes in their individual rooms or had statues of the Virgin Mary on their bedside tables.[91] In the public wards of the capital, patients wore scapulars of the blessed Virgin on their chests or cross pendants.[92]

Religious administrators, Catholic sisters, priests, servants and patients, through their combined efforts, contributed to sustain a material and visual environment connected to the divine. In her study of the Catholic sickroom, Carmen Mangion argues that 'a spiritual atmosphere [was] considered integral to Catholic understanding of a healing environment'.[93] In both religious and lay public institutions, the chapel and the consecrated objects marking out the lived-in space had thus both a spiritual and therapeutic function; they were a link to God and tools of a religious discipline that aimed to heal, if not the body, at least the soul. They invited patients to subscribe to a Catholic moral regimen centred on obedience, bodily discipline, prayer and sacramental events. And despite their principled opposition to a religiously suffused medicine, lay hospital administrators were not above harnessing Catholic moral authoritarianism for their own purpose of social discipline.

The block hospital: towards the modern institution of the twentieth century

In the late interwar period, Belgian hospitals underwent a total reconfiguration of their physical form. A new solution for large urban hospitals engaged in acute care, teaching and research came with the advent of the 'block hospital', now arranged vertically rather than horizontally. This architectural revolution had started decades earlier in the United States and the United Kingdom, where multistorey hospital towers were often installed in upscale commercial districts. Belgium's hospital landscape, however, changed slowly. The Superior Health Council originally disapproved of this new building type. Its eventual institutionalisation was the product of a determined Belgian medical profession and powerful foreign influences.[94]

The first 'block' hospital in Belgium was the new St-Pierre Hospital. In 1919 and 1920, professors from the Université Libre de Bruxelles sought the help of the Rockefeller Foundation to erect a new university hospital in the capital. Among them was Antoine Depage, who had favourably impressed the Foundation during the First World War with the setting up of his Hôpital de l'Océan on the Belgian coast.[95] The conditions imposed by the Rockefeller Foundation led to the development of a common project between the Foundation, the university and the local city government. The project focused mainly on the total rebuilding of the old St-Pierre Hospital in the heart of Brussels's working-class neighbourhood Les Marolles.[96] The hope was to create an institution 'completely modern in spirit, in the supports and facilities at its disposal, and in the opportunities it offers', as well as to 'position Brussels as a centre of medical progress'.[97] Inspiration for the building and managing of the new hospital was gathered from a long study trip to various establishments in the United States, Canada and the United Kingdom. The president of the Rockefeller Foundation also insisted that the hospital director and nurse in charge of the records do their training overseas.[98]

When it opened in 1935, the new St-Pierre Hospital had a bed capacity of 610. Its central building spread over seven floors (including the ground floor and the basement floor). It housed thirteen outpatient clinics, two large departments of general medicine and surgery on the second and third floors, four specialised departments and a maternity ward. All were equipped with laboratories, classrooms and operating rooms. The building also housed a large admission area, an emergency room (ER), an X-ray department, a social services department and a rooftop solarium.[99] Many new medical institutions such as the Jules Bordet Institute in Brussels (1939) or the University Hospital of Ghent (1937–70) followed this lead and adopted the new plan (Figure 7.4).

There were, of course, scientific reasons behind these radical transformations in hospital layout. Hygienic standards and practices shifted as the understanding of infection progressed. The dangers of contagious diseases were soon mitigated by the marketing of penicillin and other antibiotics. These scientific insights made the hygienic precautions of the pavilion hospital redundant: its wards appeared too vast, its ceilings too high, its buildings too distant from each other and its height needlessly restricted.[100] Up-to-date disinfection methods and a well-thought-out ventilation system were deemed

The material culture of caring and curing 265

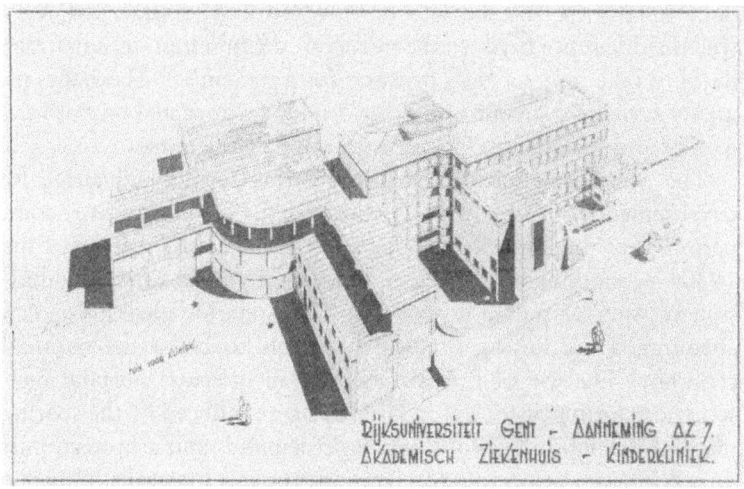

Figure 7.4 Drawing of the children's hospital (academic hospital of Ghent).

enough to ensure optimal hygiene.[101] Furthermore, makeshift army hospitals assembled during the First World War had proven that buildings made out of lighter materials such as wooden boards and concrete plates were no hindrance to safe medical practices.[102]

Other aspects of changing medical thinking and practices played into these transformations of hospital architecture. The construction of 'compact' hospitals signalled a new will, among physicians, administrators and architects, to reduce the physical and psychological distances that prevailed in the former pavilion institutions. The centralisation process initiated by monolithic hospitals meant the decompartmentalisation of hospital departments and new possibilities for collaboration between physicians. Hospital administrators wished for a more collaborative and unified medicine, mostly to mitigate the ever-growing division of medical knowledge into specialised fields.[103] The re-centralisation of hospital functions further allowed to reduce construction costs and to maximise the use of space. It also facilitated the circulation of patients and nurses within the hospital.

The nursing staff in particular benefited from the new vertical hospital, which reduced the running around required by service activity. Professional nurses felt that they should be taken into consideration by hospital planners because, more than any hospital professionals, 'they kn[e]w the distances to be travelled and [appreciated] very well the difference between the twenty or the hundred steps that one [had] to take to get a glass of water for a patient'.[104] There was no question that the layout of hospital buildings impacted on both the quality and the quantity of the work done by the nurses.

The transformation of the hospital was further influenced by developments outside of the medical realm. In the reconstruction period after the First World War and the later crisis period of the 1930s, economic imperatives, more than anything, drove the decision making of public authorities. The Superior Health Council encouraged the buying of local materials to boost the national economy. The use of Belgian concrete in interwar hospital construction, for instance, was in large measure induced by the soaring price of Belgian bricks (due to a high demand) and a protectionist duty to forego importing foreign construction materials.[105] In the 1930s, most Belgian hospital professionals came to agree on the economic superiority of block hospitals over pavilion institutions. Compact hospitals occupied smaller ground surface; not only could they be built with cheaper materials and less labour, but they also required less equipment, less maintenance work, less surveillance and less nursing and domestic personnel. They also spared hospital architects the temptation of luxurious facades and expansive architectural details. Indeed, block hospitals were characterised by a new minimalism and functionalism that were in line with the new modernist trend in architecture, a movement lead in Belgium by Gaston Brunfaut and Henry Vandevelde.[106] General technological developments such as the democratisation of electricity, the breakthrough of elevator technology and improvements in construction techniques also contributed to the achievements of modernist architects in the field of medical construction.

Social transformation

A lot of material aspects of the changing layouts of twentieth-century hospitals can be linked to major social evolutions in Belgian society, most of all, to the relaxing of class distinctions. In the mid 1940s, middle- and upper-class patients were much more comfortable with seeking medical treatment outside of their homes, in private clinics, sanatoria or specialised medical centres. But hospitals were still specifically seen as places of care for the 'economically weak'.[107] The perceived need to control and discipline the indigent hospital population, and to separate it from better-off patients, thus continued to inform hospital architecture. In the 1930s, the novel use of glass partitions allowed the nursing and medical staff to keep an eye on contagious or gravely ill individuals as much as it allowed them to monitor the inside of patient wards. In the new St-Pierre Hospital, partially glazed partition panels set up inside the patient dormitories to separate groups of beds gave the nurse continual visual access to the patients.[108] At the same time, hospital planners continued to integrate areas for paying patients into the design of public medical facilities: St-Pierre housed a thirty-three-bed wing for private patients on its fourth floor.[109]

These disciplinarian concerns decreased in intensity in the second half of the twentieth century as Belgium underwent a certain degree of social levelling. Just as in most Western societies, a series of intertwined processes impacted the social landscape of the country: the multiplication of jobs in the public and service sectors, the expansion of the middle class, universal suffrage and a democratised access to comfort and domestic technology.[110] In 1944, the decree law of 28 December introduced the national social security system for all salaried workers and offered roughly 60 per cent of the Belgian population the benefit of compulsory 'sickness-invalidity' insurance.[111] As a result, insured workers and paying patients replaced the destitute sick in the country's hospitals. In 1890, for instance, 90 per cent of the patient population of the Stuyvenberg Hospital in Antwerp was assisted by the local public welfare bureau. In 1960, this proportion was only 5 per cent.[112] In 1963, the first 'law on hospitals' guaranteed free hospital care to all social security beneficiaries.[113] By 1969 compulsory healthcare insurance was expanded to the entire population and hospitals were well on their way to become the shared referent that they are today (see Chapter 6, pp. 224–9).

As a result, the medical profession and society in general moved slowly towards a view of hospital patients as clients and no longer as recipients of public charity. In Belgian professional literature, discourses emphasising hospitals as providers of services and comparing them to hotels can be traced back at least to the 1930s.[114] But this perception grew in importance in the second half of the twentieth century. The conversion of patients into consumers parallelled the advent of the 'tower hospital' with its built-in shops and cafeterias. Concretely, the social levelling of the hospital population and a new respect for patient privacy led to the gradual elimination of large wards.[115] Hospital patient populations were no longer to be confined and disciplined.

Of course, confinement was much more difficult to do away with in the context of psychiatric architecture. But Belgian psychiatry, despite its heavily institutionalised nature and the limited impact of the local anti-psychiatric movement, underwent a process of deinstitutionalisation not entirely dissimilar to that experienced by other Western countries. If the Brugmann Institute, in the 1930s, had the first open wards of the country, the 1970s and 1980s saw the progressive opening of the whole establishment. During the latter decades, the institute's two large pavilions were replaced by smaller buildings structured around rows of individual rooms. In the same period, the Beau-Vallon asylum opened several outside residential facilities. This was a decade before the launch of the 1991 national plan to encourage the development of 'MSP' (psychiatric care houses) and 'IHP' (protected homes initiatives).[116]

The religious marking of the hospital and asylum environment also waned progressively. This was as much the result of the de-Christianisation of the Belgian population as that of the gradual replacement of religious personnel with lay trained professionals. In Antwerp, the last Catholic sisters left the Stuyvenberg Hospital in 1977.[117] As soon as the early 1930s, hospital chapels found themselves relegated to the margins of hospital locations, usually above the morgue.[118] Crosses and religious statues were now removed from sight too. These were all signs of the internal social metamorphosis of Belgian hospitals (i.e. of their transformation from charitable institutions for the poor to the technological and scientific centres that they are today).

Centralised businesses: hospitals at the end of the twentieth century

Purpose-built high-rise hospitals proved instrumental in the evolution of healthcare from a philanthropic, religious endeavour to a 'centralized business- and science-oriented service industry'.[119]

The ambition to turn hospitals into innovative institutions where patients could be treated with state-of-the art machinery and therapies incited the departure of hospitals from urban centres. The construction of modern hospitals in rural or suburban areas was part of a larger international trend. Hospitals were built in the proximity of cities and arterial roads (which allowed patients from rural areas to travel to the hospital by car) on open domains with enough acreage to allow for future expansions.[120] In Belgium, this trend was notably followed in university towns, where researchers and physicians from the (expanding) medical faculties wished to combine patient treatment with clinical research and education. In Ghent, a new academic hospital was planned on the outskirts of town during the interwar years. In Liège, an academic hospital was inaugurated in 1985 on the site of Sart-Tilman.[121] In 1975, Gasthuisberg, a new academic hospital, had opened its doors to the public in Leuven. Architecturally, these new and vast institutions consisted of a combination of several multistoreyed 'blocks'.

The continuing use of 'blocks' was encouraged by the ambitious plan to create medical centres the size of a small village. Each of these hospitals had to be built in several 'phases', which gave the impression that hospitals were located on permanent construction sites. Outsiders often perceived these large-scale institutions as labyrinths.[122] Colour-coded lines on the floor served as Ariadne's thread, helping staff, visitors and patients to navigate the maze of hallways and buildings. These huge projects and their daily upkeep, however, often led to financial and management crises. The hospitals in Ghent, Leuven and Liège all had to go through a severe financial reconstruction process in the 1980s and 1990s. This also resulted in a more autonomous governance of these institutions (whereby affiliated universities saw their influence on the management of their hospitals reduced). Due to their size and the development of increasingly complex medical technologies, late twentieth-century hospitals demanded a new form of management, closer to that of business structures.[123]

In the last decades of the twentieth century, regard for the comfort of patients, too, pointed to the new standing of hospital medicine. Locked cupboards or the private space of one's own hospital room guaranteed patient privacy. Bedside tables were no longer regularly subjected to the intrusive control of physicians and wardens. They had become small 'command centres', adorned with switches and displaying phones, remote controls, radios and individual lamps. Their function was now to satisfy the patient's recognised needs and rights to comfort and entertainment.

Conclusion

The planning, building and furnishing of a hospital is no small venture. The process requires considerable investments of time and money (a substantial part of it public) and, because hospitals must sustain the health of entire populations and came to symbolise a particular form of national achievement, it demands expertise at the forefront of scientific progress. Throughout the nineteenth and twentieth centuries, Belgian officials, architects, hospital administrators, physicians and nurses have known that they could not work in isolation. Despite its occasional protectionist tendencies, Belgium – a somewhat peripheral centre of medical progress – has always sought inspiration, expertise and help from the outside. Its agents organised research visits to French, Dutch, German, Scottish, Austrian, British and then later American facilities. They took part in international networks, made good use of international medical and architectural treaties (while trying to publish a few themselves); they sought foreign investments. As a consequence, the material history of Belgian healthcare institutions can be said to follow, in its broad outline, that of most other Western countries. Nonetheless, a certain degree of conservatism (noticeable in the late implementation of most new international trends) can be pointed out, partially due to lack of funds or religious leadership (even if the latter has shown far less resistance to scientific progress than is commonly expected).

It must be stressed, however, that the history of hospital and asylum building is international in nature. One reason for this is that it had to follow closely the rapidly evolving medical and architectural sciences, themselves the product of a constant transnational dialogue. Belgium and its neighbouring countries underwent similar processes of medicalisation and, later, deinstitutionalisation and therefore had similar architectural needs. Another reason still, has to do with non-scientific transformations. In this chapter, mutations of the material environment are shown to be driven not only by scientific progress

The material culture of caring and curing 271

and technological innovations, but also by broader social changes, as well as economic, religious, aesthetic and practical motives. Many of these developments – the slow processes of secularisation and social levelling, periods of economic depression, the advent of various aesthetic and architectural movements, etc. – impacted the materiality of the whole Western world. From pavilion hospitals, to block hospitals, to huge academic hospitals; from pavilion asylums to small late-century psychiatric units; from wooden floor and furniture to enamel, iron and glass environments; from wards with heavy religious adornments to stripped-down individual rooms, the evolution of Belgian medical institutions is in no way unique.

Some of the specificities of the Belgian case, however, should not be overlooked. The persistence of religious objects and of religious spaces inside Belgian hospitals and asylums points, for instance, to the long-standing influence of the Catholic Church in both private and public healthcare, and hints at the active role Belgian patients played in the perpetuation of this situation. The Superior Health Council also acted as a distinctively Belgian unifying force. From the mid nineteenth century on, the council sought to standardise, through the setting of national norms, the architecture and materiality of many institutions. In another area, Belgium even positioned itself as a pioneer. During the last decades of the twentieth century, the process of deinstitutionalisation signalled the loosening of the imperative of patient control that had defined most of the history of medical institutions up to that point. In Belgium, the physical opening of the institutional space and the movement towards community care had a rare precedent in Gheel's *colonie d'aliénés*. Throughout the nineteenth and twentieth centuries, Gheel embodied an internationally appealing alternative to confining institutional care, although a study of the colony's facilities shows a history not entirely free of medical authoritarianism.

By questioning the form, function, use and meaning of spaces and objects, material history challenges the two important narratives that have defined the way historians think about hospitals and asylums: the narrative of teleological medical progress and that of social control. A focus on materiality not only offers a different perspective, but it also makes room for historical actors often overlooked by traditional historiography (patients, nurses, administrators, architects and manufacturers, etc.). It shines a light on a multiplicity of points of view and, by doing so, nuances accounts of power dynamics and overly simplistic analyses of the individual and collective motivations propelling changes.

Today, much is left to explore about the materiality of Belgian hospitals and asylums. The manufacture of medical equipment and of institutional furniture, hospital construction companies, medical imagery, patient material culture, etc., are only some of the areas of institutional material culture about which historians of Belgium are still ignorant. The history of medicine in Belgium in its entirety, too, is still many steps away from its 'material turn'. Most of its subfields of research could undoubtedly benefit from a new material approach.

Notes

1. See, among others, archives from the Centre public d'action social of Bruxelles (hereafter ACPASB), St-Jean Hospital fonds, registres des surveillants, 3 and 4.
2. A. Appaduraj (ed.), *The Social Life of Things: Commodities in Cultural Perspective* (Cambridge, UK: Cambridge University Press, 1986).
3. J. D. Prown, 'The truth of material culture: history or fiction?', in *History from Things: Essays on Material Culture*, ed. S. Lubar and D. W. Kingrey (Washington, DC: Smithsonian Institution Press, 1993), 2–3.
4. Ibid., 1.
5. J. Hamlett, *At Home in the Institution: Material Life in Asylums, Lodging Houses and Schools in Victorian and Edwardian England* (Basingstoke: Palgrave Macmillan, 2015).
6. G. Adamson, 'The case of the missing footstool: reading the absent object', in *History and Material Culture: A Student's Guide to Approaching Alternative Sources*, ed. K. Harvey (London: Routledge, 2009), 192–217.
7. For example, P. Allegaert et al. (eds), *L'architecture hospitalière en Belgique* (Brussels: Ministère de la Communauté flamande – Monuments et Sites, 2005); *L'espace de vie du malade à l'hôpital*, exposition au C. H. U. André Vésale à Montigny-le-Tilleul, 17 October–11 November (Association belge des hôpitaux, 1990).
8. This association is still active today under the name Hospitium.
9. B. Majerus, 'Material objects in twentieth century history of psychiatry', *BMGN: Low Countries Historical Review*, 132:1 (2017),

149–69; S. Richelle, *Hospices. Une histoire sensible de la vieillesse. Bruxelles, 1830–1914* (Rennes: Presses universitaires de Rennes, 2019).
10 A. Adams, *Medicine by Design: The Architect and the Modern Hospital, 1893–1943* (Minneapolis: University of Minnesota Press, 2008), xxv.
11 B. Wall, *Unlikely Entrepreneurs: Catholic Sisters and the Hospital Marketplace, 1865–1925* (Columbus: Ohio State University Press, 2005), 121.
12 C. Dickstein-Bernard, 'L'initiative communale en matière hospitalière entre 1795 et 1940', in *L'initiative publique des communes en Belgique 1795–1940*, I, 12e colloque international de Spa, 4–7 September 1984 (Brussels: Crédit Communal, 1986), 375–404.
13 T. Markus, *Buildings and Power: Freedom and Control in the Origin of Modern Building Types* (London: Routledge, 1993).
14 This was a general complaint of medical professionals all over Europe. See G. B. Risse, *Mending Bodies, Saving Souls: A History of Hospitals* (Oxford: Oxford University Press, 1999).
15 J. Reinarz, 'Learning to use their senses: visitors to voluntary hospitals in eighteenth-century England', *Journal for Eighteenth-Century Studies*, 35:4 (2012), 509.
16 A. Corbin, *The Foul and the Fragrant: Odor and the French Social Imagination* (Cambridge, MA: Harvard University Press, 1986).
17 J. Guislain, *Leçons orales sur les phrénopathies, ou traité théorique et pratique des maladies mentales*, vol. 3 (Ghent: Vanderhaeghen, 1852), 344.
18 L. Wellens-De Donder, 'Enquête sur les hôpitaux d'Europe occidentale en vue de la construction et de l'agencement du nouvel hôpital Saint-Jean à Bruxelles 1828–1830', *Annales de la Société Belge d'Histoire des Hôpitaux/Annalen van de Belgische Vereniging voor Hospitaal-Geschiedenis (ASBHH/ABVGH)*, 8 (1970), 111.
19 See the Royal Navy Hospital (opened in 1762) near Plymouth, England, or l'hôpital de la Marine (1788) in Rochefort, France.
20 D. Vandevijver, 'Vers une architecture qui soigne: construction d'hôpitaux à pavillons en Belgique au 19ème siècle (1780–1914)' in Allegaert et al., *L'architecture hospitalière en Belgique*, 59.
21 A. Uytterhoeven, *Notice sur l'hôpital de Saint-Jean de Bruxelles* (Brussels: Gregoir, 1852), vi.
22 Conseil supérieur d'hygiène publique, *Instruction pour la construction et l'arrangement intérieur des hôpitaux et hospices* (Brussels: De Mortier, 1853).
23 E. Bruyneel, *De Hoge Gezondheidsraad (1849–2009). Schakel tussen wetenschap en volksgezondheid* (Leuven: Peeters, 2009), 51–54.

24 'Agentschap Onroerend Erfgoed 2020: Stuyvenberg', https://id.erfgoed. net/erfgoedobjecten/7112 (accessed 14 March 2020).
25 M. Beets-Anthonissen, 'Anvers. Hôpital Stuyvenberg' in Allegaert et al., *L'architecture hospitalière en Belgique*, 96–7.
26 Vandevijver, 'Vers une architecture qui soigne', 60.
27 ACPASB, Affaires Générales du Conseil (hereafter AGC), C394, fo. 'Fleurs, plantations'.
28 'Ordonnances concernant l'exercice de l'art de guérir en Autriche', *Gazette médicale belge*, 3 (1845), 219.
29 T. Claes and P. Huistra, '"Il importe d'établir une distinction entre la dissection et l'autopsie". Lijken en medische disciplinevorming in laatnegentiende-eeuws België', *BMGN: Low Countries Historical Review*, 131:3 (2016), 26–53.
30 C. Crommelinck, *Rapport sur les hospices d'aliénés de l'Angleterre, de la France, et de l'Allemagne* (Kortrijk: Jaspin, 1842), 10.
31 P. Allegaert et al., *Ziek tussen lichaam en geest / Malade entre corps et esprit* (Lannoo: Tielt, 2007), 21–2.
32 E. Langendries and A. van der Meersch, *Het Rommelaere complex: onderdeel van het gebouwenmasterplan voor de Gentse univerisiteit op het einde van de 19de eeuw* (Ghent: Archief RUG, 1999), 43–57.
33 'Maison d'aliénés pour hommes', *Le Messager de Gand* (31 October 1856).
34 S. Richelle, 'Hospices: lieux et expériences de vieillesses. Bruxelles, 1830–1914' (PhD diss., University of Luxembourg, 2017), 262–3.
35 'Les institutions médicales de Bruxelles', *Gazette médicale belge* 3 (10 January 1845), 11.
36 ACPASB, AGC, 126, fo. 'Le complément de mobilier – quartier des malades en construction, 1863'.
37 Uytterhoeven, *Notice*, 99.
38 On the organisational aspect of family care, see K. Veraghtert, 'Naar een moderne gezinsverpleging te Geel (1730–1860)', *ASBHH/ ABVGH*, 8 (1970), 55–73.
39 B. De Meulder, 'Het Dr. Guislaininstituut in het reformistisch architectuurlandschap. Nota's bij het ontstaan van de Gentse modelinstelling', in *Rede en waanzin: het museum Dr. Guislain in beeld en tekst*, ed. P. Allegaert and A. Cailleu (Ghent: Museum Dr. Guislain, 2001), 313.
40 J. Moran and L. Topp, 'Introduction', in *Madness, Architecture and the Built Environment*, ed. J. Moran, L. Topp and J. Andrews (New York: Routledge, 2007), 2–4.
41 D. Jaenen, 'Ouvrez les portes! Contacten tussen patiënten en 'bezoekers' in het Guislaininstituut (1857–1914)' (master's thesis, Katholieke Universiteit Leuven, 2016).

42 'Société de Médecine Mentale de Belgique: procès-verbal de la séance extraordinaire tenue à Gheel le 19 et 20 juillet 1875', *Bulletin de la Société de Médecine mentale de Belgique*, 6 (1875), 22.
43 W. Parry-Jones, 'The model of the Geel Lunatic colony and its influence on the nineteenth-century asylum system in Britain', in *Madhouses, Mad-Doctors, and Madmen: The Social History of Psychiatry in the Victorian Era*, ed. A. Scull (Philadelphia: University of Pennsylvania Press, 1981), 201–17; A. Fauvel, 'Les fous en liberté. La naissance des "colonies familiales" de la Seine', *Revue de la Société française d'histoire des hôpitaux*, 136 (2010), 16–22; A. Hushimoto, 'The invention of a "Japanese Gheel": psychiatric family care from a historical and transnational perspective', in *Transnational Psychiatries: Social and Cultural Histories of Psychiatry in Comparative Perspective c. 1800–2000*, ed. W. Ernst and T. Muller (Newcastle: Cambridge Scholars, 2010), 142–72.
44 Ministère de l'Intérieur et de l'Hygiène, *Instruction concernant les projets d'hôpitaux et d'hospices à construire en matériaux légers. Rapport du Conseil Supérieur d'Hygiène Publique* (Brussels: Ministère de l'Intérieur, 1928).
45 A. Depage, P. Vandervelde and V. Cheval, *La construction des hôpitaux. Etude critique* (Brussels: Misch & Thron, 1912), 116–67.
46 Ibid., 147–8.
47 Ibid., 122–3.
48 B. Mihail, 'L'hôpital militaire d'Ixelles. De fleuron de l'hygiénisme à chancre urbain', *Les Cahiers de la Fonderie*, 52 (2017), 18; C. Heusquin, 'L'hôpital Brugmann de l'Assistance Publique de Bruxelles', *L'Assistance Hospitalière*, 2 (1930), 57; G. Maukels, 'Hôpital Français Reine Élisabeth', *L'Assistance Hospitalière*, 3 (1931), 134.
49 See, for instance, A. Joiris, 'Le vieux Bavière au XIXe siècle, 1830–1895', *ASBHH/ABVGH*, 20 (1982), 112–23.
50 Heusquin, 'L'hôpital Brugmann', 51–91.
51 A. Bouchet, 'Histoire de la construction de l'hôpital Edouard-Herriot de Lyon', *Histoire des sciences médicales*, XX (1986), 91–2.
52 Antisepsis was introduced in the early 1880s in Brussels and in the 1890s in Liège, see C. Dickstein-Bernard, 'La pratique de la chirurgie dans les hôpitaux bruxellois au XIXe siècle', *ASBHH/ABVGH*, 19 (1981), 89–94; Joiris, 'Le vieux Bavière', 125–6.
53 Conseil supérieur d'hygiène publique, *Instruction pour la construction*, 8–9.
54 Depage et al., *La construction des hôpitaux*, 143–5; Heusquin, 'L'hôpital Brugmann', 58.
55 As was the case in the old Liège public hospital before the 1890s, see Joiris, 'Le vieux Bavière', 117.

56 Ministère de l'Intérieur et de l'Hygiène, *Instruction*, 10.
57 Ibid., 10–11; ACPASB, Affaires Générales Médicales, Personnel Médical, Chefs de service, Réunions 1899–1912, 6, rapports de la Société des Chefs de service, *Rapport sur la désinfection* par R. Verhoogen, 1–2.
58 Depage et al., *La construction des hôpitaux*, 140.
59 Ministère de l'Intérieur et de l'Hygiène, *Instruction*, 19.
60 Verhoogen, *Rapport sur la désinfection*, 2.
61 Ibid.
62 Ibid., 2–3.
63 A. Roekens (ed.), *Des murs et des femmes. Cent ans de psychiatrie et d'espoir au Beau-Vallon* (Namur: Presse Universitaire de Namur, 2014), 40.
64 Van de Vijver, 'Vers une architecture qui soigne', 63.
65 Conseil supérieur d'hygiène publique, *Instruction*, 8; Administration du service de santé et de l'hygiène du Ministère de l'Intérieur, *Instruction adoptée par le Conseil supérieur d'hygiène publique le 1er juin 1911 concernant les projets d'hôpitaux et d'hospices* (Brussels, 1911), 11.
66 Maukels, 'Hôpital Français Reine Élisabeth', 135.
67 Heusquin, 'L'hôpital Brugmann', 59–60.
68 B. Majerus, *Parmi les fous: Une histoire sociale de la psychiatrie au XXe siècle* (Rennes: Presse Universitaire de Rennes, 2013), 50–51.
69 Depage et al., *La construction des hôpitaux*, 163.
70 A. Goossens-Bara, 'De l'admission des malades payants dans les Hôpitaux des Commissions d'Assistance Publique', *L'Assistance Hospitalière*, 2 (1932), 55.
71 P. Bonenfant, 'Note historique', *L'Assistance Hospitalière*, 2 (1932), 63.
72 Goossens-Bara, 'De l'admission', 56.
73 Ibid., 56.
74 Roekens, *Des murs et des femmes*, 39–40.
75 V. Leclercq, 'Guérir, travailler, désobéir: une histoire des interactions hospitalières avant l'ère du patient autonome (Brussels, 1870–1930)' (PhD diss., Université Libre de Bruxelles, 2017), 105–8.
76 Joiris, 'Le vieux Bavière', 115.
77 Ibid.
78 On the prostitute quarters in St-Pierre, see De Ganck, 'Cultiver la différence. Histoire du développement de la gynécologie à Bruxelles (1870–1935)' (PhD diss., Université Libre de Bruxelles, 2015), 189–201.
79 ACPASB, Papers of the director of the St-Pierre Hospital (hereafter PDHSP), soins aux malades, fo.251, table 'répartition des salles'

(30 January 1914), letter from Dr Bayet to the Conseil Général, 4 November 1905.
80 ACPASB, AGC, 132, fo. 'la plainte des nommées R. & R. à charge de M. le directeur de l'hôpital Saint Pierre', letter from Isabelle R. and Jeanne R. to the Public Prosecutor, 1 February 1892.
81 Leclercq, 'Guérir, travailler, désobéir', 79.
82 Ibid., 270.
83 Richelle, 'Hospices', 138.
84 N. Ghijs et al. (eds), *Het Onze-Lieve-Vrouwehospitaal te Oudenaarde en de zusters Bernardinnen: Een bijdrage tot de ontsluiting van 800 jaar geschiedenis, 1202–2002* (Ghent: Provinciebestuur Oost-Vlaanderen, 2004), 175.
85 Roekens, *Des murs et des femmes*, 41.
86 W.-H. Mansholt, 'Openbare en particuliere Ziekenhuizen', *L'Assistance Hospitalière*, 6 (1929), 271.
87 In 1908, 97.3 per cent of the patient population of Brussels public hospitals still identified as Catholic, see Administration des Hospices et Secours de la Ville de Bruxelles, *Comptes moraux de l'Administration des Hospices et Secours de la Ville de Bruxelles* (Brussels: Administration des Hospices et Secours de la Ville de Bruxelle, 1908).
88 See the St-Jean Hospital, the Charleroi Municipal Hospital or the Stuyvenberg Hospital: ACPASB, fonds iconographique, série H/ H.ST-J./8: 'Plans et vues principales de l'Hopital St-Jean à Bruxelles' (1863), 1; Depage et al., *La construction des hôpitaux*, 437; Beets-Anthonissen, 'Anvers, Hôpital Stuyvenberg', 96.
89 Leclercq, 'Guérir, travailler, désobéir', 274–87.
90 ACPASB, FDHSP, fo. 317, letter from Léonie S. to 'Monsieur le Directeur', c.1886.
91 Richelle, 'Hospices', 145.
92 Leclercq, 'Guérir, travailler, désobéir', 284–5.
93 C. M. Mangion, '"To console, to nurse, to prepare for eternity": the Catholic sickroom in late nineteenth-century', *Women's History Review*, 24:4 (2012), 662.
94 Bruyneel, *Hoge Gezondheidsraad*, 200.
95 Set up in record time inside the Hotel de l'Océan, the 'ocean hospital' in La Panne treated wounded soldiers sent back to the coast from the Yser Front. See R. Redin, *L'hôpital de l'océan. La Panne 1914–1919. Une aventure belge au cœur de la tourmente* (Brussels: Les Editions Jourdan, 2014).
96 About the construction of the new St-Pierre Hospital and the Rockefeller Foundation, see D. Guilardian, 'Saint-Pierre & Bordet: de l'art déco

au modernisme', in *Du monumental au fonctionnel: l'architecture des hôpitaux publics bruxellois (XIXe–XXe siècles)*, ed. A. Lelarge et al. (Brussels: Éditions CIVA, 2005), 75–96.
97 J.-M. Wydooghe, 'Le Nouvel Hôpital Universitaire Saint-Pierre, à Bruxelles', *L'Assistance Hospitalière*, 1 (1930), 11.
98 Guilardian, 'Saint-Pierre & Bordet', 79–81.
99 About the layout of the new St-Pierre Hospital, see Wydooghe, 'Le Nouvel Hôpital Universitaire Saint-Pierre', 11–31; Guilardian, 'Saint-Pierre & Bordet', 95.
100 'Rapports des Commissions et des Sous-Commissions: Conditions relatives aux salles qui sont nécessaires pour les soins aux malades (IIIe Congrès International des Hôpitaux, Knocke-sur-Mer)', *L'Assistance Hospitalière*, 2 (1933), 57–8, 67.
101 S. Dehaeck and R. van Hee, 'De l'hospice à l'hôpital virtuel?' in Allegaert et al., *L'architecture hospitalière en Belgique*, 22.
102 Bruyneel, *Hoge Gezondheidsraad*, 199.
103 P. Depage, 'Le Centre de diagnostic dans les Hôpitaux', *L'Assistance Hospitalière*, 6 (1929), 291.
104 C. Reinmann, 'Quelques observations sur le nombre d'Infirmières en fonction du nombre de malades', *L'Assistance Hospitalière*, 3 (1931), 191.
105 Bruyneel, *Hoge Gezondheidsraad*, 199.
106 About modernist architecture in Belgium and the influence of the Brunfaut family on the architectural landscape of Brussels and Flanders, see J.-M. Basyn et al. (eds), *Brunfaut's progressive architecture* (Brussels: CFC Editions, 2013).
107 F. Héger-Gilbert, *Déontologie Médicale* (Brussels: Maison Ferd. Larcier, 1946), 100–1.
108 J.-M. Wydooghe, 'Les Annexes indispensables d'une Salle de malades', *L'Assistance Hospitalière*, 1 (1933), 19.
109 Wydooghe, 'Le Nouvel Hôpital Universitaire Saint-Pierre', 21–2.
110 Basyn, 'Hôpital de l'entre-deux-guerres', 66.
111 M. Carlier, 'La genèse de l'assurance maladie-invalidité obligatoire en Belgique', *Courrier hebdomadaire du CRISP*, 7:872–3 (1980), 36.
112 Beets-Anthonissen, 'Anvers. Hôpital Stuyvenberg', 99.
113 Ministère de la santé publique et de l'environnement, *30 ans de la loi sur les hôpitaux en Belgique* (n.pub., 1994), 14.
114 For a deeper analysis of the subject in the US context, see N. Tomes, 'Merchants of health: medicine and consumer culture in the United States, 1900–1940', *Journal of American History*, 88:2 (2001), 519–47.
115 *L'espace de vie du malade*, 19.
116 Roekens, *Des murs et des femmes*, 169–74.

117 Beets-Anthonissen, 'Anvers. Hôpital Stuyvenberg', 98.
118 This was the case for the new St-Pierre Hospital and in Brugmann Hospital.
119 This was also an international development, see, for example, D. Theodore, S. D. Burke and A. Adams, 'Tower of power: the Drummond medical building and the interwar centralization of medical practice', *Medical Science and Medical Buildings*, 32/1 (2009), 51–68.
120 F. Danniau, 'Naar een Academisch Ziekenhuis', UGentMemorie, www.ugentmemorie.be/artikel/naar-een-academisch-ziekenhuis (accessed 14 March 2020); G. Deneckere, *Uit de Ivoren Toren. 200 jaar universiteit Gent* (Ghent: Tijdsbeeld, 2017), 134–8.
121 G. Schoefs, F. Lorant and P. Henrion, *La leçon d'anatomie. 500 and de médecine à Liège* (Liège: Now Future, 2017).
122 J. Tollebeek and L. Nys, *De stad op de berg: een geschiedenis van de Leuvense universiteit sinds 1968* (Leuven: Leuven University Press, 2005), 153.
123 L. Nys, *Van mensen en muizen. Vijftig jaar Nederlandstalige faculteit geneeskunde aan de Leuvense universiteit* (Leuven: Leuven University Press, 2016), 159–63.

Selected bibliography

Allegaert, P. et al. (eds), *L'architecture hospitalière en Belgique/Architectuur van de Belgische hospitalen* (Brussels: Ministerie van de Vlaamse Gemeenschap. Afdeling Monumenten en Landschappen, 2004).
Appaduraj, A. (ed.), *The Social Life of Things: Commodities in Cultural Perspective* (Cambridge, UK: Cambridge University Press, 1986).
Bruyneel, E., *De Hoge Gezondheidsraad (1849–2009). Schakel tussen wetenschap en volksgezondheid* (Leuven: Peeters, 2009).
Deblon, V., 'Constructing the illusion of freedom: architecture and psychiatry in nineteenth-century Belgium', *Journal of Belgian History*, 47 (2017), 84–11.
Hamlett, J., *At Home in the Institution: Material Life in Asylums, Lodging Houses and Schools in Victorian and Edwardian England* (Basingstoke: Palgrave Macmillan, 2015).
Henderson, J., Horden, P. and Pastore, A. (eds), *The Impact of Hospitals 300–2000* (Oxford: Peter Lang, 2007).
Lelarge, A., Dickstein-Bernard, C., Guilardian, D. and Le Maire, J. (eds), *Du monumental au fonctionnel: l'architecture des hôpitaux publics bruxellois (XIXe–XXe siècles)* (Brussels: Editions CIVA, 2005).

L'espace de vie du malade à l'hôpital, exhibition at C. H. U. André Vésale à Montigny-le-Tilleul, 17 October–11 November 1990 (Brussels: Association belge des hôpitaux, 1990).

Majerus, B., 'Material objects in twentieth century history of psychiatry', *BMGN: Low Countries Historical Review*, 132:1 (2017), 149–69.

Richelle, S., *Hospices. Une histoire sensible de la vieillesse. Bruxelles, 1830–1914* (Rennes: Presses Universitaires de Rennes, 2019).

Part III

Beyond physicians

8

Dis/order and dis/ability

Benoît Majerus and Pieter Verstraete

On 13 January 1966, Maria V., an ex-patient at the Institute of Psychiatry in Brussels, wrote to her former psychiatrist asking him to provide her with medication to which she was entitled as long as she was in therapy with him:

> I am a sick person who has been cared for by you. I am still sick. I do not feel good. I have vivid dreams and I turn over 30 times every night ... As long as I was taking my medicines, it was ok. Now I have run out of medication and I am sick ... I am now going to see the doctor here, but the doctor no longer wants to prescribe me any medication, he wants you to write a letter stating that he is allowed to prescribe me this medication. Please help me, because I cannot continue to live without medicine.[1]

The letter comes from a patient file kept at this Brussels psychiatric institute. For a long time, histories of mental illness and histories of disability were mainly based on analyses of medical theories as described in scientific journals, textbooks, conference reports, etc., and were presented as progressive narratives. In the last thirty years, the emphasis has shifted from a predominantly medical perspective to one that also tries to include the voices of people with mental illnesses and disabled people themselves.[2] Bygone medical practices are no longer represented as unilateral activities where the initiative was taken only by the doctor, the nurse or another professional and where the targeted individuals passively underwent treatment, rehabilitation or special education. In adopting this new historical approach, historians turned towards neglected source material. As well as handbooks, academic journals, conference proceedings and laws, they drew on a variety of ego-documents and visual source material.

Personal letters and diaries are probably the best known of these sources, but historians also have made use of more tangible material such as works of art, demographic data like birth or death certificates and furniture or garments to underpin this historiographical reorientation.[3] All of these examples can easily be criticised for being too subjective, socially biased and intimately bound to particular contexts. That is of course true. But what is also true is that these sources have given rise to more nuanced and balanced views on what it was to be re-educated in the past, what it meant to be diagnosed as mentally ill and how people tried to align established medical knowledge with personal and/or collective convictions. In short, these new sources have helped to reveal the agency of the patients and individuals that were cared for and/or placed in special education initiatives.

Introducing readers of this book on Belgian medical history to the history of psychiatry and the history of disability simultaneously might seem to be an insurmountable task. Previously, even though several authors have tried to bring the two fields of study together,[4] they have largely remained separate with regard to the topics examined, the journals and conferences where research results are presented, as well as the methods used to explore the past. Indeed, while the history of disability mainly originated from the fruitful efforts of disability activism and critical academic theory in the 1960s and 1970s and has explicitly rejected a purely medical approach towards disability, the history of psychiatry seems to have followed a different historiographical pathway and is still largely situated within medical history.[5] To further problematise this combined discussion of the history of psychiatry and disability, one also can refer to the various conceptual and existential realities that lie behind the notions of illness/syndrome and disability: people diagnosed with mental illnesses or disabled people encounter different bureaucratic challenges, bodily realities and/or societal prejudices.

Despite these historiographical, epistemological, linguistic and existential differences, several reasons nevertheless seem to justify a combined discussion of the history of disability and the history of psychiatry. First, regardless of the manifold discussions about when and why the two categories became separated, there is a widespread and well-accepted narrative that in pre-modern times individuals with physical and mental disabilities were not distinguished from one another and were seen as forming part of the wider community of 'poor people'.[6] The histories of mental illness and disability, however, have more in common than their mere shared origins on the margins of society. Second, it can be observed that the historiographical traditions dealing with psychiatric illness and disability seem to have developed more or less in the same direction in the last twenty years. For just like the history of disability, the history of psychiatry has evolved from a merely encyclopaedic and Whiggish overview of important (and primarily male) doctors and medical inventions to a nuanced and critical approach that also reserves an important place for the voices of those with mental illnesses and takes into account broader social, political and cultural developments.[7]

In light of these general affinities between the historiography of psychiatric illness and disability, this chapter will examine the Belgian history of mental illness and disability by analysing the importance attributed to boundaries. Generally speaking, one can state that there first of all existed a phase that can be described as one in which boundaries are set up and human beings are increasingly classified, segregated from one another or gathered into subgroups. The second and third phases demonstrate an increasing unease with this tendency to demarcate and relegate. These phases are characterised by a desire first to cross and later even to blur the lines of the boundaries established in the first phase.

For a thorough understanding of what follows, three preliminary remarks should be made. First, it is remarkable that although the history of Belgian psychiatry can draw on a rather elaborate tradition, the history of disability in Belgium previously seems to have attracted much less attention from historians.[8] Second, concerning the terminology used, this chapter will speak in terms of disabled people and people with mental illnesses. At times, however, when historical terminology is used, certain terms will be placed in quotation marks. Third, and here the particular nature of the Belgian case immediately becomes clear, the history of disability and psychiatry cannot be written only by referring to doctors. Given the widespread presence of other groups of professionals such as religious orders, social workers, psychologists and pedagogues, a theoretical framework needs to be developed that overcomes the shortcomings associated with a too narrow interpretation of history in terms of medicalisation.

Establishing boundaries

Issues related to disability and mental illness began to be problematised in Belgium towards the end of the eighteenth century, just as in many other European countries. That is not to say that those who could not hear, see, walk or think in a rational way had not attracted particular attention before. Their differences already had been shaped to a certain extent by divergent religious and medical traditions.[9] Despite their particular status, however, the institutionalisation of these individuals remained rather limited. There were places where the poor and the sick were assembled, such as almshouses (*godshuysen* or *dullhuysen*).[10] However, the majority of disabled people and people with mental illnesses lived in the midst of the community in which they grew up. The tendency to segregate them from society and enclose them within the confined walls of an institution occurred to a large extent at the same time as Belgium's independence in 1830. The newly founded Belgian state was convinced that good governance required a detailed description of the population. The Belgian government therefore instigated several statistical enquiries shortly after its independence that led to a better overview of the prevalence of deafness, blindness and mental illness.

With regard to mental illness, in the 1840s the Belgian government asked three experts – Edouard Ducpétiaux, Joseph Guislain and Maurice Sauveur – to draw up a report on the 'mental institutions in the kingdom'. The report concluded that regulations needed to be introduced for the field, which led to the adoption of two laws, one in 1850 and one in 1873, creating a specific institution, the 'mental asylum', and specific professions, 'alienists' and psychiatric keepers. While the latter remained in virtual obscurity until the 1960s, when specific associations were set up, the role of the alienist soon gained professional recognition via two standard means: the establishment of a medical society in 1869,[11] the Belgian Phreniatric Society (Société phréniatrique belge, subsequently the Société de Médecine Mentale de Belgique), and the launch of two scientific journals, the *Bulletin de la Société de Médecine Mentale de Belgique* in 1872 and the *Journal de Neurologie et d'Hypnologie* in 1896 (see Chapter 5, p. 179). Nevertheless, this seemingly early specialisation should not disguise the fact that the field did not develop in a linear way. Psychiatry struggled for recognition in universities. It was some time before psychiatric education became standardised. Throughout the nineteenth century, courses were introduced in Belgian universities only to disappear a few years later. The Catholic University of Leuven was the only higher-education institution to provide a degree over time[12] – probably to some extent because of the important role of religious congregations in psychiatric care. Throughout the nineteenth century, psychiatrists also explored alternative approaches, which are often forgotten today but at the time were considered as viable options: hypnosis, 'pedotechnics', social defence and eugenics.

Just as with psychiatric disorders, statistical enquiries contributed to a heightened awareness of disability and to ever-more strident calls for institutionalisation and professionalisation. Again, it was Sauveur who was asked to map out the prevalence of blindness and deafness in the newly established country.[13] Although when the results were published, institutes for people with sensory disabilities already existed in Brussels and Ghent, the statistical overview led to the emergence of several others as well as the identification of new categories, like deaf-blindness. Indeed, Sauveur's report demonstrated that in Belgium, several deaf-blind individuals existed. In response to this finding, the founder of the Institute for the Deaf and Blind in Bruges, the Flemish priest Charles-Louis Carton, decided to take in the only deaf-blind person who was deemed to be receptive to education, Anna Timmerman.[14]

The use of statistical graphs, tables and figures to clearly illustrate the numbers of disabled people and people with mental illnesses transformed these issues into matters of public concern. What these numbers also catalysed was the idea that state intervention was necessary. But while statistical practices undoubtedly played an important role in the emergence of a more professionalised system for the care and instruction of disabled people and people with mental illness, other developments also need to be taken into account. These demonstrate that institutionalisation cannot solely be explained by referring to the activities of the medical profession. Several other groups of professionals, such as priests, statisticians and pedagogues, also recognised the value of an institutional approach.

Driven by God, money and the lure of work

As in other European countries, the emergence of institutes for deaf and blind people can be seen as part of a broader transformation of how religion and economics were interconnected throughout the Middle Ages. For a very long time indeed, it was common in Western societies to see blind individuals, for example, asking for alms. In return for the money given, the beggars would pray for the soul of the generous benefactor. Although this traditional exchange of money for religious well-being began to be questioned by people like Juan Luis Vives as early as the sixteenth century, it only became more seriously problematised towards the end of the eighteenth century.[15] As a consequence of this general transformation, many of the first handbooks on deaf and blind education reserved an important place for the issue of begging and directed educational efforts towards a vocational outcome (to replace the occupation of begging) for poor disabled people, or a pleasant pastime for disabled people who were wealthy.[16] In line with this European trend, the emergence of educational institutes for deaf and blind people in Belgium also demonstrates this problematisation of existing begging practices. In 1785 in Liège, for instance, Constantin de Hoensbroeck issued a call for essays that focused on the following topic: 'On the means of caring for blind people of both sexes and occupying them with light work of which they are capable, either by grouping them in a public establishment or by providing them with occupations and care at home that will keep them from begging.'[17]

Religion also played an important role in the emergence of a widespread network of care and educational institutions for disabled people and people with mental illnesses. In Belgium, the majority of institutes founded in the nineteenth century were the result of the initiative taken by religious actors/congregations from the early days onwards (see Chapter 2, p. 68). This can partly be explained by the liberal nature of the Belgian government, which consequently decided to intervene as little as possible in the field of charity and social care. This certainly applies to institutionalised care for disabled people. Towards the end of the nineteenth century, the large majority of existing institutes for deaf and blind people were founded and led by members of religious orders.[18]

The same religious predominance can be observed for the care of the mentally ill. The 1850 Mental Treatment Act placed the treatment of psychiatric patients in the hands of private entrepreneurs, and this did not change with the 1873 law. Alongside private secular institutions, religious congregations soon stepped up to the task. Following the periods of French and Dutch rule in Belgium (1794–1814 and 1815–30, respectively) under which the Catholic Church suffered considerably, it subsequently began to recover, especially via the creation of several religious congregations[19] that were involved in teaching and healthcare, particularly psychiatry. These congregations soon came to dominate the field. The first report by the Standing Committee of Psychiatric Asylums (Commission permanente d'inspection des établissements d'aliénés) emphasised that just 27 per cent of establishments housing psychiatric patients had lay keepers; the vast majority of subordinate staff were exclusively or primarily provided by religious congregations. Moreover, twenty-five years later, in 1876, religious staff took care of 74 per cent of psychiatric patients. This high proportion also reflects the fact that even establishments administered by municipal hospice boards (*commissions d'hospices*) or laypeople assigned most supervisory tasks and treatment to congregations.[20] There are several reasons for this. First, it represented a continuation of past practices that were only briefly interrupted by the French Revolution: the involvement of religious communities in treating the poor and sick was typical of the future Belgian territories in the eighteenth century.[21] The other reasons can be divided into ideological and financial dimensions: both the Catholics and the liberals, the two dominant political parties at the time, wanted to restrict the role of the state in the charity sector (albeit for different reasons), and the daily costs of asylums run by religious congregations were much lower than those of institutions run by lay staff. Before the First World War, in Geel, a chief nurse was paid around 1,450 francs, a Mother Superior 600, a nurse around 1,000 and a nun 400.[22]

The politics of ignorance

Although the economic and religious reasons underpinning the emergence of institutionalised care for people with psychiatric illnesses and disabilities are already well known, recent authors have also pointed towards the influence of broader political developments. 'Political' here refers to the different and changing ways of wielding power over others. Towards the end of the eighteenth century, partly as a result of the process of secularisation, it was thought that good governance was dependent on detailed knowledge about the lives and the behaviours of a nation's citizens. Several factors complicated this approach, such as solitude. The value of solitude, for example in religious practices, was increasingly called into question. Solitary people were 'problematic'. One category of people identified with solitude was profoundly deaf people, as it was hard to understand what they were talking about when they communicated using sign language.[23] Several of the early articles on the need to educate profoundly deaf people and blind people alluded to this solitary state. In an anonymous contribution to the *Encyclopaedia Britannica* of 1778, which later was identified as being written by Thomas Blacklock, the political relevance of blind people was referred to in terms of their numbers: blind people were not to be neglected, as they constituted a relatively large proportion of the population. More important, however, according to the author, was the unfortunate nature and the limited capacity to live an active life of blind people who had not received any kind of education or instruction.

This reference to the unfortunate character of non-educated profoundly deaf people and blind people arose time and again throughout the nineteenth century. In Belgium, there is also abundant source material to be found that underlines the importance of the 'unfortunate' trope for the newly established legitimacy of special education. One revealing example is the autobiographical letters that were sent by several pupils at the Institute for the Deaf and the Blind in Bruges to their director Charles-Louis Carton when they graduated. In all of these ego-documents – which were probably commissioned by those in charge of the institute themselves – reference was made to how the pupils thought about the world and about others before having benefited from the positive influence of the education provided at the institute. Louise Ryspeert, for instance, a profoundly deaf girl born in 1844, wrote the following about how she thought about death before entering the institute:

> Mr. Carton, my thoughts about death may perhaps make you laugh. The coffins gave me a sense of horror; I felt sorry for the dead: 'No, I never want to die,' I thought. 'The dead may not come to life anymore,' they might be stifled in their coffin or remain dead in the

absence of food and drink ... I thought that one died when one got a thick neck; I was careful not to eat too much, and all morning I touched my neck to feel whether it was not yet too thick.[24]

By referring to how she thought about the world before entering the institute, Louise underlined the importance of education in ridding her of her irrational and 'uncivilised' thoughts. Although it is not known whether the director made use of these letters, for example in fundraising campaigns, the practice itself demonstrates one of the many ways in which the expertise of particular professionals – in this case, members of religious orders – was promoted and intimately linked to the idea of the institute.

Following a different pathway, one can argue that treatment for people with mental disabilities, at least internationally, arose from the same preoccupation with people's inner thoughts. In France, indeed, the first institutionalised approaches towards children with mental disabilities were the result of the application of phrenological thinking and craniometry practices. Following a long and heated discussion about whether 'idiocy' should be considered as a form of mental illness, the famous psychiatrist Esquirol decided that this was not the case, firmly stating that: 'Idiocy is not a disease, it is a state in which the intellectual faculties have never manifested themselves or have not been able to develop themselves.'[25] Esquirol's definition largely contributed to the established distinction between mental illness and mental disability or intellectual/learning disability. The former refers to a situation where the person is said to require psychiatric treatment. The latter refers to children/adults who need special or inclusive educational programmes.

Despite this early nineteenth-century differentiation between mental illness and disability, the first separate educational initiatives for 'feeble-minded' children only emerged in the 1830s and 1840s, stimulated by the work of Edouard Séguin and French phrenologists such as Belhomme, Voisin and Delasiauve.[26] In Belgium, it was not until 1852–53 that a separate section for mentally disabled children was set up in the psychiatric institute of the Brothers of Charity in Ghent. In the wake of the new legal framework introduced in 1850 that laid down the obligation to provide education to those who could benefit from it, the institute decided to set up *Kinderkoer*, where those who were thought to be receptive to the beneficial influence of education would be educated.[27] In reality, however, children with severe mental disabilities could still frequently be encountered within the confines of a psychiatric institution until well into the twentieth century.

'Pillarisation' and the advent of compulsory education

While the aforementioned religious, economic and political factors clearly played a role in the history of disability and the history of mental illness in Belgium, the discussions about compulsory education in the nineteenth century only seem to have affected the history of disability, even if the discussion on moral treatment can also be viewed in this context. In Belgium, however, the debate remained primarily an intellectual one; it had no real influence on the daily practices of alienists and nurses and the experiences of psychiatric patients.

The rise of special education towards the end of the nineteenth century cannot be understood without including the discussions surrounding the introduction of compulsory education. While in other European countries such as France, the introduction of special classes and schools for so-called feeble-minded children (*enfants retardés*) almost immediately followed the introduction of compulsory education, this was not the case in Belgium. Indeed, the Belgian law that made education for children compulsory was introduced relatively late, in May 1914, whereas the first classes/schools for 'feeble-minded' children had already been founded in Brussels and Antwerp towards the end of the nineteenth century.[28] Therefore, the idea that the introduction of compulsory education forced a large number of children who could not attain required educational standards to attend schools cannot be applied to the Belgian context.

Nevertheless, one should not forget the typically Belgian context of 'pillarisation', which also had a huge impact on the educational landscape. Towards the end of the nineteenth century, the various ideological struggles around schools and schooling – for instance the First School War in 1878 – led to a situation where the majority of children were already going to school. Teachers were therefore confronted with children who had learning difficulties well before the introduction of compulsory education.

While the introduction of compulsory education did not have a huge impact on the care of people with mental illness, it should nevertheless be noted that many proponents of special education for 'feeble-minded' children had a medical background. Doctors such as Auguste Ley and Ovide Decroly played a huge role in the emergence of special schools in Brussels and Antwerp, respectively, around 1900.[29] What is important to note, however, is that these educational activities started to form a kind of institutionalised subfield within the setting of psychiatric care structures.

Taken together, the aforementioned economic, religious, political and educational factors gave rise to a professionalised network of care and educational initiatives. One of the main outcomes of these initiatives was that an ever-increasing number of disabled people and people with mental illnesses became differentiated and institutionalised. Shortly after the turn of the twentieth century, Belgium had six institutes for 'the blind', ten institutes for 'the deaf and dumb', one institute for physically disabled people and several special education classes for 'feeble-minded' children. In 1912, figures from the Standing Committee for the Inspection of Institutions of Alienated Persons referred to 54 psychiatric institutions with approximately 16,000 patients.[30]

The advent and promotion of an institutional approach towards disabled people and people with mental illnesses in Western Europe almost immediately led to counter-initiatives and criticism. Sometimes these initiatives arose within the institute; sometimes they were taken by individuals who did not have specific connections to a particular institution. A good case in point is the nineteenth-century German *Verallgemeinerungsbewegung* (generalisation) movement.[31] Proponents of this movement emphasised the fact that an institutional approach would never lead to a situation where all disabled children were educated in special schools or institutes. Instead, they argued for the integration of disabled children in regular schools as well as an overhaul of teacher training institutes. Although it is unclear to what extent the *Verallgemeinerungsbewegung* led to heated discussions and specific initiatives in Belgium, it is clear that several counter-initiatives paralleled the aforementioned institutional approach.

In what follows, two specific examples of these counter-initiatives will be introduced. The first refers to a long-standing tradition of family care for people with psychiatric disorders. The other looks at the emergence of rehabilitation in the context of the First World War. Both examples demonstrate that the development of an institutional approach did not lead to a situation in which the institute was completely cut off from the rest of the world or where there was no room for more societal care practices. On the contrary, it seems that, at least in the Belgian context, the walls of the institute have always been porous, and the institutional approach has needed to be justified time and again against alternative notions of care, education and treatment.

A disruptive care practice: the Geel colony

When the asylum system faced the first wave of criticism in Europe in the second half of the nineteenth century, many referred to the family colony of Geel as an alternative, a place where the 'insane' lived 'as a family and in freedom', to quote the subheading of a French book published in 1867. And a hundred years later, when a second wave of criticism hit psychiatry in the Western world, Geel was again hailed as a solution: it is not surprising that an American research project, the Geel Family Care Research Project, was launched at a time when anti-psychiatry was seriously undermining psychiatric legitimacy: 'As always, the regime at Geel is alluring, holding out the hope that its ancient practices can still serve as a model for an alternative system of psychiatric care in the community.'[32]

Twice in a century, Geel was held up in international networks on public and mental health (see Chapter 4) as an alternative for dealing with madness, which was traditionally structured through a medical approach, psychiatry and a specific space, the asylum (Figure 8.1). The legend of St Dymphna in the Late Middle Ages inspired the creation of a pilgrimage site in Geel, a village near Antwerp, for those seeking treatment for psychiatric disorders. From the thirteenth century onwards, the families in this village began taking patients into their homes, via a system coordinated by the canons at the Church of St Dymphna. When the Belgian government began introducing regulations for institutions to treat the mentally ill in the 1840s, questions were raised about what would happen to Geel.

Dis/order and dis/ability 295

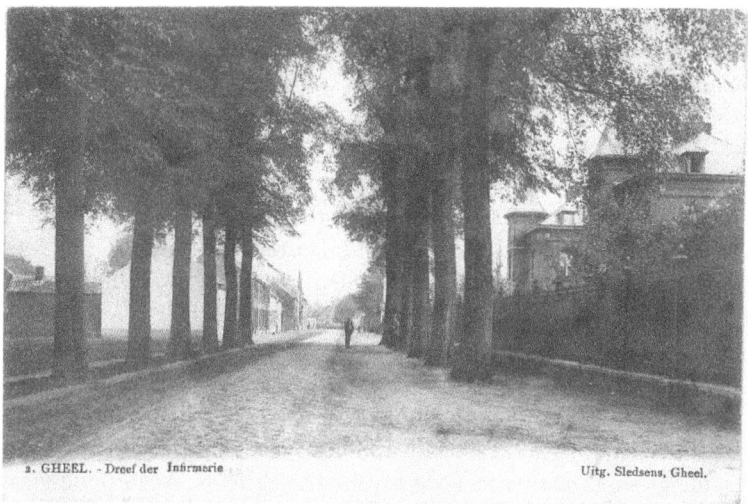

Figure 8.1 Geel – Drève de l'Infirmierie. Postcard.

Unlike other countries such as France, where similar setups did not survive the establishment of the nation state – which brought with it a system of biopolitics that conferred the task of managing psychiatric patients on medical specialists – the Belgian government decided to acknowledge the existence of this system for treating the mentally ill by creating a 'state-run colony for the family-based treatment of mental problems' in 1850.[33] Although this involved a degree of 'medicalisation' – the decision to assign patients to households was now in the hands of a doctor – it was a long way from the general tendency to intern patients in asylums that characterised most of the systems introduced in the latter part of the nineteenth century.

However – and this is a point that is often raised – Geel did not welcome all psychiatric patients. 'Raging madmen or madwomen' and 'senile' patients were not accepted. The town of Geel was divided into sectors, each administered by a doctor. Regulation was introduced to clarify the rights and duties of host families, who could be stripped of their permission to take in patients if they failed to comply. Finally, a patient record was created for each person treated in Geel. So although the mid nineteenth century represented a break with previous centuries, with the state partly taking back control via doctors and the considerable sway they held over patients and especially their families, the situation in Geel remained unusual in that the patients living there enjoyed relative freedom.

While patient numbers varied considerably over the nineteenth and twentieth centuries – from 850 in the early 1860s to more than 3,000 by the beginning of the Second World War – they remained high, despite a significant fall after the Second World War, with 1,700 patients in the late 1960s. In this rural town, patients represented up to a quarter of the population: their presence was seen as a normal part of everyday life. Accounts of people walking in town and engaging in conversation with passers-by, not aware that they were talking to patients, can be found in most reports about Geel, both in the Belgian and European mainstream press and in debates on the treatment of psychiatric patients. Anthropological work in the 1970s showed a more ambiguous picture. Lodgers were accepted in the public sphere, as the following notes from an anthropologist's notebook describing a march by a brass band show: 'A middle-aged resident, rather small in stature, accompanies the brass band to the side of the road: he waves his arm to the rhythm of the music ... This patient wears a smart suit, very neat. His tie is rather improvised and he wears shabby, inelegant shoes on his feet. He thus accompanies the brass band, approximately at the same level as the drum major, on the side of the road, but slightly in front of the road.'[34] His presence was tolerated for the whole march. But at the same time, lodgers were segregated in cafes, where they were not integrated into 'normal' social circles and were not members of local associations, despite no explicit rules banning them from membership.

Geel became the focus of attention during the contentious discussions about psychiatry in the late nineteenth century, which looked at issues such as the role of psychiatry and 'no restraint' and notions of 'recovery' and 'chronicity'. It was described by some as a place 'that could help asylums get rid of incurable patients who were taking up room and preventing them from carrying out their real mission as hospitals dispensing treatment'.[35] But Geel's management did not agree with this vision, which reduced it to a centre for the chronically ill, and used statistics to argue that recovery figures were just as good as in other asylums in Belgium, if not better.

For Geel's opponents, the relative lack of doctors, more liberal regulation and less direct supervision all ran counter to the paradigm on which psychiatry had developed and gained professional recognition: the asylum as a place that protects psychiatric patients from the abuse they suffer in their local communities. The many visitors to Geel even pointed to a 'lack of science',[36] an assertion Geel's supporters countered by emphasising that the isolated conditions within closed asylum structures were medically counterproductive for psychiatric patients.

Although other countries introduced similar systems – Veldwijk (1886) in the Netherlands, Dun-sur-Auron (1892) in France and Uchtspringe (1894) in Germany – Belgium was unique in the Western world for the sheer number of psychiatric patients treated via this system. No other country had such a high proportion of psychiatric patients living with families: in 1900 in Belgium, nearly 3,000 patients were hosted by families (mostly in Geel) out of a total of 16,300 psychiatric patients interned.[37]

While Geel was held up as a model for theoretical discussions among alienists, the system also had a considerable economic impact in several areas, from the local to the transnational level. For the families hosting patients, it often brought considerable economic benefits. In a region of Belgium with little industrial activity, accepting patients, most of whom could be given farming work to do, provided host families with regular additional income because of the allowances they were paid. But in times of high inflation – especially during the two world wars – it was no longer economically advantageous to take in patients, and the institution had difficulties finding host families. Similarly, if the required medical checks became too restrictive, families sometimes opted out. The interest from local communities was often matched by a desire from Belgian town and city councils to reduce costs: they had to pay a significant proportion of the expenses required for psychiatric patients and could make savings by placing them in Geel rather than in asylums. This economic model was even appealing to neighbouring countries: in 1938, of the 3,000 'boarders' in Geel, 754 came from the Netherlands.[38]

When the asylum model came under increasing scrutiny in the 1960s, Geel (and to a lesser extent Lierneux[39]) was the focus of much attention. At a time when Geel itself was experiencing difficulties – with the industrialisation of agriculture and the need for fewer labourers, the number of willing host families began to dwindle – for many it was seen as an exemplary model for community-based psychiatry that should be developed. L'Equipe, the first sector-based mental health service in Belgium, set up in 1963, can clearly be seen as a continuation of Geel – and not just because its first director, Jean Vermeylen, was born in Geel and his psychiatrist father worked there.[40]

In/out: the challenge of re-education and reintegration

A second example of the porous nature of boundaries can be found at the beginning of the twentieth century. At the outbreak of the First World War, Belgium had a well-established network of care and educational institutes for disabled people, but the state largely remained in the background.[41] This hands-off approach drastically changed through the war years, 1914–18, in response to the impact of the new industrialised warfare. With the sheer scale of the conflict and the introduction of new military weapons such as toxic gases, machine guns and tanks, the First World War destroyed the minds and lives of millions of men and women.[42] Belgian military forces were affected too, and as early as 1915 the Ministry of War decided to open a professional rehabilitation institute for those soldiers who had one or more amputated limbs, had lost their sight or had other bodily problems.[43]

Although at this time only disabled soldiers were said to fall under the responsibility of the state, this radical shift in the government's attitude towards disabled people would have a lasting effect on the overall relationship between the state and disabled people. Alongside religious congregations and other private initiatives, the state increasingly became an important player in the development of overall care and educational system for disabled people. The First World War also had an impact on the vocabulary used to speak about disabled people. The pension system, for instance, set up by the state to financially remunerate the sacrifice made by disabled soldiers, undoubtedly contributed to the spread of thinking in terms of percentages when dealing with disabled individuals. But although shell-shocked soldiers were considered as 'invalid' soldiers

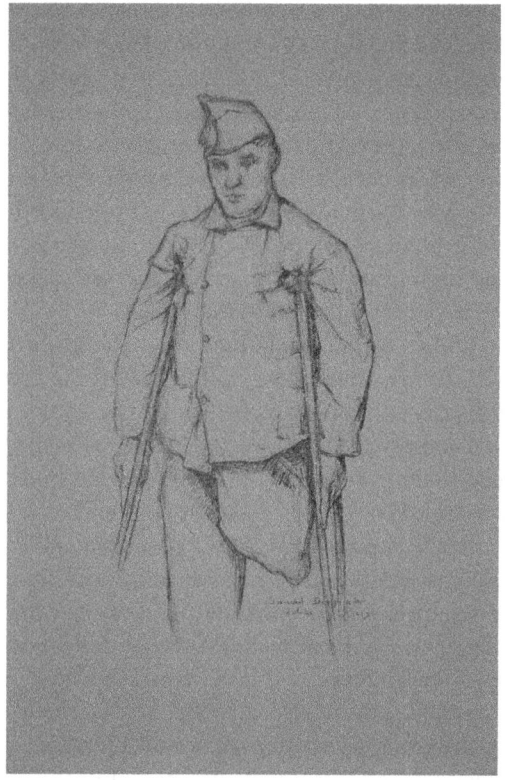

Figure 8.2 'Invalide' – drawing by Samuel De Vriendt, dated 1923, Woluwé.

at that time, the Great War had a much less significant impact on post-war Belgian psychiatric developments (Figure 8.2).[44]

As well as reconfiguring the position of the state towards disabled people, the Great War also had an impact on existing care practices in another area, in that it emphasised the importance of work. Preparing pupils for a life of work in the community had already been on the agenda of educational institutes for some time. The Great War, however, clearly highlighted the importance of work as part of care and educational practices. The main aim of the war-related rehabilitation discourse was to restore invalid soldiers to full fitness in economic terms, to restore their bodily powers and desire to work. On top of that, the fact that these individuals were adult men also opened up a relatively new field, that of adult special education. Again, this was not completely new, since during the nineteenth century several initiatives had also been launched to expand care and education to those pupils who graduated from institutes for 'the blind' and 'the deaf and dumb'.[45] But these initiatives mostly occurred within the confines of the institutes. What becomes clear when we look at what happened in the context of care for blind people is that in the immediate aftermath of the war, four organisations were set up and were almost entirely dedicated to caring for adult blind individuals.[46]

Given the impact of the rehabilitation discourse on the nature of and approach to care practices, it can be seen as the culmination of an idea that had been fermenting for some time within the confines of educational and psychiatric institutes, namely that the scope of the institute needed to be expanded, both geographically and existentially. Another example taken from the history of disability can further illustrate this point: the major debate between oralism and manualism in issues related to deaf education. Just like in other Western European countries, Belgium was confronted with increasing criticism for the use of sign language in educational institutes.[47] Influenced by eugenicist thinking, sign language had been associated with 'animal' and immoral behaviour. It was also claimed that teaching deaf people to communicate using sign language would ultimately harm them, since once they left the institution they would not be able to communicate with speaking people in society. Reflecting these and other arguments, it was decided at an 1880 conference of directors of Western institutes for deaf people that from that moment onwards sign language would be prohibited in deaf institutes.

Recent historical research has demonstrated that the move from manualism to oralism should not be interpreted as a radical shift but as a gradual process. This was also the case for Belgian institutes that provided schooling for deaf pupils, such as at the Ghent Institute for the Deaf-Mute. In an unpublished document, Sister Ghislena Spillemaekers described the separation between pupils who were still allowed to use sign language and those who were not:

> Given the fact that one already needed to tackle a shortage of available rooms [before the introduction of the oral method], achieving the separation depended on considerable cooperation and foresight,

vigilance, surveillance and extra sacrifice from the staff ... As the number of speaking pupils rose, they were given more premises, but the glass doors along which they could have come into contact with the elderly [those who still were allowed to sign] were always carefully covered with curtains.[48]

The gradual move from manualism to oralism represents a broader evolution in which people increasingly started to question the role and the actual functioning of psychiatric and disability institutes. More and more attention was directed to the conditions of those living outside the institute. What people learned in institutes and how they were cared for of course remained important, but these aspects were increasingly accompanied by questions as to how life in the institute would eventually lead to a more or less successful life in society itself. The central place attributed to work in these discourses, however, sometimes stands in stark contrast with the lived realities of the disabled people themselves. One example is what happened with the Belgian war-blinded, who, just like other physically disabled soldiers, were retrained for a new trade or profession.[49]

Among the eighty-eight officially recognised Belgian blinded soldiers, some were able to fulfil the high expectations to be found within the discourse of rehabilitation, but some who were not. Isidore van Vlasselaer, for instance, was described in a personal file that can be found at the Royal Archives in Brussels as a courageous man of good moral character.[50] According to the author of the report, he seemed perfectly happy at home and occupied himself with his son's studies. He would have been happy to go to Brussels to be retrained at the Royal Institute for the Belgian War-Blinded were it not for the fact that he would have to leave his wife and son behind. The report stated that if circumstances allowed, Van Vlasselaere would voluntarily come to Brussels.[51] The life of the blinded soldier Julien Dhont, however, was very different as it was described as extremely painful, both morally and physically: 'He enjoys all his intelligence, he hears everything but no longer knows how to communicate by any means with the outside world: he cannot express a desire or make known his physical needs either orally or in writing.'[52] As well as demonstrating the existential challenges raised by the institutional approach, these two references to the personal lives of two Belgian war-blinded soldiers also make another point clear, namely the fact that education and educational qualities were increasingly affected by decision-making processes that gave rise to official and powerful statements about individuals' futures. Based on this kind of expertise, several groups of professionals would very soon start to compete with one another to safeguard or expand their sphere of activity.

Blurring boundaries

Ever since an institutionalised network of care and education structures for disabled people and people with mental illnesses emerged in the early 1800s, the envisioned boundaries have continuously been subject to criticism. Although these critical voices and activities led to a substantial number of initiatives that ultimately established bridges between society and the institutional archipelago, until the 1960s the care, education and treatment of disabled people and people with psychiatric disorders remained dominated by an institutional approach. Just like in other countries, the legitimacy of the institution was increasingly questioned, leading not only to a crossing of institutional boundaries but also to a blurring of the borders that separated the institution from society. While, to a certain extent, scholars have already begun to examine these processes on an international level and for other countries, there is little to no information available about Belgium. It nevertheless seems a promising and necessary field of study given the trend towards inclusion that started in the late 1970s and early 1980s, as well as the sometimes ahistorical interpretations of this movement. The second half of the twentieth century is often presented as a monolithic period in which people with psychiatric illnesses and disabilities were finally taken out of institutes. While to a certain extent this holds in Belgium for disabled people, the hypothesis runs into difficulties when applied to care infrastructures for people with mental illnesses. Special educational initiatives have indeed been increasingly criticised, and eventually this movement led to the introduction of the M-Decree in the Flemish-speaking part of Belgium in 2015. This decree stipulates that children with special educational needs should in principle be educated in mainstream schools and not relegated to a system of special schools. Although the story of the introduction of this inclusive approach towards the education of disabled people remains to be written, it seems to be very much in line with other innovative care practices that have been introduced for disabled people. One of these is the introduction of the personal assistance budget (see Chapter 6, p. 232), which will be described in what follows.

While the introduction of the M-Decree in 2015 and the development of the personal assistance budget did indeed seem to confirm the trend towards more inclusive approaches to care and special education, they do not tell the full story. There is of course much more to say about the second half of the twentieth century. Not only did particular segregational approaches continue to exist, but it is also important to point out that some inclusive practices, as well as some of our historical interpretations of these inclusive practices, seem to misguide us. A good case in point here is the deinstitutionalisation movement. Just like in other countries, Belgium too was affected by ideas inspired by the international antipsychiatry movement. However, when one takes a closer look at how the precise numbers of beds that were available in psychiatric institutions between 1960 and 2000 developed, it seems logical to conclude that these ideas led to the increased inclusion of people with psychiatric illnesses. Taken together, the numerical approach to psychiatric inclusion in Belgium and the stories behind the introduction of the personal assistance budget seem to necessitate more complex frameworks if we are to understand the particularities of the history of special care and education initiatives in the second half of the twentieth century.

Deinstitutionalisation ... and its limits

Just like in other Western countries, the role of institutions – whether schools, barracks or hospitals – was strongly contested from the 1960s onwards in Belgium. The iatrogenic nature of asylums and institutes for disabled people was particularly emphasised. Several organisations were particularly vocal in their criticism, the most well known being the Groupe d'Études pour une Réforme de la Médecine (GERM), a think tank for medical reform, and Groupe information asiles (GIA), an information group on asylums.

Strongly inspired by a similar group set up by Michel Foucault and others in 1972 in France, GIA was composed of doctors, nurses, psychologists, social workers and asylum patients. Psychiatrists had lost their monopoly: not only did other professionals contest their knowledge, but also patients whose accounts had long been considered as proof of their condition were now taken seriously. It was the first time that former psychiatric patients (*ex-psychiatrisés*, as they called themselves) had become publicly involved in this field. They were able to contribute their unique experience and expertise, which was particularly valued in this movement. The former psychiatric patients in GIA were members of the Mouvement de libération des marginaux mentaux (Movement for the liberation of marginalised psychiatric patients).

Nevertheless, the idea of deinstitutionalisation remained problematic. The number of beds in psychiatric institutions decreased very slowly from 27,303 in 1958 to 25,536 in 1973 and 23,220 in 1982. The high level of institutionalisation made Belgium an exception inside Europe.[53] Belgium was also witnessing significant growth in other institutions that housed patients previously interned in psychiatric asylums – 'oligophrenic patients' (now referred to as mentally disabled people) and elderly people. There was a significant increase in medical-educational establishments for mentally disabled patients from the 1960s onwards. Between 1972 and 1979, they doubled in number and their capacity rose from 18,000 to 25,000 patients.[54] While this led to the removal of disabled patients from psychiatric asylums, where they had represented a significant proportion of the population,[55] the patients were transferred to other institutions (Figure 8.3).

The same was true for elderly people. The general inspector for asylums in the Ministry of Public Health, Edmond Bruyninckx, estimated in 1957 that a third of interned patients were aged over seventy.[56] In this area too, the 1970s saw an increase in capacity but also a change in the nature of the care offered. First, there was an increase in new institutions for elderly people – in the early 1970s, the Belgian government planned not only for the addition of 4,500 beds for elderly people over a seven-year period,[57] but also for the creation of new institutions for geriatric psychiatry. Second, rest homes, which had a capacity of almost 60,000 beds in 1970, were gradually turned into nursing homes so that they could house a more fragile elderly population.

Dis/order and dis/ability 305

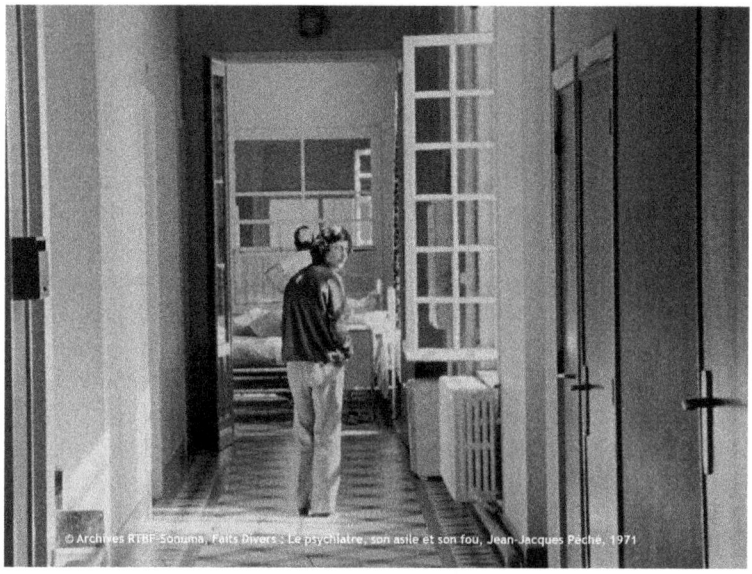

Figure 8.3 Excerpt from the 1971 television programme 'Faits divers' about the Lovenjoel Psychiatric Hospital.

Rather than deinstitutionalisation, a more appropriate term would be 'transinstitutionalisation', even if other less institutionalised structures were also beginning to emerge. In Belgium, the latter were essentially organised within the CSM network (Centres de santé mentale or mental health centres). In addition to these centres, other more radical alternatives to institutional psychiatry were starting to be developed. While this was not exclusive to Brussels,[58] the Belgian capital did see a large number of initiatives of this nature. This can probably be explained by the absence of a strong Catholic influence – which had a particularly restrictive effect in Flanders – and the wave of protest led by the Université libre de Bruxelles.

These CSMs demonstrate how the idea of deinstitutionalisation can be seen as part of the broader sweep of the history of psychiatry in the twentieth century. They developed from the Ligue nationale belge d'hygiène mentale (National Belgian League for Mental Hygiene), which was set up in 1923. Inspired by a movement launched by a former psychiatric patient, Clifford Beers, in the United States in 1908, the league promoted treatment outside the confines of institutions and encouraged the notion of 'mental health'. The League was involved in several prevention campaigns (tackling drug addiction, diagnosing 'abnormal' children, etc.) and opened dispensaries – there were eleven in Belgium as of 1933. After the war, from 1953 onwards, the Belgian government began funding these dispensaries, and in 1975, a new legislative framework gave greater clarity to their role and incorporated them into a broader public health policy similar to the sectorisation policy pursued in France.

In 1972, 32 CSMs for adults were affiliated to the league, offering treatment for more than 8,000 adults in Belgium. Compared with the 25,000 patients in psychiatric establishments, this figure was certainly not negligible. Over the following decade, the number of centres quadrupled – by the late 1970s, Belgium had 135 CSMs – but there was a distinct regional imbalance. While the situation in Brussels reflected the standards laid down in the royal decree adopted in 1975, with one centre for 50,000 inhabitants, Flanders lagged behind – of the 113 centres planned, there were only 59.[59]

The League stipulated four categories of services that CSMs should provide: 'medical services', 'psychological services', 'social services' and 'psychotherapy and rehabilitation'.[60] We will look in more detail at how they worked in practice by examining two of the Brussels-based institutions, those in Anderlecht and Saint-Gilles. These two centres emphasise the heterogeneous nature of CSMs. The Anderlecht-based L'Equipe, set up very early on in 1961, became a key centre in terms of the diversity of services it provided (aftercare, day care, occupational rehabilitation, occupational therapy, etc.), and also its role as a flagship institution. It served as a benchmark in the 1970s and 1980s for advocates of the CSM system. It produced a considerable volume of highly visible scientific research, which helped legitimise this social approach to psychiatry. The centre in Saint-Gilles was set up fourteen years later and was essentially just a consultation centre.

But the two institutions did have some points in common. They were both based in urban areas, unlike most psychiatric establishments, which tended to be situated in the countryside or on the outskirts of towns. This urban setting also facilitated close cooperation with other players. In its first annual report, the Saint-Gilles CSM provided a list of the bodies it worked with, which included the social workers in the Commission d'Assistance

Publique (CAP, or Public Welfare Committee), the town's police department and social services, the Little Sisters of the Assumption, the Jewish social services, the parish assistance and support group, polyclinics in the town and the Association of Belgian and Immigrant Women.[61]

The rise of neo-liberal care practices

Another way to illustrate the tendency not just to cross borders but also to blur them is to take a closer look at the introduction of the personal assistance budget in the Flemish region of Belgium. The personal assistance budget revolutionises the traditional care structure by directly giving a certain amount of money to disabled people that they can use to pay for the help they need. Since the money can be used to pay for care in an institution, this new approach cannot be put on a par with deinstitutionalisation. However, what is undoubtedly involved in the introduction of this new scheme is a reversal of the traditional relationship between expert and patient. The personal assistance budget is based on the idea that there is no better expert than the disabled person. He or she knows best what is best for him or her.

The introduction of the personal assistance budget in Belgium can only be understood when seen in the context of what happened in the United States during the 1970s, when Edward Roberts, who was paralysed after contracting polio when he was fourteen years old, started his studies at the University of California, Berkeley.[62] Roberts experienced a huge number of practical issues as he used an iron lung. This huge machine that took over his respiratory functions made it impossible for him to rent a regular student room on campus. The solution that was sought for Roberts, being lodged in the campus hospital, eventually led to the foundation of the Center for Independent Living, an organisation that continued to call for a reorganisation of existing care structures for disabled people in the light of values such as autonomy, emancipation and participation.

It was Roberts's Center for Independent Living and its corresponding ideas that eventually, after passing through Sweden, affected the Flemish care landscape in the 1980s. Midway through the decade, two disabled Flemish people, Jan-Jan Sabbe and Luc Demarez, asked to meet with the Swedish professor Sven-Olof Brattgard to talk about the concept of *Fokuswonen*. Unfortunately, Brattgart could not meet them as he was sick, so Sabbe and Demarez needed to reorganise their study trip. In the end, they met Adolf Ratzka, who had taken up Roberts's ideas and introduced them to Sweden. Inspired by this meeting, in 1987 the two decided to organise a day to explore the issue of housing for disabled people. Ratzka was invited but cancelled at the last minute because of illness. His lecture, however, which was entitled 'Opstand van de verzorgden', was read aloud and not ignored, with a summary being published in a leading Belgian journal. One of the issues that caught the attention of the journalist was the idea of personal assistants: 'These are not nurses, educators, helpers or people who think they know better than the disabled person what is good for them and how everything has to be done. No, assistants are employees who carry out tasks according to the wishes of the disabled employer.'[63]

The first experiments with the personal assistance budget that were conducted in the early 1990s should not, of course, be interpreted in the sense that disabled people had previously never occupied the position of employer. Instead, what the introduction of the independent living idea brought about was an official recognition of the informal status of employer. The first steps towards the official introduction of the personal assistance budget were taken in 1992 when a steering group, Cliëntgebonden budget, was founded. However, it was not until 1995 that Minister Wivina Demeester started a one-year experiment to give twenty disabled people an individual budget each that they could use to pay for the care they needed.

The government's reluctance was not well received by several groups of disabled people. Through lawsuits and public demonstrations, they fought for their right to make autonomous decisions about what kind of care they needed and how this care should best be organised.[64] One example is the lawsuit filed by Jan-Jan Sabbe in 1989 against the Public Centre for Social Welfare (OCMW), which did not want to cover the additional living costs caused by his disability. Another example is the protests by the public action group Genoeg gerold! on 18 November 1994. That day, Minister Wivina Demeester gave a lecture at an academic gathering that focused on 'integration by means of technical aids'. Given the problems with reimbursement of such measures – as a result of the system organised by Demeester's ministry – several groups of disabled people found it highly ironic that she had come to speak at this event, and they therefore disrupted her presentation.

The outcome of these and many other events was that disabled people – at least in theory – stopped being seen as dependent, passive and 'pathological' individuals. Instead, the voices they raised, the actions they organised and the allies they mobilised time and again emphasised the fact that they were people like anybody else. While their pleas were heeded on several sides, it is also important to note that their voices were coupled with a new neo-liberal conception of care.

Conclusion

The Belgian history of disability and mental illness can be written as a complex and often contradictory narrative of boundaries. Just like in many other Western countries, approaches to physical disability and mental illness – the lived realities connected to the terms, as well as the terms themselves – are the outcome of several eighteenth-century processes that led to the problematisation of particular lifestyles. Not being able to see, hear, walk or think in a 'logical' way was increasingly seen as a problem that should be taken care of in a professional context where appropriate care, education and instruction could be given. The boundaries that were established in order to gather and contain the people concerned were manifold and clearly present: one can think of the tangible brick walls that enclose an institute, the straitjackets used in psychiatric asylums and the material obstacles encountered by disabled people who wanted to participate in society. However, this list should also include non-tangible boundaries such as widespread attitudes of pity and the dominant views on how we 'should' communicate with one another. All of these boundaries are real and have shaped the lives of disabled people and those with psychiatric disorders as well as those who can be identified as professionals.

And these boundaries have never been radically removed. People have always looked out for cracks in the walls, for openings that would enable them to transgress the boundaries or explore more societal care practices. In contrast to what is often implicitly accepted, these crossings of boundaries have always paralleled the very establishment of the boundaries themselves. What the Belgian case study described here also makes clear is that although these boundaries were transgressed from the moment they were established, their legitimacy has been increasingly challenged from the 1960s onwards. While many other scholars have already described this in some detail, what our Belgian case study makes clear is that the outcome of these processes can and should be analysed critically. A common understanding of deinstitutionalisation, for example, cannot be found by exploring the history of mental illness in Belgium. When one considers the neo-liberal empowerment of disabled people that was and is implied in the introduction of the personal assistance budget, several critical questions can immediately be raised.

While the very presence of boundaries, the reality of their transgression and the counterproductive consequences of the critical movements that originated in the 1960s are of course not unique to the Belgian context, there are nevertheless various aspects that do make the Belgian case study unique. First and foremost, unlike other European countries deaf and blind people were almost always taken care of in the same institutions. Second, religious communities played a huge role in Belgium, and state involvement came at a relatively late stage compared to other Western countries. Third, the history of special education cannot solely be understood by means of the existing historical frameworks, which mainly focus on the introduction of compulsory education in order to explain the emergence of special schools.

Notes

1 'Ik ben een zieke die bij u verzorgt is geweest. Ik ben nog steeds ziek. Ik voel mij niet goed. Ik droom 's nachts. Draai mij wel 30 keer rond in een nacht ... Nu zoolang ik mijn medicamenten innam ging het nog. Maar nu heb ik geen medicamenten meer en nu be ik ziek hoor ... Ik ga nu hier naar de dokter maar de dokter wil mij geen medicamenten meer voorschrijiven, hij verlangt een brief van u waarin staat dat hij

mij die medicamenten mar voorschrijiven. a.u.b. Wilt u mij helpen, want zonder medicamenten kan ik hensch niet verder'. Archives du CPAS, Institut de Psychiatrie, Ancienne Série, no. 13500. The name of the patient has been anonymised.
2 A. Bacopoulos-Viau and A. Fauvel, 'The patient's turn: Roy Porter and psychiatry's tales, thirty years on', *Medical History*, 60:1 (2016), 1–18.
3 B. Majerus, 'Material objects in twentieth century history of psychiatry', *BMGN: Low Countries Historical Review*, 132:1 (2017), 149–69. See also S. De Veirman, 'Deaf and disabled? (Un)employment of deaf people in Belgium: a comparison of eighteenth-century and nineteenth-century cohorts', *Disability and Society*, 30:3 (2015), 460–74.
4 See, for instance, L. Bradley, 'A mad fight: psychiatry and disability activism', in *The Disability Studies Reader*, ed. L. J. Davis (New York: Routledge, 2013), 115–31; B. Linker, 'On the borderland of medical and disability history: a survey of the fields', *Bulletin of the History of Medicine*, 87:4 (2013), 499–535; and S. Gilman, 'Madness', in *Keywords for Disability Studies*, ed. R. Adams, B. Reiss and D. Serlin (New York: New York University Press, 2015), 114–19.
5 For a good introduction to (the history of) disability history, see, for instance, C. J. Kudlick, 'Disability history: why we need another "other"', *American Historical Review*, 108:3 (2003), 763–93. For the history of psychiatry, see G. Eghigian (ed.), *The Routledge History of Madness and Mental Health* (London: Taylor & Francis, 2017).
6 The best-known example of this approach probably is Michel Foucault's *Le grand renfermement*, which is situated in the second half of the seventeenth century. Although heavily criticised, the gist of Foucault's argument has been taken up by other scholars like Henri-Jacques Stiker, who in his book *A History of Disability* discusses at length the historical category of 'the poor'. M. Foucault, *Histoire de la folie à l'âge classique* (Paris: Plon & Stiker, 1961); H.-J. Stiker, *A History of Disability* (Ann Arbor: University of Michigan Press, 1997)
7 See, for instance, the introductory chapter to P. K. Longmore and L. Umansky (eds), *The New Disability History: American Perspectives* (New York: New York University Press, 2000).
8 For a recent overview of the history of psychiatry, see the special issue of the *Journal of Belgium History*, 4 (2017). No comprehensive academic overview of the history of disability in Belgium has been published yet. The interested reader can find bits and pieces that zoom in on particular fragments, such as a history of deaf people, an introduction to the rehabilitation of physically mutilated First World War soldiers, the impact of the Great War on the emancipation of blind people in Belgium in the interwar period and an analysis of the visual representation of

'mentally retarded' patients at the Guislain institute. See L. Raemdonck and I. Scheiris, *Ongehoord Verleden. Dove frontvorming in België aan het begin van de 20ste eeuw* (Ghent: Fevlado-Diversus, 2007); C. van Everbroeck and P. Verstraete, *Verminkte stilte: De Belgische invalide soldaten van de Groote Oorlog* (Namur: Presses universitaires de Namur, 2014); P. Verstraete, 'Remastering independence: the re-education of Belgian blinded soldiers of the Great War, 1914–1940', *Educacio i Historia*, 19:31 (in press); and P. Devlieger, I. Grosvenor, F. Simon, G. van Hove and B. Vanobbergen, 'Visualising disability in the past', *Paedagogica Historica*, 44:6 (2008), 747–60. The different levels of attention from historians can also be appreciated by taking a closer look at how heritage is dealt with. In the case of mental illness, Belgium has a well-known cultural institution that focuses on the history of psychiatry from an artistic point of view (Museum Dr Guislain). Although there are also several museums dedicated, for instance, to the history of blind or deaf people in Belgium, these are much less well known by the general public.

9 For an overview of medical literature concerning profoundly deaf people and blind people, see, for instance, C. Guyot and R. T. Guyot, *Liste littéraire philocophe ou catalogue d'étude de ce qui a été publié jusqu'à nos jours sur les sourds-muets; sur l'oreille, l'ouïe, la voix, le langage, la mimique, les aveugles etc. etc.* (Amsterdam: N. V. Boekhandel & Antiquariaat B. M. Israël, [1842] 1967).

10 In Bruges, for example, a home for fourteen blind individuals is thought to have been founded in 1304 by Count de Béthune. In memory of this event the city of Bruges organises a *Blindekensprocessie* every year. There is little to no information to be found with regard to the blind inhabitants of that charitable institution, however. Anon., *Oorsprong & vermaerdheyd der Kappelle van O.L.V. van het blinde lieden Gasthuys, gezeyd Blindekens, binnen Brugge, Ter oorzaek van den vij-honderd-jarigen jubilé, den 15 augustus 1815* (Bruges: Weduwe De Moor en Zoon, 1815).

11 This was the second association of specialists to be created in Belgium. See K. Velle, *De nieuwe biechtvaders: de sociale geschiedenis van de arts in België* (Leuven: Kritak, 1991), 112.

12 B. Majerus, 'Een fragmentarische geschiedenis van de Belgische psychiatrie (19de – 20ste eeuw)', *Geschiedenis der geneeskunde*, 14:2 (2010), 92.

13 D. Sauveur, *Note sur la statistique des sourds-muets de la Belgique* (Brussels: n.pub., 1835). One of the publications where the impact of Sauveur's statistical overview on the emergence of education for disabled people can be seen is the journal that was published in 1837

and 1838 by Charles-Louis Carton, the founder of the Institute for the Blind and Deaf in Bruges: *Le sourd-muet et l'aveugle*.
14 P. Verstraete and Y. Söderfeldt, 'Deaf-blindness and the institutionalization of special education in 19th century Europe', in *Disability History Handbook*, ed. M. Rembis, K. Nielsen and C. Kudlick (Oxford: Oxford University Press, 2015), 265–80.
15 For a good discussion of government action towards the poor, see G. Procacci, *Gouverner la misère. La question sociale en France 1789–1848* (Paris: Seuil, 1993). Applied to the history of disability, see P. Verstraete, 'The politics of activity: emergence and development of educational programs for people with disabilities between 1750 and 1860', *History of Education Review*, 38:1 (2009), 78–90.
16 See one of the first essays on the education of blind people that was published by Valentin Haüy in 1784: *Essay sur l'éducation des aveugles*. In the opening chapter of the essay Haüy clearly states that the main goal of the educational institute was: 'Pmo. Pour occuper agréablement ceux d'entr'eux qui vivent dans un état aisés Sdo. Pour arracher à la mendicité ceux qui ne sont point avantagés des faveurs de la Fortune, en leur donnant des moyens de subsistance; & rendre enfin à la société leurs bras ainsi que ceux de leurs conducteurs' (7–8) ('First of all, to pleasantly occupy those of them who live in a well-to-do state. Second, to snatch from begging those who do not benefit from the favours of fortune, by giving them means of subsistence; and finally give back to society their arms and those of their conductors.')
17 'Sur les moyens d'entretenir les aveugles des deux sexes et de les occuper utilement par un travail léger et dont ils soient capables, soit en les rassemblant dans un établissement public, soit en leur procurant chez eux des occupations et des secours qui les mettent à l'abri de la mendicité'. G. Claes, *Blindenonderwijs en blindenzorg in België (1835–1880)* (Leuven: Niet gepubliceerde licentiaatsverhandeling, Faculteit Letteren en Wijsbegeerte, KU Leuven, 1972), 16.
18 It should be noted that the Belgian practice of housing deaf and blind people together in a single institution is rather atypical when compared to other European countries.
19 Between 1800 and 1892, eleven male and seventy-one female congregations were created in Belgium. See C. Dhaene and L. Dhaene, *Sint-Jozef Kortenberg. Van 'Maison de Santé' tot Universitair Centrum. 145 jaar zorg voor geesteszieken, 1850–1995* (Kortenberg: Universitair centrum Sint-Jozef, 1995), 26.
20 *Onzième rapport sur la situation des asiles d'aliénés du Royaume (1874–1876)* (Brussels: Fr. Gobbaerts, 1878), 8.

21 W. van Waesberghe, 'Het Belgische Krankzinnigenbeleid in de XIXde eeuw', *Annales de la Société Belge d'Histoire des Hôpitaux et de la Santé publique*, 22 (1984), 80–1.
22 'Asiles – colonies d'aliénés de Gheel. Personnel. Fixation du taux des traitements, ainsi que du taux moyen des émoluments tenant lieu de supplément de traitement (15 mai 1912)', in *Recueil des circulaires, instructions et autres actes émanés du ministère de la justice ou relatifs à ce département* (Brussels: n.pub., 1912), 194–7.
23 For this line of thought, see P. Verstraete, 'Savage solitude: the problematisation of disability at the turn of the eighteenth century', *Paedagogica Historica*, 45:3 (2009), 269–89; and Y. Söderfeldt and P. Verstraete. 'From comparison to indices: a disabling perspective on the history of happiness', *Health, Culture and Society*, 5:1 (2013), 249.
24 Letter from Louise Ryspeert to Charles-Louis Carton, Bruges, 19 April 1862 (Charles-Louis Carton Archives, Bruges), n.p.
25 Esquirol (1818) in Bourneville, *Recueil de mémoires, notes et observations sur l'idiotie* (Paris: Imprimerie topographiques des enfants, 1891), 152.
26 P. Verstraete, 'The taming of disability: phrenology and bio-power on the road to the destruction of otherness in France (1800–60)', *History of Education*, 34:2 (2005), 119–34.
27 M. van Walleghem, *Ontwikkeling van de basisfuncties bij jonge mentaal gehandicapte kinderen* (n.pub., 1973); and V. Massin and B. Majerus, 'Des psychiatres et des enfants: Une histoire belge autour du congrès de 1937', *Revue d'histoire de l'enfance 'irrégulière'. Le Temps de l'histoire*, 18 (2016), 149–66.
28 For more detailed information about the introduction of compulsory education in Belgium, see M. De Vroede, 'De weg naar de algemene leerplicht in België'. *BMGN*, 75 (1970), 141–66.
29 See, for instance, A. van Gorp, *Tussen mythe en wetenschap: Ovide Decroly (1871–1932)* (Leuven: Acco, 2005).
30 *Quatorzième rapport sur la situation des asiles d'aliénés du Royaume (1892–1911)* (Brussels: J. Goemaere, 1913), 64–5.
31 A. Leonhardt (ed.), *Hörgeschädigte Schüler in der allgemeinen Schule: Theorie und Praxis der Integration* (Stuttgart: W. Kohlhammer Verlag, 2009).
32 W. Parry-Jones, 'The model of the Geel lunatic colony and its influence on the nineteenth century asylum system in Great Britain', in *Madhouses, Mad-Doctors, and Madmen: The Social History of Insanity in the Victorian Era*, ed. A. Scull (Philadelphia: University of Pennsylvania Press, 1981), 201–17, at 213.

33 In 1884, the Belgian government created a second family settlement, this time in French-speaking Belgium, in Lierneux. However, this colony never reached the same size and fame as Geel: *Lierneux 1884–1984: psychiatrie d'hier et d'aujourd'hui* (Herstal: Impr. de la Province de Liège, 1985).
34 'Un pensionnaire d'âge moyen, plutôt petit de taille, accompagne la fanfare au bord de la chaussée: il agite le bras au rythme de la musique … Ce patient porte un costume de bonne coupe, très soigné. Sa cravate est plutôt improvisée et il porte aux pieds des chaussures grossières, peu élégantes. Il accompagne ainsi la fanfare, à peu près à hauteur du tambour-major, sur le côté de la chaussée, mais légèrement devant la chaussée'. E. Roosens, *Des Fous Dans La Ville? Gheel (Belgique) et Sa Thérapie Séculaire*, Perspectives Critiques (Paris: PUF, 1979), 73–4.
35 E. Régis, *Précis de Psychiatrie* (Paris: Gaston Doin, 1907), 34.
36 *Sixième rapport de la Commission permanente d'inspection des établissements d'aliénés: 1859* (Imprimerie de M. Hayez, 1861), 123.
37 W. van Waesberghe, 'Het Belgische Krankzinnigenbeleid in de XIXde eeuw', *Annales de la Société Belge d'Histoire des Hôpitaux et de la Santé publique*, 22 (1984), 84.
38 J. Rathé, G. Goris and G. Vandercruys, *De Duitsers kwamen niet: de lotgevallen van de Joodse patiënten in de Geelse kolonie (1940–1945)* (Geel: MGraphics, 2011), 21.
39 *Lierneux 1884–1984*.
40 J. Vermeylen, 'Né à Geel', in *Histoire et institution, les 20 et 21 octobre 1995. Rencontres préparatoires au congrès organisé à Bordeaux par l'Union Internationale d'Aide à la Santé Mentale en juin 1996* (Brussels: L'Equipe, 1995), 5.
41 One of the contexts where the government already displayed a degree of awareness concerning disability issues was the army. It was known that many men had become (partially) blind after contracting a disease in the army. Another example is of course the debates that were held with regard to work injuries. See J. Vandendriessche, 'Ophthalmia crossing borders: Belgian army doctors between the military and civilian society, 1830–1860', *BTNG: Journal of Belgian History*, 46:2 (2016), 10–33; and J. Deferme, J., 'De schuld van het toeval: de Belgische wet op de arbeidsongevallen (1903) als een breekpunt in het parlementaire sociale denken', *Tijdschrift voor sociale geschiedenis*, 27:1 (2001), 57–76.
42 For some introductory works on the connection between the First World War and disability, see J. Bourke, *Dismembering the Male: Men's Bodies, Britain and the Great War* (London: Reaktion Books, 1996); D. Cohen, *The War Come Home: Disabled Veterans in*

Britain and Germany, 1914–1939 (Berkeley: University of California Press, 2001); and D. A. Gerber (ed.), *Disabled Veterans in History* (Ann Arbor: University of Michigan Press, 2000).
43 P. Verstraete and C. van Everbroeck, *Verminkte stilte: de Belgische invalide soldaten van de Groote Oorlog* (Namur: Presses Universitaires de Namur, 2015).
44 Ruben Debusschere, 'De militaire psychiatrie in België voor de Eerste Wereldoorlog: verkenning van een discipline in wording' (master's diss., KU Leuven, 2013).
45 Moreover, in the nineteenth century various initiatives were also taken that were directed solely towards disabled adults. A good example of this is Pasteur's rehabilitation initiative for mutilated miners, introduced around 1900 in the region of Charleroi. See P. Pasteur and L. Caty, *L'assistance aux estropiés par la création d'écoles d'apprentissage et d'ateliers. Rapport à la députation permanente du conseil provincial* (Frameries: Impr. Provinciale Dufrane-Friart, 1907).
46 Licht en liefde, Brailleliga, Algemeen Vlaams Blindenverbond and Oeuvre National des Aveugles.
47 D. Baynton, D., *Forbidden Signs: American Culture and the Fight against Sign Language* (Chicago: University of Chicago Press, 1996).
48 'Daar men om deze scheiding te verwezenlijken maar over de te voren reeds onontbeerlijke lokalen kon beschikken, werd daartoe van het toenmalig personeel veel overleg en vooruitzicht, groote wilskracht, waakzaamheid, toezicht en verdubbelde opoffering vereischt ... Naarmate de klappers in getal toenamen, kregen zij meer lokalen tot hunne beschikking, maar de glazen deuren langs dewelke zij met de ouderen zouden hebben kunnen in aanraking komen waren altijd zorgvuldig met gordijntjes behangen.' Unpublished document, Archives of the Sisters of Love, Ghent.
49 The blinded soldiers were initially cared for in the French Institute for the Blind in Amiens. Given the negative impact of this situation on their morale, they were soon transferred to the Port-Villez rehabilitation institute. In 1919 a special Royal Institute was founded for them in Boitsfort; it remained open until the last blinded soldier was rehabilitated (1921).
50 Personal file of Isidore van Vlasselaere/Archives of the Royal Palace/ Archives of Queen Elizabeth no AE 806/ Brussels.
51 Ibid.
52 Confidential file on Julien Dhont/Queen Elizabeth Archives no. AE 806/Archives Queen Elizabeth/Royal Archives/Brussels.
53 Helena Medeiros, David Mcdaid, Martin Knapp, MHEEN Group and Judit Simon, 'Shifting care from hospital to the community in

Europe: economic challenges and opportunities', *MHEEN II Policy Briefing*, 4 (2008), 10.
54 *Annuaire statistique de la Santé Publique* (Brussels: Ministère de la santé publique et de la famille, 1979), 240.
55 In Beau-Vallon, an asylum for approximately six hundred patients, the category 'oliogophrenia, idiocy, imbecility, mental retardation' accounted for 36 per cent of patients between 1961 and 1970. L. Lacroix and A. Roekens, 'Des patientes, des vies', in *Des murs et des femmes. Cent ans de psychiatrie et d'espoir au Beau-Vallon*, ed. A. Roekens (Namur, Presses Universitaires de Namur, 2014), 74.
56 E. Bruyninckx, 'Considérations sur le problème des vieillards atteints de troubles mentaux', *Acta Neurologica et Psychiatrica Belgica*, 7 (1957), 537–50.
57 'Troisième âge', *Bulletin d'information pratique pour la santé mentale*, 9 (January 1971), 14.
58 In Leuven, Passage 144, a non-medicalised institution, inspired by Ronald Laing and the International Philadelphia Association, is supported by criminology professor Steven de Batselier. When the academic authorities of the Katholieke Universiteit Leuven threatened to dismiss Batselier, several student demonstrations were held to support him. AMSAB-ISG, APL-B, box 141, affaire Steven De Batselier, De Batselier S. and M. Lietaert Peerbolte, Passage 144: terug naar de baarmoeder (Antwerp, Soethoudt, 1979). In Antwerp, a group of psychiatrists, lawyers, caregivers and former patients gathered together to publish the magazine *Spuit*, which was in print from 1975 to 1980. Interview conducted on 15 February 2016 with Sam Landuyt.
59 J. Orenbruch, C. Bastyns, I. W. Domb and M. Toledo, *La nouvelle politique psychiatrique belge*, vol. 1 (Brussels, 1979), 350.
60 *La folie parmi nous – Pour une politique de la santé mentale*, coll. 'La revue nouvelle', 10 (1973), 334.
61 AMSAB-ISG, APL-B, box 140, rapport d'activités du Centre de Santé Mentale Sectorisé de Saint-Gilles (1975), 7.
62 For an introduction to the history of polio, see W. Gareth, *Paralyzed with Fear: The Story of Polio* (Basingstoke: Palgrave Macmillan, 2013).
63 Artikel uit De Standaard (1988), cited in A. Looten, *Een geschiedenis van het persoonlijk assistentiebudget in Vlaanderen, 1987–2001* (Leuven: Niet-gepubliceerde Masterproef, Faculteit Psychologie en Pedagogische Wetenschappen, KU Leuven, 2001), 25.
64 For some stories about the disability protests, see S. Barnartt and R. Scotch, *Disability Protests: Contentious Politics, 1970–1999* (Washington, DC: Gallaudet University Press, 2001); J. Shapiro, *No Pity: People with Disabilities Forging a New Civil Rights Movement*

(New York: Three Rivers Press & Fleischer, 1994); and D. Zames and F. Zames, *The Disability Rights Movement: From Charity to Confrontation* (Philadelphia: Temple University Press, 2001).

Selected bibliography

Devlieger, P., Grosvenor, I., Simons, F., Geert van Hove, G. and Vanobbergen, B., 'Visualising disability in the past', *Paedagogica Historica*, 6 (2008), 747–60.
Dewinter, J., Verhulpen, M. and Croes, L., *75 jaar Sint-Kamillus Bierbeek – Een baken in het zorglandschap* (Bierbeek: Universitair psychiatrisch centrum Sint-Kamillus, 2008).
Dhaene, C. and Dhaene, L., *Sint-Jozef Kortenberg. Van 'Maison de Santé' tot Universitair Centrum. 145 jaar zorg voor geesteszieken, 1850–1995* (Kortenberg: Universitair centrum Sint-Jozef, 1995).
Majerus, B., 'La désinstitutionnalisation psychiatrique: un phénomène introuvable en Belgique dans les années 1960 et 1970?', in Alexandre Klein, Hervé Guillemain and Marie-Claude Thifault (eds), *La fin de l'asile? Histoire de la déshospitalisation psychiatrique dans le monde francophone* (Rennes: Presses Universitaires de Rennes, 2018), 143–55.
Majerus, B., *Parmi les fous. Une histoire sociale de la psychiatrie au 20e siècle* (Rennes: Presses Universitaires de Rennes, 2013).
Majerus, B. and Roekens, A., 'Being crazy in Belgium', *Journal of Belgian History*, XLVII (2017), 4.
Massin, V. and Majerus, B., 'Des psychiatres et des enfants: Une histoire belge autour du congrès de 1937', *Revue d'histoire de l'enfance 'irrégulière'. Le Temps de l'histoire*, 18 (2016), 149–66.
Roekens, A. (ed.), *Des murs et des femmes: cent ans de psychiatrie et d'espoir au Beau-Vallon* (Namur: Presses Universitaires de Namur, 2014).
Scheiris, I. and Raemdonck, L., *Ongehoord verleden. Dove frontvorming in België aan het begin van de 20ste eeuw* (Ghent: Fevlado Diversus, 2007).
Stockman, R., *Geen rede mee te rijmen* (Sint-Martens-Latem: Museum Dr. Guislain, 1989).
Van Ertvelde, A., Verstraete, P. and Depicker, M., 'Meerstemmig feestgedruis: Een terugblik op vijftig jaar tewerkstelling van personen met een handicap, 1967–2017', in M. Carlier and F. Maes (eds), *Naar een duurzame en inclusieve arbeidsmarkt. Evidence-based practice and practice-based evidence* (Ghent: SKRIBIS, in press).
Van Waesberghe, W., 'Het Belgische Krankzinnigenbeleid in de XIXde eeuw', *Annales de la Société Belge d'Histoire des Hôpitaux et de la Santé publique*, 22 (1984), 69–96.

Van Walleghem, M., 'Het *ontstaan van de zorg voor* zwakzinnigen in België', in M. Depaepe and M. D'hoker (eds), *Onderwijs, opvoeding en maatschappij in de 19de en 20e Eeuw. Liber amicorum prof. Dr. Maurits de Vroede* (Leuven: Acco, 1987), 165–74.

Verstraete, P., 'Remastering independence: the re-education of Belgian blinded soldiers of the Great War, 1914–1940', *Educacio i Historia* (in press).

Verstraete, P. and Van Everbroeck, C., *Verminkte stilte. De Belgische invalide soldaten van de Groote Oorlog* (Namur: Presses Universitaires de Namur, 2014).

9

Medicine, media and the public

Tinne Claes and Katrin Pilz

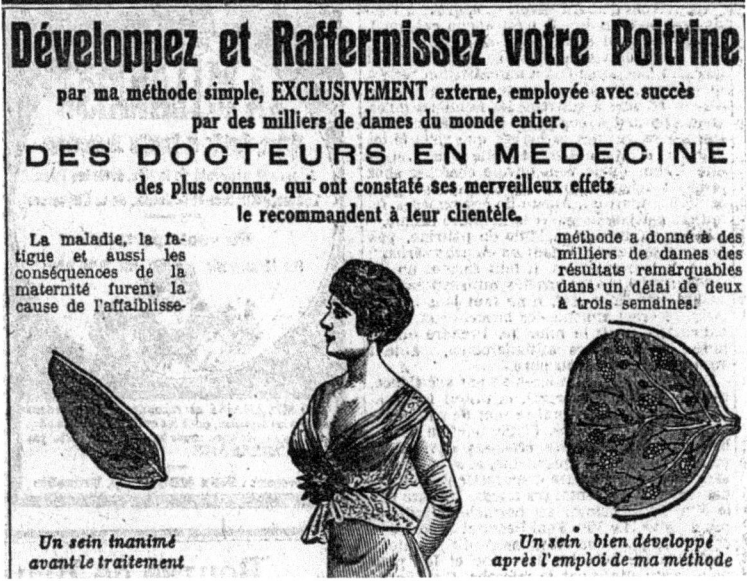

Figure 9.1 Newspaper advertisement for a 'breast-enhancing' product, *Le Peuple*, 19 May 1914, p. 6.

The newspaper advertisement in Figure 9.1 from 1914 promised women a way to 'develop and firm their chest'.[1] The seller provided expert evidence in order to convince customers – namely, two images contrasting the internal anatomy of the breast before and after treatment, accompanied by references from 'very well-known doctors of medicine'. The advertisement seems to reflect a well-known historiographical narrative, emphasising the growing influence of medicine in the nineteenth and twentieth centuries. First, it suggests that medicine had become the most authoritative field of knowledge regarding the body and health. Second, it illustrates the increasing impact of medicine in society: a preference for large, firm breasts – the beauty ideal – was represented as a medical issue, and the strategic use of medical images suggests that laypeople were familiar with visual depictions of anatomy. Yet the advertisement also complicates grand narratives of professionalisation and medicalisation, for it shows that 'quacks' also claimed medicine as a privileged site of knowledge for their own commercial agenda, and indeed often created their professional identities by copying mainstream physicians.

Over the past two decades, philosophers and historians of science have replaced the model of diffusion, according to which knowledge was created by scientists before moving to the public sphere, by a model of circulation, according to which knowledge was constructed by mutual interactions between the scientific and the public domain. Building on Bruno Latour's notion of actor-network theory or Nicholas Thomas's account on material exchange, historians of science, most importantly James Secord, argued that knowledge production in itself should be seen as a process of communication and exchange.[2] As a result of this theoretical shift, historians have questioned the dichotomy between the scientific and the popular, instead looking for connections between them.[3]

In a similar vein, historians have shown that the sharp antagonism between 'official' and 'alternative' medical beliefs was not a historical reality, but a cultural construct that did not match the practices of patients and practitioners. They have argued that 'professional' physicians could not monopolise medicine: not only treatments, but also different views of health co-existed and complemented each other on the medical market. Furthermore, as the advertisement above suggests, not only 'professional' physicians made use of a medical discourse to bolster their credibility.[4] In fact, studies have shown that experts of all kinds, ranging from academics to natural healers, mothers or priests, were dependent on their audiences for recognition of their authority.[5] To sum up, static divides – between the scientific and the popular sphere, between the expert and the lay public, and between orthodox and heterodox medicine – were nuanced by a more multifaceted interpretation of knowledge production, ascribing a more active role to historical actors outside of the academic world.

Yet Belgian historiography regarding the permeable boundaries between the scientific and the popular is still in its infancy, although recent mass digitisation projects of primary sources such as newspapers and magazines could certainly facilitate research along these lines.[6] The history of public manifestations of medicine is mostly confined to short chapters in edited volumes, monographs or doctoral dissertations. In these works, the history of popularisation is mostly a sidetrack to contextualise the actual topic of study, be it a general history of medicine or a history of homosexuality, adolescence or anatomical models.[7] Only a handful of articles have accorded sustained attention to the history of popularisation.[8] Apart from the work of Evert Peeters and Anne Hilde van Baal, the picture is equally bleak for the history of 'alternative' medicine.[9]

As there exists no comprehensive Belgian monography on the history of popular medicine or science, historians are dependent on general works discussing British, French, German or other European contexts.[10] Although these studies are useful to indicate broad evolutions, such as the importance of the hygienist movement or the rise of mass media, their findings do not always fully apply to the Belgian sociopolitical context. From existing case studies we know that local specificities are crucial to understand the transformation of medical knowledge. For example, Peeters has suggested that humoral representations of the body adhered to the worldview of many Catholic physicians in Belgium, and that this might explain both the popularity of holistic therapies such as hydrotherapy, and why academic physicians continued to pay lip service to the humoral theories until well into the nineteenth century.[11] Another example considers the state interference towards mass media. Public television retained a factual monopoly until 1989. In Flanders, scientific programmes took centre stage in programming despite a lack of popularity. As these programmes served political goals, namely the emancipation of the Flemish people and the cultural integration of the Dutch linguistic region, viewing figures were not television makers' primary concern.[12]

Yet international movements and media were also quintessential for the popularisation of medicine in Belgium, as the market was too small to sustain original large-scale productions. The 'carriers' of medical knowledge, whether magazines, exhibitions, movies or other forms of media, often came from abroad. In the nineteenth century, for example, Belgium was so well known for its *contrefaçon* (counterfeit) publishing, that scholars have argued that it held the 'monopoly of the French book', as French literary and scientific works travelled the world through Belgian copies.[13] In her work on popular anatomical atlases, Veronique Deblon has shown that anatomists and editors made compilations combining the 'best of' French and German medical images, and adapted and enriched them with extra information. Rather than simply reprinting international works, they turned them into 'Belgian' editions and tailored them to the needs of the intended audience.[14] In a similar vein, recent literature has highlighted Belgium as a 'European leader in organizing international action against depravity in film', despite its lack of a commercially strong domestic film industry – a reality that also impacted the creation and distribution of medical and public health films.[15] As will become evident throughout this chapter, other manifestations of medical knowledge should likewise be interpreted within a system of exchange: 'foreign' knowledge changed according to local norms and customs, and in ways that were dependent on the intended audience.

In order to thematise this tension between the local and the global, this chapter focuses on the media through which medicine circulated, in particular models displayed in health exhibitions and medical films. A perspective based on Secord's concept of circulation allows us to elucidate context-specific trajectories of knowledge, recognising that views regarding the body and health travel and shift in meaning. This approach allows us to decentralise grand narratives on medicalisation and professionalisation, and to place the medical patient and consumer at the centre of our attention. We do not interpret popular medicine as a body of knowledge, but rather as the relationship between science and the public. We interpret this relationship as a mutual one: medical knowledge was not simply transferred from the scientific to the public domain, but was transformed and adapted between the scientific and the popular spheres. By drawing attention to these modifications and interpretations of medicine, we give lay audiences agency in the historical narrative: they transform from passive recipients into active actors and consumers, who have the agency to interpret, choose from and respond to different views of the body and health.

Even though this chapter mainly focuses on health exhibitions and medical films, it is certainly possible to study other audiovisual media in a similar vein. Within media studies, virtually all forms of knowledge communication (radio programmes, lectures, magazines, posters, charts, slides, advertisements and so on) have been analysed as a dynamic process, using the same key questions. In a nutshell, the question of 'what' is being communicated is always dependent on a simultaneous understanding of 'how', 'where', 'when', 'by whom' and 'for whom'.[16] In our view, historians can learn a lot from such a media approach. Until now, Belgian historiography has mainly focused on 'products' of popular medicine, most notably posters, leaflets and manuals, newspapers and magazines.[17] Studies mostly have neglected the process of communication that is inherent to these media. Audiences have rarely received any attention. The same holds true for actors such as publishing houses, manufacturers and sponsors. In our view, it is time to change this. If we want to write histories of popular science that transcend boundaries between different cultural spheres, geographic localities or time spans, we should not interpret primary sources as finished products but as ongoing processes.

This chapter consists of two main parts: one on health exhibitions, the other on medical films. Within both parts, three questions structure our narrative. First, we clarify the model of circulation by focusing on the movement of knowledge between different places, cultural domains and disciplines. Then, we turn to the question of expertise. We complicate the narrative of professionalisation by drawing attention to the diverse ways in which popular medicine was given credibility, and by looking at collaborations between professional physicians and other actors. Lastly, we draw attention to the agency of the audience. We argue that historians should treat the lay public as an active actor by contrasting curatorial or directorial aims with actual visitors' responses.

Health exhibitions

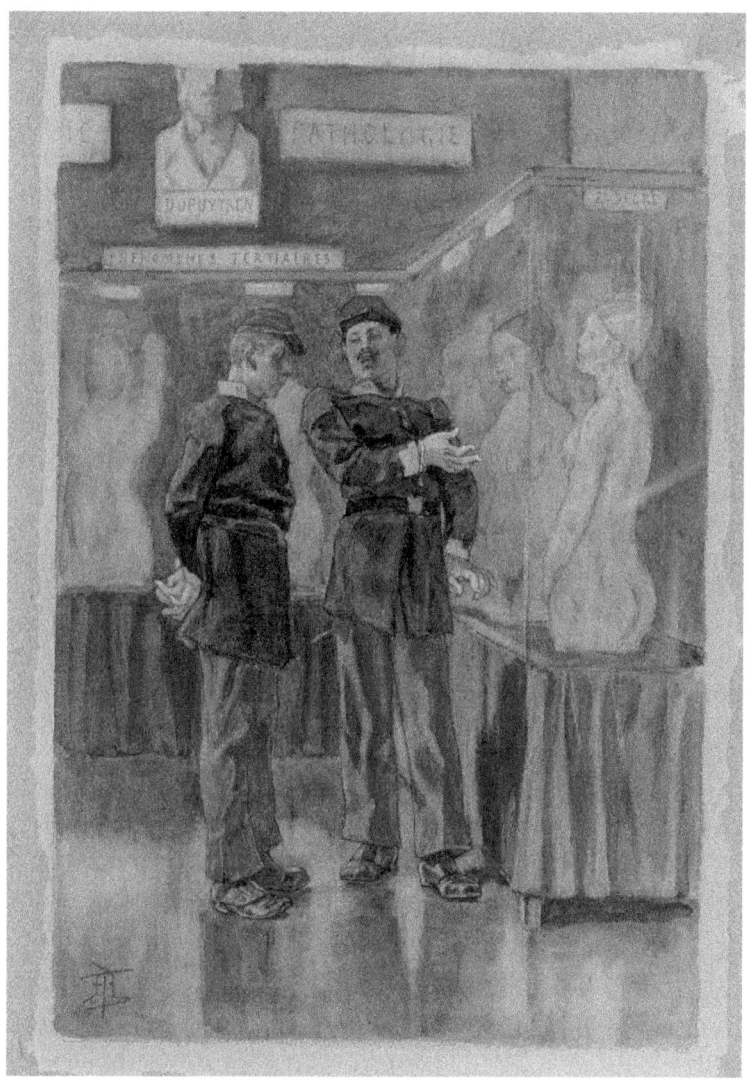

Figure 9.2 Félicien Rops, *La Leçon d'hygiène*. Série des Cent légers croquis, 1878–81.

In *La leçon d'hygiène* (ca. 1878–81), the Belgian painter Félicien Rops depicts two military men visiting a hygiene museum (Figure 9.2). They are looking at wax models illustrating the symptoms of syphilis. One soldier appears to be explaining the displayed disease; the other is blushing uneasily. Health exhibitions such as the one depicted by Rops were a common phenomenon. Itinerant, often international, collections on the body and health toured around Belgium from the 1840s onwards.[18] In the early twentieth century, a provincial hygienist museum was established within this tradition in Mons.[19] Temporary and travelling exhibitions also continued to exist. In the 1930s, for example, the Belgian Red Cross organised the exhibition *De Mensch* (The Human Being) in the Egmont Palace in Brussels.[20] Health and hygiene were important topics in the world fairs.[21] Today, Gunther von Hagens carries on the tradition by touring the world with spectacular displays of plastinated bodies, bearing both explanatory labels with medical information and quotes about mortality from religious and philosophical sources.[22]

These exhibitions reached ever wider audiences. Around 1860, anatomical museums moved from coffee houses or shopping arcades (venues of bourgeois entertainment) to the fairground. Aligning themselves with both the prophylactic aims of the emergent hygienist movement and the cultural ideal of educating the people, proprietors of popular museums lowered their entrance fees in order to 'allow the working man to visit their collections'.[23] Aside from workers, they targeted other high-risk groups in the battle against epidemics. Soldiers, who not coincidentally took centre stage in Rops's painting, could often visit health museums at half price, as it was, perhaps justifiably, believed that their lifestyle put them at risk of 'the venereal peril'.[24]

Yet the visual display of pathological models, many of them depicting the results of venereal disease, was not considered to be appropriate for everyone. Until well into the twentieth century women could only visit anatomical museums separately. This was both because their presence would make male visitors feel uneasy and in order to protect their modesty. Women received a censored and gendered view of the body and health (see Chapter 1, p. 40). For instance, models depicting genital organs or venereal diseases were removed from display, and maternal tasks were emphasised and grounded in anatomical 'facts'.[25] Yet these separate visits also generated possibilities for women, as they created job opportunities for female guides and thus possibly paved the way for female proprietors. At least in Belgium, it was not unusual for wives of museum owners to take over the anatomical museum after their husband's death.[26] In fact, international studies have stressed the importance of women for the circulation and popularisation of science in general, thus disrupting the idea that women were excluded from science during the nineteenth century.[27]

Children, too, only gradually gained access to health exhibitions. From the 1890s onwards, a few popular anatomical museums represented themselves as suitable and didactic for family outings, offering reduced rates for children.[28] Schools became attractive customers after 1895, when health education became a compulsory part of the curriculum.[29] The provincial hygiene museum of Mons and the *De Mensch* exhibition, for instance, tried to attract schools by emphasising their didactic potential in the first half of the twentieth century.[30]

Things in motion

Having discussed a few general characteristics of health exhibitions – what, when and for whom – we now turn to the question of circulation. In historiography, there has been a tendency to discuss different types of health exhibitions separately.[31] As an unintended consequence of this approach, the differences between these institutions have been overly emphasised. In this section, however, we focus on the circulation and (re)interpretation of objects *in between* different types of exhibitions, such as itinerant anatomical museums, academic collections and provincial hygiene museums. When studying the trajectories of museum objects, three forms of movement come to the fore: between different countries, between university museums and popular collections and between private and public exhibitions. A focus on 'things in motion', rather than on 'snapshots' of things in specific case studies, allows historians to elucidate both the circulation and, perhaps more importantly, the transformation of medicine across borders and cultural domains.[32]

First, health exhibitions provide an insight into the dynamics between the international and the local (see Chapter 4, p. 135). Nineteenth-century popular anatomical museums were international phenomena. Most of them, for instance the museums of Kahn, Prauscher and Spitzner, came from abroad and toured across Europe. The objects on display were international as well, ranging from French or German anatomical models to specimens from colonial contexts.[33] In later exhibitions, too, objects were exchanged across borders. On the world fairs, for example, didactic objects from several countries were displayed in the same pavilion.[34] In 1938, the Red Cross arranged the move of the 'see-through man' from the hygiene museum of Dresden to Brussels. This anatomical model entirely made from glass, enabling viewers to see organs, nerves and blood vessels, was one of the most popular models of the time and toured the international exhibition circuit as a symbol of Aryan superiority and modernity.[35]

Yet despite their international character, health exhibitions did change per country, and even per city. Research has shown that curators of itinerant collections accommodated their displays to the interests and sensitivities of the public. Local doctors were, for example, asked to review the collection on its scientific merits, and supposedly obscene objects were occasionally removed from display at the request of the local police, suggesting that the authority and decency of international collections had to be confirmed locally.[36] These mechanisms persisted well into the twentieth century. In newspapers from 1938, for instance, reviews by Belgian physicians and professors, as well as by King Leopold III, had to confirm the quality of the exhibition *De Mensch*.[37] Moreover, international studies have shown that visitors' responses to exhibitions could differ profoundly depending on the particular context.[38] The study of the content of, and response to, health exhibitions across borders thus appears to be a fruitful area of research, enabling historians to see the continued importance of local contexts in an era in which the organisation of science became international. Contemporary research on the different responses to *Body Worlds* – provoking the 'anger of Christians' in Germany while being welcomed as 'a wonderful educational vehicle' in the United States – might provide inspiration for this type of research.[39]

Objects also moved between the university and the fairground. Hieke Huistra has shown that universities in the Netherlands closed their anatomical collections for general audiences around 1850.[40] A similar evolution took place in Belgium, although universities continued to open their doors for lay audiences on public holidays.[41] Significantly, popular itinerant museums started to tour across Belgium (and the Netherlands) around the same time. These collections were inspired by their, now inaccessible, academic counterparts. The Spitzner museum, for example, was modelled after the Museum Dupuytren, the anatomical museum of the Faculty of Medicine of Paris.[42] Most popular museums displayed medical models that were also part of university collections, such as anatomical wax models by Louis Auzoux or Jules Baretta. Even objects that contemporary critics occasionally described as 'sensational', such as the display of criminals' or celebrities' skulls, were also part of university collections. The anatomical museum of Liège, for instance, contained a collection of skulls of decapitated convicts, while the University of Leuven possessed an anatomical preparation and plaster cast of the brains of the famous writer and poet Guido Gezelle.[43]

Lastly, the contents of private or temporary exhibitions, and official museums, were strikingly similar. To name but a few examples, although politicians claimed that the provincial hygiene museum of Mons, which opened in 1911 and still constitutes a blind spot in research, offered a sober and serious, less 'sensational', display of knowledge, the collection does not appear to have differed from those of fairground museums. For instance, 148 models depicting the results of venereal disease were placed in a separate room inaccessible for children – a practice reminiscent of the display of controversial models in *cabinets reservés* in fairground museums.[44] In 1938, several newspaper reports compared the *De Mensch* exhibition to the Spitzner museum, again suggesting that a focus on similarities and exchanges would be a fruitful approach for historians.[45]

Doctors, showmen and expertise

Strict divisions between the 'academic' and the 'popular' are equally hard to maintain when we consider interactions between physicians and proprietors of popular health exhibitions. Curators from popular collections positioned themselves within the medical community. Many of them called themselves physicians (even if they had no medical training), and guided visitors around in white doctor's coats. In doing so, they constructed medicine as an authoritative field of knowledge regarding the body: when it came to health and disease, physicians received expert status.[46]

Even the *enfants terribles* of the popular scene used a medical discourse to bolster their credibility. A well-researched example is the case of Constant Crommelinck, who occasionally gave lectures on health and the body in mid-nineteenth-century Belgium, sometimes in popular anatomical museums.[47] Even though important medical journals such as *Le Scalpel* refuted his holistic views of the body as 'quack' medicine, Crommelinck continued to call himself a doctor. Crommelinck remained, arguably, the most popular medical lecturer for over twenty years, showing that alienation from academic medicine did not necessarily lead to the downfall of popular scientists (or museums). In the end, one's recognition as a medical expert did not depend on professional opinions, but on the judgement of the audience.[48] A similar argument was made in studies on hydropaths and other contested healers. Although many 'alternative' practitioners questioned the effectiveness of mainstream therapies, they used scientific knowledge, networks and institutions to strengthen their authority.[49]

In general, however, the relations between the medical community and proprietors of popular museums were friendly in Belgium; unlike in Britain and other European countries, where physicians increasingly denounced popular museums as sensationalist and obscene establishments.[50] The Musée Spitzner, for instance, was appreciated for decades by both the medical community and local authorities.[51] Physicians regularly organised lectures on public hygiene within the museum. Medical practitioners, students and nurses could visit at a reduced price. In 1926, the city council of Antwerp gave Spitzner a fairground stand at the Sinksenfoor for the following three years because 'the museum is managed in a decent way, and its collections have a good reputation in the local medical community'.[52] In fact, the extraordinarily lengthy existence of popular anatomical museums in Belgium suggests that they were seen as effective institutions for a long time. The Spitzner collection, for example, toured the big Belgian cities from the 1880s until as late as the 1960s. When it was increasingly considered to be outdated for medical education, it gradually became a museum on the history of medicine.[53]

One reason for the continued existence of popular medical exhibitions was their embeddedness in local politics. From the twentieth century onwards, as local and federal authorities began to see health education as their responsibility, politicians increasingly collaborated with private institutions. In the words of Onghena, popularisation became part of 'conscious, urban politics'.[54] In 1933, for instance, Madame Spitzner proposed the Brussels aldermen for public health to work systematically together in order to establish a city museum for social hygiene.[55] This example also points to the importance of the proprietor, as Madame Spitzner's continuous efforts to promote her collection as important to public health – seeking collaborations with health organisations, city councils and schools – was perhaps the most important reason that her museum continued to exist.

The stance of the twentieth-century medical establishment was ambiguous. On the one hand, physicians criticised the 'sensational' nature of 'pseudoscience' that was so seemingly hard to control and administer. The medical community occasionally rejected popular exhibitions – not only fairground museums, but also world fairs and the aforementioned exhibition *De Mensch* – as they turned 'serious' science into a consumer good.[56] On the other hand, physicians participated in what they called 'the education of the people'. By organising public lectures on practical themes, most importantly on hygiene topics, they attempted to stimulate the public's moral and intellectual development.[57]

Discipline and agency

Several historians have underlined the disciplinary or moralising aspects of health exhibitions. Inspired by the Foucauldian notion of 'biopolitics', they have argued that these exhibitions were meant to discipline the visitor's gaze, body or behaviour. When discussing the 'strategies' of nineteenth-century hygienism in Belgium, Karel Velle, argued that medical advice had 'other motives than the advancement of health', as it was imbued with cultural norms and values.[58]

In more recent international research, too, the disciplinary aspects of health exhibitions were an object of scrutiny. Michael Sappol argued that popular museums represented disease as a natural enforcement of moral law, and Elizabeth Stephens called anatomical displays a 'disciplinary technology, requiring one to regulate one's body and its practices in accordance with cultural norms'.[59] Underpinning these interpretations was the grand narrative of medicalisation, according to which the authority of physicians grew while more and more previously religious or social norms and values were becoming grounded in medicine and the body.

It is true that the programmatic aim of prevention went hand in hand with moralisation in health exhibitions. The late nineteenth-century battle against venereal disease, for instance, led to an idealisation of traditional conjugal ethics. Sexual acts outside of faithful heterosexual relationships (i.e. marriage) were condemned as irresponsible and unhealthy. In the introduction of the exhibition catalogue of the Musée Consael, the proprietor proudly stated that many young men had changed their promiscuous lifestyle after viewing the objects on display. In the same museum, several models allegedly showed the 'pathological results' of sexually deviant behaviour, ranging from masturbation to homosexuality or prostitution.[60] More generally, popular representations of disease were, and still are, imbued with notions of right and wrong, of responsibility and guilt. In the nineteenth-century popular anatomical museum, kidney disease was represented as the stubborn alcoholic's fate; today, the display of smokers' lungs in the *Body Worlds* exhibits or printed images on cigarette packs might convince smokers to change their ways.

Curators of health exhibitions thought three-dimensional models were particularly suitable for conveying these preventive and moralising messages to a broad audience. Not only did visual representations of disease enable illiterate visitors to learn about the symptoms of diseases, realistic depictions of impaired bodies also allowed for identification. The pathological model had to function as a conditional, future self: a scary outcome of behaviour that should be changed. Through identification, pathological models were meant to create a shock that would lead to a permanent change of mentality. In the words of the catalogue of the Spitzner Museum, the horror evoked by pathological models would 'perpetuate' the lessons of the museum 'in our memory'.[61]

Yet fear was not the only emotion that exhibitions evoked. Inspired by the history of emotions, historians have shown that curators' intentions did not always match visitors' responses.[62] Regarding anatomical displays specifically, historians have pointed at erotic responses from visitors, especially in an era during which visual representations of naked bodies were rare. Anna Maerker, for instance, has found that the glass cabinets containing anatomical models of female genitalia in the Specola Museum in Florence had to be replaced more regularly than other display cases, presumably because visitors touched them.[63] One could wonder why the soldier in Rops's painting is blushing: is he afraid he might have contracted a venereal disease, or is he distracted by the graphic and three-dimensional display of naked women?

Health exhibitions could not only be titillating. They could also be pleasant rather than instructive or boring. Indeed, some contemporary critics worried that health exhibitions were 'sensationalist', meaning that science was made subordinate to entertainment. In the words of one reviewer of the *De Mensch* exhibition, visitors 'would leave the exhibition with the same attitudes they entered' because they did not go to the exhibition to learn, but to have fun.[64] In Stijn Bussels and Bram van Oostveldt's research on the 1894 world fair in Antwerp, the emotion of 'boredom' took centre stage. In their view, the world fair did not evoke admiration or pleasure, but disinterest and fatigue. As visitors had gotten used to large-scale spectacles in the preceding decades, the world fair had lost much of its appeal. Yet Bussels and Van Oostveldt also drew attention to curators' responses, arguing that they increasingly changed visual displays for experiments and performances, allowing for a more active kind of spectatorship.[65] Similar stories of interaction and dialogue hold true for health exhibitions. In response to criticism regarding the pornographic nature of their displays, for instance, proprietors of popular anatomical museums developed ways to discipline their visitors. They organised guided tours in order to gain control of visitors' interpretation of the museum or placed explicit models in *cabinets reservés* – separate rooms that were inaccessible for working-class audiences and women.[66]

To sum up, the history of health exhibitions shows the value of an approach based on circulation. A focus on interaction not only enables historians to nuance their understanding of the boundaries between 'science proper' and 'popular science', but also allows for a more active interpretation of audiences. Visitors of health exhibitions did not passively soak up the knowledge on display, but had the agency to respond in unintended ways. In the next section, we will show that similar mechanisms were at play in the medical film industry. By looking at the production and reception of movies regarding health, specifically the film *Un ennemi public* (1937), we will further emphasise the importance of non-medical actors and contexts for the circulation of medical knowledge.

Medical films

The camera initially pans over the lavish Palais de Justice, the emblem of national power built under the now notorious King Leopold II, before it leads the film spectator to the narrow streets of the working-class district the 'Marolles'. The film *Un ennemi public*, produced in 1937,[67] depicts a view on urban everyday life in Brussels (Figure 9.3). The film was cinematographically interpreted by documentary filmmaker Henri Storck, and sponsored by representatives of the national public health circle, such as the physician, professor and social reformer René Sand, and the Ligue Nationale belge contre la tuberculose.[68] The film, which was directed at a working-class audience, depicts the life of a factory worker: his family life, the insanitary housing situation in the metropole and the challenging physical work in the printing factory, are all part of the main narration. *Un ennemi public* was in the first instance produced to communicate knowledge regarding tuberculosis, which was at the time seen as both a social and an epidemic disease. Storck and his sponsors wished to raise awareness, and to mobilise support for public health measures aimed at prevention.[69]

Today we may be used to seeing surgical operations in reality TV formats introduced with the trigger warning 'viewer discretion advised'. Fictional TV shows, such as *Emergency Room* and *Grey's Anatomy*, lead their viewers through dramatic episodes about common and rare diseases, modern diagnostic technologies and operations, exploring the lives of both doctors and patients in the microcosmos of the clinic. Whereas these documentaries and fictional dramas are an integral part of today's programming

Medicine, media and the public 335

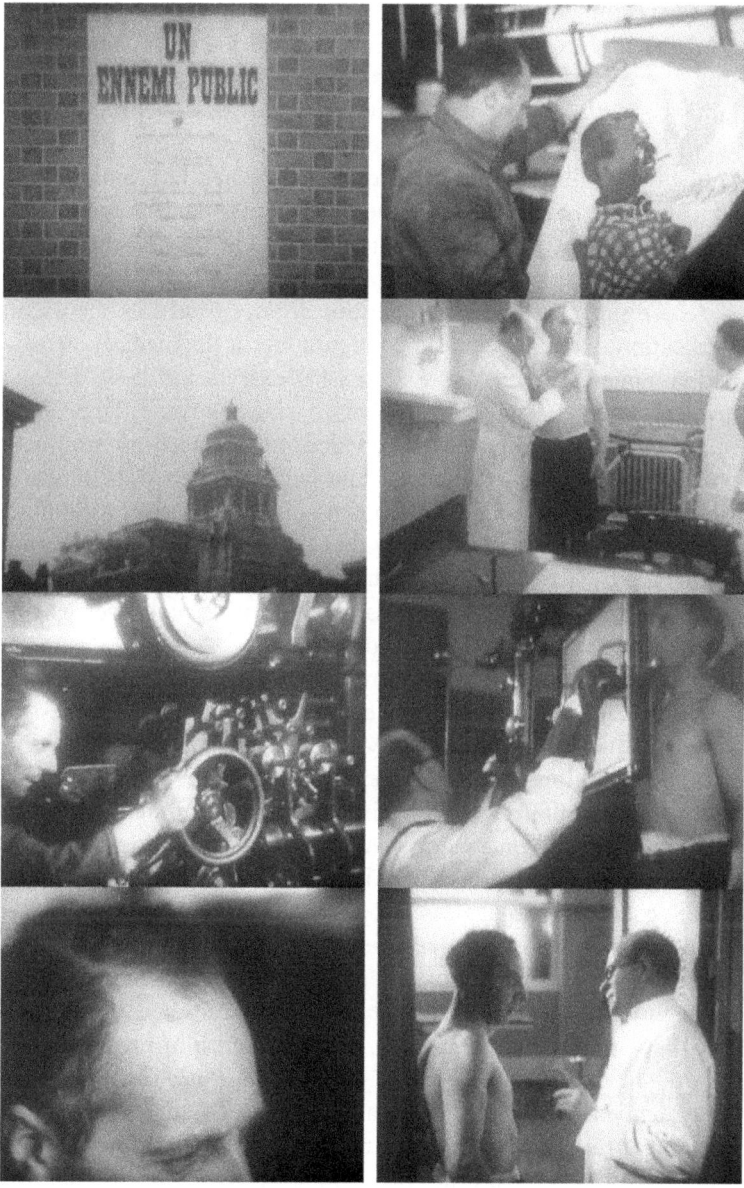

Figure 9.3 Film stills of the public health film on Tuberculosis *Un ennemi public* (1937), 35 mm, b/w, sound, ca. 15 min.

for television, radio and digital broadcasting, their origins have until recently been a blind spot in medical historical and media study research.[70] After the First World War, the growing film industry with an increased attention for health programmes against epidemics and social disease engendered a new genre: the public health film. Films on topics such as general hygiene, sexual education, venereal disease, tuberculosis and malaria prevention gained popularity in the 1920s, notably in Europe and the United States.[71]

As a result, there were contentious debates regarding the useful application, composition and configuration in the medical, artistic and commercial film worlds as to what extent, and how, delicate medical subjects should be shown to cinemagoers.[72] Depending on the topic, screenings were divided into projections for men, women and children. Films on infant hygiene, birth and childcare, were commonly intended for women only and sex education films were appropriated for specific audiences too. Similarly to offering soldiers exclusive visits to health exhibitions on venereal disease, film scenes depicting male genitals affected with syphilis were exclusively shown to male military audiences.[73]

Explicit clinical depictions were rather rare in health or popular-scientific films, and if used they were contested by moral, aesthetical and scientific commentators.[74] Much like tuberculosis films, venereal disease films tried to address a broad public by introducing different social milieus and life circumstances, framing the topic of risk in a storyline that made viewers empathetic. Films conveyed the message that everyone could be put at endemic, epidemic and hygiene risk, regardless of one's gender, social status or race. Whereas addressed audiences were the targeted consumers in this context, the various early cinematographically depicted forms of health and disease were still exclusively outlined by medical scientists, public health officers, teachers and film professionals. Yet, the health educators' intentions to change public ideas on the body, hygiene, sexuality, health and sickness, could not be fulfilled without turning to the targeted public itself. In addition, medical experts had to turn to other professionals, as they were often neither knowledgeable of filmmaking techniques, nor experienced public health promoters.[75]

Between the clinic and the public cinema

The invention and vast improvement of imaging techniques, such as photography and cinematography, as well as of medical imaging techniques, such as X-ray and microscopic photography, led on to new considerations regarding how to use them as tools for medical and public education and research at the end of the nineteenth century (see Chapter 5, p. 184). European film producers were eager to promote the importance of a scientific affiliation with the newly introduced cinematograph. Professional filmmakers wanted to collaborate with physicians in the production of public health films in order to diversify and advance their professional repertoire. Clinicians were further using film as a life-like medical record, evidencing their research practices. The oldest preserved Belgian medical films, held in the Cinémathèque Royale de Belgique, are part of a collection of clinical short films that date back to 1905. They were produced by Arthur van Gehuchten, a neurologist and professor at the Université catholique de Louvain, who established the university's neurology chair and clinic.[76]

Presumably inspired by the work of the Romanian neurologist Gheorghe Marinescu, Van Gehuchten started to film patients with so-called *maladies nerveuses* resulting in movement disorders, like Parkinson's and Huntington's. He recorded them in different settings: outdoors, in the garden of the clinic and in his so-called *cage de verre*,[77] a gallery-like laboratory that functioned as an indoor film studio.[78] As uncontrollable movements were hard to describe in words, neurologists were (next to surgeons) the leading specialists using film for research and education. Much like medical models, rare clinical cases served as a 'celluloid archive' that could be reused and reproduced with the cinematograph. Whereas in most cases Van Gehuchten operated the camera himself, his early film series encouraged other medical specialists – namely neurologists, psychologists and psychiatrists, such as his son Paul van Gehuchten at the Université catholique de Louvain, Ovide Decroly in Brussels, Ludo van Bogaert in Antwerp and Léon Laruelle in Brussels – to collaborate with professional camera operators including Antoine Castille.[79]

Although clinical films were not intended for public viewing, questions regarding how to show patients in a 'scientifically' and 'aesthetically' appealing way were at times as controversial as for public health films. The filming of nude patients, for instance, was constantly challenging medical and lay audiences. In the early 1920s, health films often included clinical reels from patients in order to make them visually impactful and effectively disturbing.[80] Unlike elsewhere in Europe, clinical research and teaching films appear to have been mainly produced by individual neuroscientists or others occupied with mental health (see Chapter 8, p. 334). From the early twentieth century onwards, university professors in Belgium bought and used foreign educational films, notably surgical films, for their courses. While centralised national film departments in other European countries were systematically collaborating with university clinics and public health educators for the production of films in disciplines such as surgery and gynaecology, the market for, and interest in, these initiatives, was absent in Belgium until the interwar period.[81]

The earliest clinical films were quite isolated as they were issued by individual medical researchers and teachers. Although they were intended only for scientific venues, they were also projected beyond their original purpose. For example, the French surgeon Eugène-Louis Doyen had filmed surgeries and showed them at medical meetings. Interestingly, Doyen's films were also accessible for public and private screenings, and were widely advertised and distributed in Brussels.[82] After critics had denounced him for using film as a tool for self-promotion, Doyen had learnt that copies of his surgical films were leaked to non-scientific distribution channels, such as public fairgrounds, and were sold to well-known film producers without his consent.[83] This case had demonstrated the risks of the new medium, and further challenged the standing of medical educational films.[84] This example of problematic circulation between clinical and public spaces appears to have led to a decline in the production of surgical films. Extracted from their original purpose of educating medicine in the clinical projection room, clinical films allegedly became sensationalist or voyeuristic, as lay audiences paid to see the body turned inside out, the blood gushing, the patient exposed. More generally, the controversy concerning the leaking of the Doyen films appears to have impacted the position of the medical community, which neglected the possibilities of film for public health until the end of the First World War. Another reason for this reluctant attitude towards film was its connotation with occult magic, an association that blurred the boundaries between science and spectacle.[85]

When public health themed films finally found their way to the public in the late 1910s through screenings in public venues such as schools, factories, fairs and army camps, filmmakers preferred purely fictional re-enactments over 'real' footage, or at least enriched information with fictional elements that made scientific knowledge easier to comprehend for lay spectators.[86] Public lectures, microscopic images and other visual displays of bodily processes and medical examinations were contrasted with the counterexample of bad housing and labour circumstances.[87] In the first half of the twentieth century, Belgian public health films, much like elsewhere in Europe, focused on topics such as hygiene, childcare, epidemics and occupational accident protection. Educational hygiene films mostly considered social diseases and epidemics, such as alcoholism and tuberculosis, and were aimed at high-risk groups, such as industrial workers, but also military men and veterans, mothers, children and, in colonial contexts, indigenous people.[88] Realised by different public health departments these films were prepared and executed by professional and clinical film directors. This specific genre is therefore an optimal source for discussing interdisciplinary, intercultural, scientific and public, institutional and visual questions regarding how concepts of the healthy and the diseased body could be conveyed in motion as well as in still pictures.[89]

The extensive Belgian collection of public health films circulating in the early twentieth century is almost entirely composed of French and American national hygiene films that were distributed by Belgian health prevention and public film organisations.[90] In the tradition of films such as *Le dispensaire antituberculeux* (France, 1917),[91] *La visiteuse d'hygiène* (France, ca. 1925),[92] and *Les Maladies Sexuelles et leurs Conséquences* (France, 1923), the public health films that are conserved in Belgian archives took over corresponding film elements regarding the state of the art narratives, displaying content, form and aesthetic styles common for public films about tuberculosis and venereal disease. The films discuss hygiene behaviour regarding nutrition, housing and the workplace, and show statistics of epidemics and possible relief and treatment.[93] Despite the existence of a vivid documentary film culture in Belgian cinema from the 1920s onwards, with directors such as Charles Dekeukeleire and Henri Storck as important figures, it was not unusual for small countries without a strong film industrial infrastructure to use international movies before turning to the production of local films, notably regarding specific genres such as hygiene film.[94]

In fact, *Un ennemi public* was the first official, nationally produced public health film.[95] The lack of a local film production scene makes one wonder about the extent to which Belgian films were considered to be important as identificatory media tools, as authorities argued in other European countries, such as France, Germany, the United Kingdom, Italy and Austria.[96] A representative number of foreign hygiene films were distributed and circulated in Belgian cinemas or other projection venues, and the press regularly received and reported of these films. In contrast, prior to the production of *Un ennemi public*, the value of domestically produced health films was underreported. Health propaganda supporters, such as René Sand, frequently promoted the motion picture as a promising medium for communicating health prophylaxis and educating a public mass audience on treatment and self-monitoring (see Chapter 4, p. 151). Nonetheless, as they referred to the existing French film productions, there does not appear to have been an explicit institutional desire for national production.[97] This can be explained by a lack of budget and infrastructure in the 1920s, a decade characterised by both an economic crisis and a relative lack of political authority over health matters. In this context, it was hard to compete with the French and the American educational film market as it was easier and cheaper to buy existing international films, and appropriate them for distribution and screenings in Belgian cinemas, also with the insertion of translated intertitles.[98]

Professional filmmakers, medical film directors and expertise

Cinematography developed in scientific spaces: the first motion pictures, whether as (pre-cinema) serial photographs, chronophotographs or cinematic films were created by natural scientists or technophiliacs, being therefore self-evidently part of the scientific sphere.[99] Yet these mechanically produced images immediately caught the public's attention: X-rays and microscopic photography, as well as motion pictures, were projected in, and circulated between, scientific and public spheres.[100] In the interwar years, the medical community debated about using film as scientific evidence, while a few scientists and physicians began to use the medium for public health education.

Questions regarding 'the good educational film'[101] emerged in Europe after the First World War, when the film industry as well as the educational film movement were supported in a more systematic way. A growing community was interested in the conception, production and distribution of health films despite the fact that they were less profitable than entertainment movies. Public health films, issued by national health departments, were interdisciplinary collaborations between professional filmmakers, politicians and physicians. The alliance of well-known filmmakers and directors brought together by Storck and Sand can be seen as a classic example in view of European health film policy.[102]

Commercial filmmakers increasingly collaborated with representatives from the medical community.[103] Documentary filmmakers, such as Storck and Castille, worked with physicians, such as the psychologist and progressive educator Ovide Decroly and neurologist Léon Laruelle from the 1920s onwards.[104] In this way, the link between film and science, already imagined by the Lumière brothers, was finally established.[105]

The case of Storck, who individually took action to produce public health films, shows that national debates on medical filmmaking as a tool for public education could be promoted and stimulated by various actors, who interacted with each other. Professional filmmakers not only interacted with physicians, but also with producers and the intended audience, whether this was a population of 'health consumers' or students training to be physicians. Storck's efforts to promote these films were not exclusively grounded in the wish to better citizens' health, but were also a strategical attempt to better his standing with national authorities and to secure his future career as a filmmaker. The transformation of the film medium into a channel of health-related information engendered various questions regarding the interaction between viewers and health film producers.[106]

Discipline and agency: viewers as consumers?

In national and international debates regarding how best to convey public health knowledge to lay audiences, physicians and health authorities were outlining what composers should know about the topic of their films and about the targeted audience and their struggles in life. In order to make films effective, so it was believed, abstract medical knowledge, for example regarding bacteria, had to be made as legible as possible for a viewing audience that lacked prior knowledge.[107]

Until well into the 1930s and 1940s, audiences did not play an active role in the filmmaker's decision-making process. Public viewers' reactions and feedback at screenings were taken into consideration but were only debated within an expert-driven network. Systematic surveys or interviews were only erratically conducted. However, as consumer advocacy became more important – both in general and in relation to medical care – market research for public health productions gained ground.

Production notes of hygiene films suggest that debates between filmmakers and sponsors not only considered the question of how to convey a scientific moral message, but also of how sociopolitical narratives could be implemented through film.[108] Cinema appealed to those trying to popularise public health information following institutional agendas and health marketing narratives. But the actual transdisciplinary collaboration of those involved in film production was more complex than expected. For instance, a representative of the Ligue Nationale belge contre la tuberculose, who corresponded with Storck about the tuberculosis film production, wished to prominently film the building of the Ligue in Schaerbeek and insert the Cross of Lorraine, the symbol for the 'crusade' against tuberculosis. Storck diplomatically declined the request, because viewers would easily recognise camouflaged advertising and often did not react well to this kind of 'in-your-face' propaganda.[109]

Film narratives attempted to speak to the public's emotions in order to inform them about the prevention or treatment of disease. This could mean reaching the viewer with emotions of disgust, shock, reassurance or solidarity.[110] Filmmakers tried to make the viewer feel like a potential patient. Citizens were not only addressed as film consumers, but also as modern health consumers. Visual practices of health promotion and disease prevention had to produce a new way to think about the body and health. Epidemics were often discussed in terms of individual behaviour and risk. Disease was represented as self-inflicted; its treatment as one's own responsibility.[111] As the emphasis was on the individual, this meant that social and structural problems – such as limited workers' rights or bad housing – were neglected. The underlying message was that for those who were instructed, and did not take the expert's advice seriously, disease could be framed as being one's own fault.[112]

Whereas this emphasis on individual responsibility was commonly left uncriticised by reviewers, they did suggest that filmmakers had to know the lives and struggles of targeted spectators. In an essay entitled 'Does Cinema Appear as Educationally or Morally Corruptive?'[113] written in 1934, Victor de Ruette, inspector for *'des Etablissements pour malades mentaux et enfants anormaux du Royaume'* ('institutions for the mentally ill and abnormal children of the kingdom') stated that the different contexts of the potential viewers, distinguished by their profession, urban or rural origin, confession, gender, race and age, should be taken into account when evaluating hygiene and public health films. In de Ruette's view, however, physicians remained the most suitable evaluators of such films since they would be able to judge the educational and psychological value of different narratives and visual displays.

Conforming with the international contemporary debate on the so-called good and immoral as opposed to the 'morally corruptive' cinema, de Ruette elaborated that the most crucial task for health educational films should be to exclusively claim film as an educational rather than an entertaining medium. The point of this was to prevent the supposed moral and physical decay of 'the' public. Illiterate rural and colonised populations, who did not have the same access to public education as citizens in the metropole, were considered to be important target groups. In addition, a crusade against illiteracy was globally pronounced with the help of educational films, which would reach and inform viewers who were not able to read books or access formal education. The cinematic image was considered to be a suitable vivid didactic media that could visualise complex phenomena hard to describe in words.[114]

Un ennemi public is a classic example of combining scientific images with fictional narrative: micro-cinematographic displays of tuberculosis pathogens or authentic shootings from Belgian clinics and sanatoria were intertwined with fictional scenes. The scene in which the protagonist visits a doctor and attends an X-ray examination in the clinic was staged at the actual hospital rooms of the St-Pierre university clinic in Brussels.[115] On set the film staff was instructed by the hospital's technicians on how to operate the X-ray device.[116] The shooting location was thus 'real', but the character of the doctor was interpreted. In other European health films, it was common to feature real patients, doctors and members of clinical staff to underline the immediate reality of medical risk and care.

Storck had suggested a private physician as consultant, who should arrange terms with the Ligue Nationale belge contre la tuberculose. The logistics of all participating and funding parties proved to be difficult. The production was more time-consuming since not all parties agreed on who should be the primary decision-making authority. Storck was increasingly dissatisfied with the way in which the production had unfolded. At some point, in a letter to one of his fellow film peers, Storck minimalised his impact on the final film, as he criticised the lack of artistic freedom during the production.

The storyline and impact of *Un ennemi public* appeared to lose importance throughout its production. Whereas the film was originally intended for a large audience, the producers were ultimately content to be able to screen the film in representative settings. Political officials, journalists and other distinguished members of Belgian society were invited to the premiere. Invited officials and press reported gushily about the successful, both morally and educationally valuable, film.

Afterwards, *Un ennemi public* was screened in local cinemas in the city, periphery and countryside, and was made accessible to all ages and sexes. Yet the public audience was less enthusiastic, as often was the case for educational films.[117] The lacking commercial outlet was anticipated, but the failure in popularity by the targeted viewing population was still frustrating for the producers and health officials. The impact was, rather, to be found in the interaction between participating producers and public addressees.[118] Viewers were often fed up with the moral tone or the disgusting motion pictures of diseased body parts. Young cinemagoers preferred exotic travelogues, crime stories and adventurous western films to 'boring' educational films. Even after introducing more representative forms of evaluation through conducting surveys and collecting statistical data, the actual educational impact on public health film viewers was criticised and doubted.

Experienced hygiene film producers suggested that educational films should be 'easily understood, visually impressive, sensual, appealing or when needed deterrent', but principally they should be relatable, convincing and at least capable of raising interest. In turning to humorous film elements and introducing microcinematographic images they thought they could minimise the risk of boring their audiences. Tuberculosis films tried to combine a moral tone with humour. In *Un ennemi public*, for instance, the white-coated doctor talked to his blue-collar patient in a conventional scientific paternalist manner, but nevertheless comic ways are used to attract viewers (indeed, the actors and extended film cast often came from comedy backgrounds).[119] Despite the growing concern with the public's response, it was always an expert authority that transformed medical knowledge for a public audience. Even though interactions between the public and the professional sphere were increasingly sought after, they remained hierarchical.

Conclusion

The second half of the twentieth century is often represented as a period in which the gap between the scientific and the public sphere grew – an evolution that was confirmed by the rise of mediating actors, such as the science journalist.[120] However, this chapter shows that specialised 'mediators', such as curators, guides or film directors, have played an important role in the spread and transformation of medical knowledge since the nineteenth century. Similarly, the years in between 1945 and the emergence of anti-authoritative movements in the late 1960s are often characterised as the golden age for alliances between politics, media and science.[121] Yet this phenomenon, too, can be compared to earlier initiatives from city councils or public institutions, such as the Ligue nationale belge contre la tuberculose.

Audiences were never mere passive consumers of knowledge. In the nineteenth century, just as today, they had the agency to choose from and adapt different views of the body and health, and could respond to them in unintended ways. Sometimes their reactions incited popularisers to change their ways. The role of the audience has grown further in times of broadcasting media. The systematic acquisition of data on visitors' and viewers' reactions became pivotal for health-related market research and media programming. When one takes into account that television programmes, for instance, can be dismissed if they do not reach good viewing figures, the power of the audience becomes hard to deny.[122] Since the digital era, democratic accessibility of websites and databases, such as YouTube, Wikipedia, medical trial sites or health and fitness apps monitoring physiological data, are easier to consume than ever before, and have given rise to reflection and criticism regarding the status of experts in science communication.[123] US surveys in the late 1990s showed, for instance, that most of the respondents were getting healthcare information from television before they would consult doctors. Magazines, journals, newspapers, radio and, most importantly, the Internet have become crucial media for seeking medical advice.[124]

From all this, it is clear that the popularisation of medicine was, and is, not a top-down process, but rather the result of exchanges between different actors, ranging from physicians to carnies, from film directors to working-class audiences, from politicians to television producers. Knowledge was not simply diffused by scientists, but transformed as different actors interacted with each other. Even if the relationship between the scientific and the public sphere was hierarchic, interactions were mutual. Not only did popularisers enter (or pretended to enter) in alliances with scientists to bolster their authority, scientists also actively pursued rapprochements with larger audiences in order to enhance their own. Until today, the reach and public relevance of one's scientific work is an important argument for the legitimation of research and its funding.

Belgium appears to be a particularly interesting case to study these instances of circulation. As the market was often too small for original productions, there was room for international institutions. Yet in order to attract Belgian audiences, these foreign players (whether curators of health exhibitions, moviemakers or others) did have to adapt themselves to local tastes and sensitivities. The boundaries between the scientific and the popular sphere, too, appear to have been more permeable than in other countries. The example of the Spitzner Museum suggests that Belgian politicians were particularly enthused by collaborations with commercial institutions.

To conclude, it is time to revise our big pictures and the place of popularisation within them. The idea of 'professionalisation' does not account for the continued importance of lay experts, and 'medicalisation' was not a mere top-down process but was at least in part initiated by lay audiences and patients, who sought medical knowledge and treatments themselves.[125] As Huistra's research on the Netherlands has shown, recent mass digitisation projects might provide us with the right tools to grasp the history of popularisation in all its complexity.[126] It is now possible to complement more traditional sources, such as medical journals or parliamentary discussions, with a systematic study of newspapers, ego-documents and popular magazines. Historians are better equipped than ever to elucidate both the roles of different actors in the popularisation process and the circulation of ideas. Popularisation was not a monologue but a conversation: let us study it as such.

Notes

1 'Développez et raffermissez votre poitrine', *Le Peuple* (19 May 1914).
2 B. Latour, *Pandora's Hope: Essays on the Reality of Science Studies* (Cambridge, MA: Harvard University Press, 1999); N. Thomas, *Entangled Objects: Exchange, Material Culture, and Colonialism in the Pacific* (Cambridge, MA: Harvard University Press, 1991); J. A. Secord, 'Knowledge in transit', *Isis*, 95:4 (2004), 654–72.
3 J. R. Topham, 'Rethinking the history of science popularization/ popular science', in *Popularizing Science and Technology in the European Periphery 1800–2000*, ed. F. Papanelopoulou et al. (London: Routledge, 2009), 1–20.
4 F. Huisman, 'Shaping the medical market: on the construction of quackery and folk medicine in Dutch historiography', *Medical History*, 43:3 (1999), 359–75.
5 J. Vandendriessche, E. Peeters and K. Wils, 'Introduction: performing expertise', in *Scientists' Expertise as Performance: Between State and Society, 1860–1960*, ed. J. Vandendriessche, E. Peeters and K. Wils

(London: Pickering & Chatto, 2014), 1–13. On lay actors claiming medical expertise, see W. Ruberg, 'Mother knows best: the transmission of knowledge of the female body and venereal diseases in nineteenth-century Dutch rape cases', in *The Transmission of Health Practices, c.1500 to 2000*, ed. M. Dinges and R. Jütte (Frankfurt: Franz Steiner Verlag, 2011), 35–48.

6 The Royal Library of Belgium started the digitisation of newspapers in 2004. A selection of newspapers can be accessed through their website at www.belgicapress.be (accessed 20 February 2018). Several medical journals are also being digitised, cf. www.kbr.be/fr/impress (accessed 20 February 2018).

7 K. Velle, *De nieuwe biechtvaders: de sociale geschiedenis van de arts in België* (Leuven: Kritak, 1991); W. Dupont, 'Free-floating evils: a genealogy of homosexuality in Belgium' (PhD diss., University of Antwerp, 2015); L. Di Spurio, *Du côté des jeunes filles: Discours (contre-)modèles et histoire de l'adolescence féminine* (Brussels: éditions de l'université libre de Bruxelles, 2020); C. Pirson, *Corps à Corps. Les Modèles anatomiques entre art et médecins, 1699–2008* (Paris: Mare & Martin, 2009).

8 S. Onghena, 'Professor, wat kunt U ons vertellen? Wetenschapsprogramma's tijdens de pioniersjaren van de Vlaamse televisie, 1953 – ca. 1970', *Tijdschrift voor Geschiedenis*, 125:2 (2012), 217–32; S. Onghena, 'Tot lering en vermaak: wetenschappelijke kinderboeken van Belgische uitgevers in de tweede helft van de negentiende eeuw', *De Gulden Passer*, 89:2 (2011), 211–37; T. Claes and V. Deblon, 'Van panoramisch naar preventief. Populariserende anatomische musea in de Lage Landen (1850–1880)', *Negentiende Eeuw*, 39:3/4 (2015), 287–306; K. Wils, 'Tussen wetenschap en spektakel. Hypnose op de Belgische theaterscène, 1875–1900', *Tijdschrift voor mediastudies*, 20:2 (2017), 54–73. An ongoing interuniversity project looks at the history of the use of the 'magic lantern', including for science popularisation, see www.uantwerpen.be/en/projects/b-magic (accessed 19 March 2020).

9 E. Peeters, *De beloften van het lichaam. Een geschiedenis van de natuurlijke levenswijze in België, 1890–1940* (Amsterdam: Bert Bakker, 2008); A. H. van Baal, *In Search of a Cure: The Patients of the Ghent Homeopathic Physician Gustave A. van den Berghe 1837–1902* (Rotterdam: Erasmus, 2008).

10 For example, K. Knight, *Public Understanding of Science: A History of Communicating Scientific Ideas* (London: Routledge, 2006); P. Bowler, *Science for All: The Popularization of Science in Early-Twentieth-Century Britain* (Chicago: University of Chicago Press,

2009); D. Raichvarg and J. Jacques, *Savants et ignorants: une histoire de la vulgarisation des sciences* (Paris: Seuil, 1991); S. Nikolow (ed.), *Erkenne Dich selbst! Strategien der Sichtbarmachung des Körpers im 20. Jahrhundert* (Cologne: Böhlau, 2015).

11 E. Peeters, 'Questioning the medical fringe: the "cultural doxy" of Catholic hydrotherapy in Belgium, 1890–1914', *Bulletin of the History of Medicine*, 84:1 (2010), 92–119.

12 Onghena, 'Professor', 225–30.

13 J. Hellemans, 'Les contrefaçons belges au Québec ... Au temps où le livre français était belge', *Documentation et bibliothèques*, 57:3 (2011), 169–77.

14 V. Deblon, 'Imitating anatomy: recycling anatomical illustrations in nineteenth-century atlases', in *Bodies Beyond Borders: Moving Anatomies, 1750–1950*, ed. K. Wils, R. De Bont and S. Au (Leuven: Leuven University Press, 2017), 139–61.

15 R. Molhant, *Les Catholiques et le Cinéma: Une étrange histoire de craintes et de passions. Les débuts: 1895–1935* (Brussels: OCID), 19; J. Trumpbour, *Selling Hollywood to the World: U.S. and European Struggles for Mastery of the Global Film Industry, 1920–1950* (Cambridge: Cambridge University Press 2001), 211–13; D. Biltereyst and D. Treveri Gennari (eds), *Moralizing Cinema: Film, Catholicism, and Power* (New York: Routledge, 2014).

16 On the value of such a media-approach, see J. Leach, 'Science communication', in *The Handbook of Communication History*, ed. P. Simonson et al. (London: Routledge, 2013), 289–301.

17 K. Velle, *Lichaam en hygiëne* (Ghent: MIAT–KRITAK, 1984); K. Velle, 'Bronnen voor de medische geschiedenis: de Belgische medische pers (begin XIXde eeuw–1940)', *Annalen van de Belgische vereniging voor de geschiedenis van de hospitalen en de volksgezondheid*, 23–4 (1988), 66–119; W. H Helfland, 'Some one sole unique advertisement': public health posters in the twentieth century, in *Imaging Illness. Public Health and Visual Culture*, ed. D. Serlin (Minneapolis: University of Minnesota Press, 2010), 126–42.

18 Pirson, *Corps à Corps*, 163–205; Claes and Deblon, 'Van panoramisch', 287–306.

19 Province de Hainaut, *Musée d'Hygiène: nouveau catalogue illustré* (Mons: Charleroi Imprimerie provinciale, 1925).

20 Roode Kruis, *De mensch: tentoonstelling Egmont-paleis, Brussel, 1–31 oktober 1938: catalogus* (Brussels: Roode Kruis van België, 1938).

21 G. Convents, 'Van de verburgelijking van het populair vermaak tot amusement voor iedereen', in *De panoramische droom: Antwerpen en de wereldtentoonstellingen 1885, 1894, 1930*, ed. M. Nauwelaerts,

C. Terryn and P. Verbraeken (Antwerpen: Uitgeverij Antwerpen 93 vzw, 1993), 236–47.

22 E. Stephens, 'Inventing the bodily interior: écorché figures in early modern anatomy and Von Hagens' *Body Worlds*', *Social Semiotics*, 17 (2007), 313–26.

23 Claes and Deblon, 'Van panoramisch', 301.

24 L. Nys, 'De grote school van de natie. Legerartsen over drankmisbruik en geslachtsziekten in het leger, 1850–1950', in *Degeneratie in België 1860–1940: Een geschiedenis van ideeën en praktijken*, ed. J. Tollebeek, G. Vanpaemel and K. Wils (Leuven: Leuven University Press, 2003), 79–118.

25 'M. Spitzner', *La Chronique* (20 July 1878); 'Een bezoek aan het anatomisch museum', *Vooruit* (4 September 1921).

26 For instance, Madame Consael and Madame Spitzner inherited their late husbands' museum.

27 Knight, *Public Understanding*, 182–96; M. Rossiter, 'Women and the history of scientific communication', *Journal of Library History*, 21:1 (1986), 39–59.

28 'Le Musée Castan', *La Chronique* (3 March 1892).

29 Velle, *Lichaam en hygiëne*, 63–4.

30 'Door beter weten naar gezonder leven', *De Gentenaar* (22 June 1938).

31 G. Achten et al., *Grand Musée anatomique du docteur Spitzner: 1856–1896* (Brussels: Musée d'Ixelles, 1979); N. Poot, G. Vanpaemel and S. Waelkens, *Een walvis in de stad. De collecties van de Leuvense Faculteit Wetenschappen* (Leuven: Lipsius, 2014).

32 We borrow the term 'things in motion' from A. Appadurai, 'Introduction: commodities and the politics of value', in *The Social Life of Things: Commodities in Cultural Perspective*, ed. A. Appadurai (Cambridge: Cambridge University Press, 1986), 3–63.

33 Claes and Deblon, 'Van panoramisch', 292; Pirson, *Corps à Corps*, 163–205.

34 'La société médicale allemande de Paris', *La médecine à l'exposition l'universelle de 1867* (Paris: Germer-Baillière, 1867).

35 Roode Kruis, *De Mensch*, 8. On the Glass Man, see K. Fiss, *Grand Illusion: The Third Reich, the Paris Exhibition and the Cultural Seduction of France* (Chicago: University of Chicago Press, 2009), 73–5.

36 Claes and Deblon, 'Van panoramisch', 287–306.

37 'De tentoonstelling De Mensch of het geheim van het leven', *De Gentenaar* (1 October 1938).

38 A. Maerker, *Model Experts: Wax Anatomies and Enlightenment in Florence and Vienna, 1775–1815* (Manchester: Manchester University Press, 2011).

39 F. Hutton, *The Study of Anatomy in Britain, 1700–1900* (London: Pickering & Chatto, 2013), 133; L. Schulte-Sasse, 'Advise and consent: on the Americanization of Body Worlds', *BioSocieties*, 1:4 (2006), 369–84.
40 H. Huistra, 'Weg met pottenkijkers! Hoe het publiek verdween uit het Leids anatomisch kabinet', *Negentiende Eeuw*, 34:3 (2010), 193–208.
41 City Archives Ghent, 335, Musées de l'université de zoologie et d'anatomie comparée: ouverture au public 1919–20.
42 Pirson, *Corps à Corps*, 163–205.
43 T. Claes, 'De onwetendheid baart de ziekte. Het populaire anatomische museum als een plaats van preventie en moralisering', in *Vesalius: het lichaam in beeld*, ed. G. Vanpaemel (Leuven: Davidsfonds, 2014), 139–45.
44 Province de Hainaut, *Musée d'Hygiène*, 100.
45 J. D., 'A propos de l'exposition de l'Homme, organisée par la Croix Rouge de Belgique', *La Libre Belgique* (5 October 1938).
46 Pirson, *Corps à Corps*, 197.
47 Deblon, 'Imitating anatomy', 115–37; T. Claes, 'Alternative anatomy: the popular lectures of Constant Crommelinck in Brussels (1850–1880)', in Wils et al., *Bodies Beyond Borders*, 139–61.
48 Vandendriessche et al., 'Introduction', in *Scientists' Expertise as Performance*, 1–13.
49 Peeters, 'Questioning the medical fringe', 92–119.
50 A. W. Bates, 'Dr Kahn's museum: obscene anatomy in Victorian London', *Journal of the Royal Society of Medicine*, 99:12 (2006), 618–24.
51 Pirson, *Corps à Corps*, 197–8.
52 City Archives Brussels, ASB IP II 2581, Letter from City Council of Antwerp to City Council of Brussels, 27 September 1926.
53 Achten, *Grand musée anatomique*.
54 S. Onghena, 'Spektakelstukken. De mise-en-scène van de wetenschap in de Belgische stad, 1890–1914', in *Tussen beleving en verbeelding: de stad in de negentiende-eeuwse literatuur*, ed. I. Bertels et al. (Leuven: University Press Leuven, 2013), 43–69, at 44.
55 City Archives Brussels, ASB IP II 3333, Letter from Madame Spitzner to City Council of Brussels, 27 December 1933.
56 J. D., 'A propos de l'exposition de l'Homme', 2.
57 Onghena, 'Spektakelstukken', 61–5.
58 Velle, *Lichaam en hygiëne*, 101.
59 E. Stephens, 'Inventing the healthy body: the use of popular medical discourses in public anatomical exhibitions', in *The Body Divided: Human Beings and Human 'Material' in Modern Medical History*, ed. S. Ferber and S. Wilde (Ashgate: Farnham, 2011), 223–38, at 236.

60 T. Consael, *Museum voor ontleed-, volken- en ziektenkunde: gids van den bezoeker, bevattende de noodige en juiste aanduidingen en uitleggingen van ons verzameling* (Brussels: Lefèvre, 1885).
61 P. Spitzner, *Katalogus van het groot anatomisch museum van dr. P. Spitzner* (n.pub., n.d.).
62 S. Alberti, 'Objects and the museum', *Isis*, 96:4 (2005), 559–71. On Belgium, see L. Nys, *De intrede van het publiek: Museumbezoek in België, 1830–1914* (Leuven: Leuven University Press, 2012), 219–50.
63 Maerker, *Model Experts*, 128–33.
64 J. D., 'A propos de l'exposition de l'Homme', 2.
65 S. Bussels and B. van Oostveldt, 'De Antwerpse wereldtentoonstelling van 1894 als ambigu spektakel van de moderniteit', *Tijdschrift voor Geschiedenis*, 125:1 (2012), 5–20.
66 Claes and Deblon, 'Van panoramisch', 302.
67 H. Storck, *Un ennemi public*. Ligue Nationale belge contre la tuberculose. sound film. b/w 15 min (Belgium, 1937).
68 Archives générales du Royaume (AGR), Brussels, Section Prophylaxie de l'Oeuvre Nationale Belge de Défense contre la Tuberculose, founded in the 1920s, Dossier: Min. Santé Publique, Adm. Hygiène Publique, 1482, Buhl Committee 117.
69 R. Sand, 'Le programme de la médecine sociale', *Vers la santé*, 3 (1922), 497–506; K. Ostherr, *Cinematic Prophylaxis: Globalization and Contagion in the Discourse of World Health* (Durham, NC: Duke University Press, 2005).
70 Cf. Chapter 'Television', in *Cultural Sutures: Medicine and Media*, ed. L. D. Friedmann (Durham, NC: Duke University Press, 2004), 197–262.
71 Cf. D. Cantor, 'Uncertain enthusiasm: the American Cancer Society – public education and the problems of the movie, 1921–1960', *Bulletin of the History of Medicine*, 1:81 (2007), 39–69; C. Bonah, D. Cantor and A. Laukötter (eds), *Health Education Films in the Twentieth Century* (Rochester, NY: University of Rochester Press, 2018).
72 Cf. Ostherr, 'Cinematic prophylaxis'.
73 C. Bonah, 'A word from man to man: interwar venereal disease education films for military audiences in France', *Gesnerus: Swiss Journal of the History of Medicine and Sciences*, 72:1 (2015), 15–38.
74 Cf. K. Pilz, 'Aufklärung? Abschreckung? In der mit Sexualität gespannten Atmosphäre des Kinos? Sexualität in Wiener klinischen und populärwissenschaftlichen Filmen der Moderne', in *Sexualität und Widerstand. Internationale Filmkulturen*, ed. A. Basaran, J. B. Köhne, K. Sabo and C. Wieder (Vienna: Mandelbaum, 2018), 54–76.

75 M. S. Pernick, 'Thomas Edison's tuberculosis films: mass media and health propaganda', *Hastings Center Report*, 8:3 (1978), 21–7, 25.
76 G. Aubert, 'Arthur van Gehuchten takes neurology to the movies', *Neurology*, 59:10 (2002), 1612–18; T. Lefebvre, 'À la découverte d'Arthur van Gehuchten', *Bulletin de la Sémia*, 1 (2002), 7. His filmed cases were partly published posthumously in A. van Gehuchten, 'Les Maladies Nerveuses' (Leuven: Librairie Universitaire, 1920), 532–44.
77 P. van Gehuchten, *L'œuvre scientifique de Arthur van Gehuchten* (Brussels: Impr. des Sciences, 1973).
78 G. Marinesco, 'Application du cinématographe à l'étude des troubles de la marche dans les maladies nerveuses', *Journal de Neurologie*, 18 (1900), 316; A. van Gehuchten, 'Coup de couteau dans la moelle lombaire', *Le Névraxe*, 9:2 (1907), 208–32.
79 Medical film collections: Achives de la Cinématèque Royale de Belgique, Brussels, Arthur van Gehuchten (Archives UCL, Louvain 1905–1914); Private Archive Institute Born-Bunge, Antwerp, Ludo van Bogaert (Instituut Born-Bunge, Antwerp, 1934–50).
80 Cf. A. Laukötter, 'Vom Ekel zur Empathie. Strategien der Wissensvermittlung im Sexualaufklärungsfilm des 20. Jahrhunderts', in *Erkenne Dich selbst! Strategien der Sichtbarmachung des Körpers im 20. Jahrhundert*, ed. S. Nikolow (Cologne: Böhlau, 2015), 305–19.
81 As was the case in Germany, France and Austria. Cf. K. Pilz, 'Medicine in motion: early medical filmmaking shaping clinical specialisation, public health and visual modernity in Vienna and Brussels' (PhD diss., Université libre de Bruxelles and Universität Wien, 2020).
82 'Annonce films Doyen', *Cinéma-Revue-Belge. Journal hebdomadaire de la Cinématographie et de toutes les industries qui s'y rattachent*, 12 (1912), 8–9.
83 Quoted by Desjardin in *Contrefaçon artistique des cinématographies du Dr Doyen* (21–2), in T. Lefebvre, *La chair et le celluloïd. Le cinéma chirurgical du docteur Doyen* (Paris: Brionne, Jean Doyen éditeur, 2004), 54.
84 L. Haesaerts, 'Le Cinéma scientifique', in *Numéro spécial de Les Beaux-Arts publié pour l'Institut national de cinématographie scientifique de Belgique à l'occasion du IIIe Congrès de l'Association internationale du cinéma scientifique* (Brussels: n.pub., 1949), 378–92, at 368.
85 P. Väliaho, *Mapping the Moving Image: Gesture, Thought and Cinema circa 1900* (Amsterdam: Amsterdam University Press, 2010), 109.
86 Cf. P. Thevenard and C. Tassel, *Le cinéma scientifique français* (Paris: La Jeune Parque, 1948).

87 M. Cadé, *L'écran bleu: La représentation des ouvriers dans le cinéma français* (Perpignan: Presses Universitaires de Perpignan, 2004).
88 R. Sand, 'L'histoire de la médecine du travail', *Archives Belges de Médecine Sociale, Hygiène, Médecine du Travail et Médecine Légale*, 9:7 (1949), 395–420 and 484–507.
89 Cf. 'Darstellung von Krankheiten in neueren Lehr- und Kulturspielfilmen', *Zeitschrift für Ärztliche Fortbildung*, 25:13 (1928), 472–3.
90 Cinémathèque Royale de Belgique (CRB), Brussels, List/Dossier: films hygièniques.
91 L. Bourgeois, *Le dispensaire antituberculeux. L'assistance publique de Paris*, b/w 5 min. (France 1917), CRB.
92 Comité National: *La visiteuse d'hygiène*, b/w 5 min. (France ca. 1925), CRB.
93 Cf. T. Lefebvre, 'Les victimes de l'alcoolisme (Pathé – 1902). Quand le cinéma des premiers temps puise son inspiration dans le discours hygiéniste dominant', *Archives. Institut Jean Vigo – Cinémathèque de Toulouse* (May 1992); Archives de la Ville de Bruxelles (AVB), Brussels, film poster, AVB, Affiches cinéma XIII-12 'Affiche de cinéma. Les Maladies Sexuelles et leurs Conséquences. Cinéma Le Régent. Rue Neuve, Bruxelles ('Un document scientifique sensationnel ... Pour combattre un fléau il faut le connaître!')
94 F. Henrion, 'A propos de Cinéma Scientifique', *Union des anciens étudiants de l'ULB*, 334 (1966), 37–40.
95 Until then, colonial and in Belgium produced health films were nominally produced by American health officers, such as a film on venereal diseases produced in 1926, AGR, Brussels, Dossier: Min. Santé Publique, Adm. Hygiène Publique, 1482, Dossier: Cinéma/films éducatives.
96 Cf. M. Braun et al. (eds), *Beyond the Screen: Institutions, Networks and Publics of Early Cinema* (New Barnet: John Libbey, 2012); C. Taillibert, *L'Institut international du Cinématographe éducatif. Regards sur le rôle du cinéma éducatif dans la politique internationale du fascisme italien* (Paris: L'Harmattan, 1999); Z. Druick, 'The International Educational Cinematograph Institute, reactionary modernism, and the formation of film studies', *Canadian Journal of Film Studies*, 16:1 (2007), 80–97.
97 Among others such as micro-cinematographic (microscopic motion pictures) life science and surgical films, cf. B. de Pastre and T. Lefebvre (eds), *Filmer la science, comprendre la vie: le cinéma de Jean Comandon* [exhibition catalogue] (Paris: Centre national de la cinématographie, 2012).
98 Which was common also for other films in smaller countries with less commercial film industry, cf. P. Mosley, *Split Screen: Belgian Cinema*

and *Cultural Identity* (New York: State University of New York Press, 2001).
99 Cf. K. Pilz, 'Hearts and brains in motion: medical animated film as a popular and controversial medium for education and research', *Wiener Klinische Wochenschrift – The Central European Journal of Medicine*, 132 (2020), 52–6.
100 Cf. W. Benjamin, *Das Kunstwerk im Zeitalter seiner technischen Reproduzierbarkeit* (Berlin: Suhrkamp, [1936] 2010), 500.
101 Cf. E. Blaschitz, *Der 'Kampf gegen Schmutz und Schund'. Film, Gesellschaft und die Konstruktion nationaler Identität in Österreich (1946–1970)* (Vienna: Lit Verlag, 2014).
102 These collaborations were common also in the case for contemporary Germany, France and Austria.
103 Cf. O. Decroly, 'Le cinéma comme procédé d'étude et moyen d'enseignement de la psychologie de l'enfant', *Document pédotechnique* (1929), in CED, Brussels, manuscript.
104 S. Wagnon, *Ovide Decroly, un pedagogue de l'Éducation nouvelle 1871–1932* (Brussels: PIE, 2013), 141–6.
105 A. Lumière, *Notice sur le titres et travaux de Auguste Lumière Correspondant de l'Institut et de l'Académie de Médecine de 1887 à 1940* (Lyon: Imp. Léon Sézanne, 1940).
106 Cf. K. Ostherr, 'Empathy and objectivity. health education through corporate publicity films', in Serlin, *Imaging Illness*, 62–82.
107 Cf. J. Rancière, *Le destin des images* (Paris: La Fabrique éditions, 2003).
108 S. Curtis, *The Shape of Spectatorship: Art, Science, and Early Cinema in Germany*, Film and Culture Series (New York: Columbia University Press, 2005).
109 Archives de l'ULB (AULB), Fond Henri Storck, Dossier: correspondence *Un ennemi public*, letter Ligue Nationale belge contre la tuberculose and Henri Storck, spring 1937.
110 Cf. Laukötter, 'Vom Ekel zur Empathie', 305–19.
111 K. Ostherr, *Medical Visions: Producing the Patient Through Film, Television, and Imaging Technologies* (New York: Oxford University Press, 2013).
112 Pernick, 'Thomas Edison's tuberculosis films', 25.
113 V. de Ruette, 'Cinéma éducatif ou cinéma démoralisateur?', *Journal de l'Institut international du cinématographe éducatif*, 4 (1933), 290–308.
114 M. Loiperdinger, 'The social impact of screen culture 1880–1914', in *Screen Culture and the Social Question 1880–1914*, ed. L. Vogl-Bienek and R. Crangle (New Barnet: KINtop, 2014), 9–19.
115 Cf. on the history of Brussels university clinics: R. Bardez, 'La Faculté de médecine de l'Université Libre de Bruxelles: entre création,

circulation et enseignement des savoirs (1795–1914)' (PhD diss., Université libre de Bruxelles, 2015); and V. Leclercq, 'Guérir, travailler, désobéir: Une histoire des interactions hospitalières avant l'ère du "patient autonome" (Bruxelles, 1870–1930)' (PhD diss., Université Libre de Bruxelles, 2017).

116 AULB, Brussels, fond Henri Storck, production notes 1937.
117 A. Mebold, 'Just like a public library maintained for public welfare: 28mm as a comprehensive service strategy for non-theatrical clientele, 1912–1923', in *Networks of Entertainment: Early Film Distribution 1895–1915*, ed. F. Kessler and N. Verhoeff (New Barnet: John Libbey, 2007), 260–74.
118 J. Tanner, 'Populäre Wissenschaft. Metamorphosen des Wissens im Medium des Films', *Gesnerus: Swiss Journal of the History of Medicine and Sciences*, 66:1 (2009), 15–39, at 17.
119 De Ruette, 'Cinéma éducatif ou cinéma démoralisateur?', 303–4.
120 Onghena, 'Professor', 227.
121 R. Halleux and G. Xhayet, 'De ontwikkeling der ideeën', in *Geschiedenis van de wetenschappen in België 1815–2000*, ed. R. Halleux et al. (Brussels: Dexia, 2001), 15–34.
122 T. Boon, *Films of Fact: A History of Science in Documentary Films and Television* (London: Wallflower Press, 2008), 2 and 184.
123 F. Mclellan, 'Medicine.com: the internet and the patient–physician relationship', in *Cultural Sutures: Medicine and Media*, ed. L. D. Friedmann (Durham, NC: Duke University Press, 2004), 373–85.
124 Ibid., 1–5.
125 P. Conrad, 'The shifting engines of medicalization', *Journal of Health and Social Behavior*, 46:1 (2005), 3–14; S. Snelders and F. Meijman, *De mondige patiënt: historische kijk op een mythe* (Amsterdam: Bert Bakker, 2009).
126 H. Huistra, 'Experts by experience: lay users as authorities in slimming remedy advertisements, 1918–1939', *Bijdragen en Mededelingen Betreffende de Geschiedenis der Nederlanden*, 132:1 (2017), 126–48.

Selected bibliography

Anderson, N. and Dietrich, M. R., *The Educated Eye: Visual Culture and Pedagogy in the Life Sciences* (Hanover, NH: Dartmouth College Press, 2012).

Bonah, C., Cantor, D. and Laukötter, A. (eds), *Health Education Films in the Twentieth Century* (Rochester, NY: University of Rochester Press, 2018).

Bonah, C. and Laukötter, A. (eds), *Body, Capital, and Screens: Visual Media and the Healthy Self in the 20th Century* (Amsterdam: Amsterdam University Press, 2020).

Claes, T. and Deblon, V., 'Van panoramisch naar preventief. Populariserende anatomische musea in de Lage Landen (1850–1880)', *Negentiende Eeuw*, 39:3/4 (2015), 287–306.

Friedmann, L. D. (ed.), *Cultural Sutures: Medicine and Media* (Durham, NC: Duke University Press, 2004).

Onghena, S., 'Professor, wat kunt U ons vertellen? Wetenschapsprogramma's tijdens de pioniersjaren van de Vlaamse televisie, 1953–ca. 1970', *Tijdschrift voor Geschiedenis*, 125:2 (2012), 217–32.

Onghena, S., 'Spektakelstukken. De mise-en-scène van de wetenschap in de Belgische stad, 1890–1914', in I. Bertels, J. H. Furnée, T. Sintobin, H. Vandevoorde and R. van de Schoor (eds), *Tussen beleving en verbeelding: de stad in de negentiende-eeuwse literatuur* (Leuven: Leuven University Press, 2013), 43–69.

Pauwels, L. (ed.), *Visual Cultures of Science: Rethinking Representational Practices in Knowledge Building and Science Communication* (Hanover: University Press of New England, 2006).

Peeters, E., *De beloften van het lichaam. Een geschiedenis van de natuurlijke levenswijze in België, 1890–1940* (Amsterdam: Bert Bakker, 2008).

Peeters, E., 'Questioning the medical fringe: the "cultural doxy" of Catholic hydrotherapy in Belgium, 1890–1914', *Bulletin of the History of Medicine*, 84:1 (2010), 92–119.

Secord, J. A., 'Knowledge in transit', *Isis*, 95:4 (2004), 654–72.

Serlin, D. (ed.), *Imaging Illness: Public Health and Visual Culture* (Minneapolis: University of Minnesota Press, 2010).

Van Baal, A. H., *In Search of a Cure: The Patients of the Ghent Homeopathic Physician Gustave A. van den Berghe 1837–1902* (Rotterdam: Erasmus, 2008).

Vandendriessche, J., Peeters, E. and Wils, K. (eds), *Scientists' Expertise as Performance: Between State and Society, 1860–1960* (London: Pickering & Chatto, 2014).

Epilogue

Including *all* citizens of Belgium: narratives beyond the profession and the state

Frank Huisman

This volume is the impressive result of the collective efforts of Belgian (medical) historians to do at least two things: first, to put Belgium on the map of medical historiography and, second, to do so using the latest methods and approaches. With a single stroke, the Belgian field presents itself at the forefront of medical history. Not only is Belgium now ready to be included in international comparative research, but the sophisticated chapters in this volume invite us to engage in further research using the concepts and agendas of our Belgian colleagues. The editors invited me to comment on the volume and the potential of its 'new narratives'. They even suggested a title for my epilogue – 'Medicine Beyond Belgium' – implying I take the view from the rest of Europe in evaluating the Belgian case. That does not seem to be feasible, if only because similar volumes about other European countries are lacking. Therefore, I chose to approach the volume as a self-contained unit, asking questions like: what is new to these narratives? How do they relate to earlier ones? What are their strengths? What are their weaknesses? Who is the audience for these narratives? How do they affect our research agenda?

Diversity and dynamism

It has been stated ad nauseam that 'traditional' medical history was written by, for and about doctors. This led to narratives mainly appealing to their intended audience, namely stories about progress through science and about the productive collaboration between the profession and the state for the benefit of mankind. This situation profoundly changed when social historians entered the scene in the 1970s and 1980s. They claimed that health, illness and healing are not the exclusive domain of doctors but important to all of us. The way in which we understand our body and its diseases is not primarily scientific. Moreover, the healthcare system is funded by all citizens, while its organisation affects the health and wealth of all of us. Therefore, the 'new historians' claimed that it was legitimate for them to write about the medical past as well. They argued that health and illness precede medical consultation, and that cultural notions about them are all-pervasive. Physician-medical historians were held to be unduly selective and monopolistic about the medical past, appropriating a specific version of it. Qualifying their progressivist narrative as finalistic – and thus celebratory rather than analytic – and unpacking categories like science, profession and the state, the 'new historians' created new narratives. These were not just populated by medical men, but by patients, alternative healers, clergymen, women and other historical actors as well. The perspective of medical history was turned upside down – taking the patient's perspective – while its sources expanded enormously – any medium documenting the past was now deemed of potential value – and its methodological toolkit grew and diversified with every 'turn'. In their Introduction, the editors stress that the innovative character of the volume is in its attention to the multiplicity of actors, places and media. Acknowledging that physicians remain central players, they argue that roles and identities have become more complex, thus fragmenting and blurring the picture.

The agenda of the volume is to move *beyond* the state, institutions and physicians, because the 'turns' in history writing have made us aware that there are many dimensions preceding and accompanying consultation of a physician whose academic training and medical practice is regulated and overseen by the state. While the social turn pointed us to the power dimension involved in medicine and healthcare, the cultural turn made us realise that in referring to our bodies, we are moving in multivocal semantic networks. The ways in which we conceptualise our body and frame our diseases has implications for the ways in which we relate to them and act upon them. With the performative and the praxeological turns, the focus changed from idea to practice and from blueprint to action, while the material turn called to take the built environment (and objects in general) into account. Finally, the somatic turn built on anti-essentialist notions by distinguishing between sex and gender. While not doing justice to these and other turns, the point here is that they all represented a call to move away from a universalist history of ideas, and from taking a top-down (professional, male, bourgeois, Western) perspective. All 'turns' pointed to the diversity and dynamic nature of society (and therefore healthcare), calling to do justice to it in our representations of the medical past.

Many chapters in this volume are responding to this agenda of diversity and dynamism. In Chapter 1, for example, Jolien Gijbels and Kaat Wils show that even though academia was no place for women until well into the nineteenth century, medicine and healthcare have always been thoroughly gendered. But when women finally knocked on the door – around 1875 – male physicians tried to naturalise medicine as a typically male endeavour, referring women to 'caring professions' like nursing and midwifery. While the Royal Academy of Medicine argued that women were too delicate (in body and mind) or indeed too ignorant to become a physician, women dismissed this claim as an attempt to maintain and legitimise the conventional division of labour, with men on top of the medical hierarchy. Feminists were keen on claiming and redefining the female body, in order to liberate themselves and secure their place under the sun. This was by no means an easy task: for the better part of the twentieth century, female physicians had a hard time trying to set up their own practice – some of them even resorting to the colonial route, hoping to be more fortunate in the Belgian Congo. In the end, women succeeded in entering the medical curriculum and making a career as a Doctor of Medicine, but only after a long and protracted struggle in which class and gender differences often reinforced each other. In the late twentieth century, the number of female medical students exceeded that of their male counterparts. The point that Gijbels and Wils are making is that healthcare is a battlefield, and that the combatants are using all rhetorical means at their disposal to support their claims, also including medical historiography. While female voices may be difficult to find in the nineteenth century, this is not to say that they did not exist or that they did not make themselves heard. Therefore, in order to recapture the full and inclusive picture of the medical past, we need to be critical and creative in finding and interpreting our sources, sometimes reasoning 'against the grain', sometimes even using silences in the past in a productive way.

The same applies – probably even more so – to the stories that can be told about the colonial past. African indigenous healing practices continued to thrive during the colonial era. They were hardly affected by – or indeed in contact with – Western medicine. Still, the voices of Africans are hardly ever heard, because the colonial narrative has always been told by the European coloniser. The two quotes at the beginning of Chapter 3 by Sokhieng Au and Anne Cornet nicely illustrate the profound difference between both worlds: the rendering of a medical ceremony among the Bakongo in 1941 is followed by a medical report on a trypanosomiasis expedition to the Belgian Congo written almost forty years earlier. The contrast between both texts could not be bigger: while the former describes a healing ritual replete with religious offerings, chants and music firmly embedded in the local community, the latter is a technical report on a diseased woman, filled with clinical details and metrics in an attempt to objectify disease. Thus, Au and Cornet are setting the stage for a story about Western medicine and other colonial institutions. At first sight, theirs may look like a rather traditional story. However, their sophisticated introduction is putting things into perspective by pointing out that indigenous healers and Western medical practitioners were living in two separate worlds. By also reminding us that 'medicine' is defined by the disciplinary lens of scholars who are writing about it (both past and present, both physicians and historians), they succeed in avoiding the trap of Eurocentrism. Their story about state-organised medical service, missionary medicine and industrial medicine from the perspective of Belgium loses all of its 'traditional' connotations, because the reader is made aware that they are only reading one side of the story. Having said that, the authors make it abundantly clear that the Belgians were not on a humanitarian mission in Congo. Although Belgium was a latecomer on the colonial scene, it quickly and brutally caught up. King Leopold II regarded the Congo as his personal fiefdom, exploiting it ruthlessly. 'Health' was not considered to be a public good but rather a commercial or military one, with medicine helping to create a racial and gendered discourse of difference used to avoid the Congolese ever coming to be considered as Belgian citizens. Again, science was instrumental in creating binary distinctions, naturalising difference and inferiority, legitimising colonial hierarchies. Again, we realise that we should not fall into the trap of uncritically adopting 'actor's categories', and that we should never blindly follow the sources that happen to be available to us. Au and Cornet make us keenly aware that colonial archives were produced for specific commercial and military goals, not to satisfy the historical or anthropological curiosity of later generations. The story about indigenous healing practices in Africa is yet to be written.

Although medical history has long been fascinated by the ways in which 'the normal' and 'the pathological' are constructed, the focus tended to be on discursive medical practice. Disability studies challenged the exclusive right of medicine to frame disease – in body and mind – and the monopoly of the state to act upon it. Taking the patient's perspective, they broadened the scope by pointing to alternative ways of framing health and disease, and by making us aware that other groups (like priests, statisticians or pedagogues) have been involved in understanding and coping with impairment – however defined. In doing so, disability studies challenged the unilinear stories of professionalisation and medicalisation by including other voices than those of the profession and the state. In Chapter 8, Benoît Majerus and Pieter Verstraete show how this may shatter our received image of ongoing civilisation and progress through the doings of the medical profession and the state. In its attempt to create productive citizens and a healthy nation, the newly independent state of Belgium (1830) felt the need to deal with the threat 'lunatics' caused to public order and morality. The expert advice of people like Joseph Guislain led the new state to adopt legislation giving rise to the discipline of psychiatry and the building of psychiatric institutions. Next to (or even opposed to) the story about normalisation that has traditionally been told about the rise of psychiatry and its institutions, Verstraete and Majerus present two stories that may be considered as counter-narratives. Keen on showing the agency of laypeople, they tell the story of the Geel colony and that of deinstitutionalisation. Contrary to the treatment offered in asylums by professional psychiatrists, the Geel colony represented an alternative model of community care 'where the insane lived as a family and in freedom'. To the critics of the disciplinary regimes of psychiatry, the Geel colony was an example to be emulated and followed. In the 1960s and beyond, psychiatry and its institutions were heavily criticised. People inspired by the work of Michel Foucault, Ivan Illich, Thomas Sasz and Erving Goffman argued that the state had grown into a 'therapeutic state' – medicalising all 'abnormal' behaviour – creating 'total institutions' where psychiatrists took total control over someone's life. They therefore called for deinstitutionalisation: by setting the insane free, their humanity would be restored, while it would also have a healing effect on society at large. Although Verstraete and Majerus fully realise that deinstitutionalisation has its limits, by reminding us of the constructed character of the boundaries between normal and pathological and between lay and professional, they invite us to look beyond (narratives about) the profession and the state.

Another way of toning down the solid character of professionalisation and medicalisation theories is by looking at the ways in which knowledge about the body – in health and illness – circulated in society. Whoever presumes that the profession and the state were dominant and all-pervasive, will opt for a top-down perspective and a diffusion model, using 'official' sources only. However, scholars intrigued by the dynamics in the public sphere will allow for agency of laypeople, hybridity and reciprocity, also using 'grey' literature. By looking at the mediating role that health exhibitions and medical movies played in the past, in Chapter 9 Tinne Claes and Katrin Pilz intend to show that categories like 'the state', 'the profession' and 'the public' were by no means homogeneous entities. Claiming that the antagonism – and even hierarchy – between 'official' and 'alternative' medical beliefs was a cultural construct rather than a historical reality, their searchlight is on historical actors outside of academia. Arguing that popularisation was not a monologue but rather a conversation, they focus on the media through which medicine circulated in society, putting the citizen-patient-consumer centre stage. They show that exhibitions and movies moved between the university, the fairground and the cinema. Anatomical exhibitions were taken out of their context, speaking to others than to their intended audience. In these new contexts, they went for the sensational, the grotesque or the erotic rather than for educational value, leaving visitors free to respond in unintended or unexpected ways. Something similar applied for medical movies. At the same, Claes and Pilz observe that 'it was always an expert authority that prepared and transformed medical knowledge for a public audience ... Interactions remained hierarchical'. This makes one wonder how 'hybrid' the encounter between science and the public really was. Or to put it differently: are we looking at counter-narratives opposing medical discourse or rather at the elevation of laypeople to medical standards? One is inclined towards the latter: health exhibitions and public health movies – embodying the ideals and agendas of the sanitary movement – reached ever-wider audiences, especially after the Second World War. Ironically, then, the dominance of the profession and the state is confirmed in this chapter.

This is not to say however, that we can simply discard alternative actors' voices or historiographies, as Joris Vandendriessche and Tine Van Osselaer show in Chapter 2. If there is one thing preceding medical consultation, it is religion. Religion supplies answers to existential questions, giving meaning to birth, suffering and death, offering solace to believers. Therefore, religion may be regarded as a source of health and recovery. In order to understand how people have been dealing with health, illness and healing it is therefore imperative to take religion into account: without it, no medical history can claim to offer a complete story. Over the course of the nineteenth century, the Catholic Church developed into a major institution in Belgium, pervading all domains of society. By the mid nineteenth century almost half of the orders were involved in the provision of medical care, after having been suppressed under French rule. Belgium had the largest Catholic university in the world (Leuven) and even in the Congo Catholics held disproportionate power. It was a force to be reckoned with, and the Vatican always took good notice of what was going on in Belgium. This situation had developed after independence in 1830, with the constitution of the new nation state offering ample opportunity for religious orders to establish themselves. Its liberal freedoms gave free reign to the Catholic Church, making it dominant in the provision of medical care as well. However, contrary to what earlier historiography wanted us to believe, Vandendriessche and Van Osselaer stress that religiously inspired care was hardly ever at odds with medicine. They argue that medicine and religion were not in opposition with each other but coexisted and interacted with each other. This view has implications for their view on 'secularisation' as well. Rather than being simply a matter of 'less religion, more medicine', the Catholic Church remained an important force when in the late twentieth century issues concerning abortion, euthanasia, *in vitro* fertilisation and genetic screening came to be discussed. Medical ethics in Belgium tended to be dominated by Leuven academics, who attempted to mediate between medical developments and Catholic doctrine. Today, questions relating to the meaning of life, suffering and death and the goals and limits of medicine are as relevant as ever before.

Moving beyond the profession and the state

This volume opens up new vistas in other ways as well. Its chapters look not just beyond the profession and the state, but they do so by presenting a rather under-researched case: Belgium. For a long time now, the centre of gravity of European medical history has been the United Kingdom. Thanks to the generous funding by the Wellcome Trust, the field has been thriving there, as it no doubt will continue to do. Many wonderful monographs have been written about Britain's medical past, inspiring colleagues across the world. But for history to thrive, it is in need of many more national perspectives. While medicine may be an international intellectual endeavour transcending national borders, healthcare systems tend to be a product of their national context. Different political cultures produce different constellations of healthcare, while the logic of path dependency limits the extent to which national systems may derive from each other. Given the fact that there are many different national styles of healthcare, it makes sense to compare them – if only in an attempt to put any given healthcare system into perspective. Medical history is therefore in need of national narratives, as many as possible. This volume is a courageous attempt to supply just that for Belgium. And although there is some irony in the fact that these new narratives – keen on moving *beyond* the state – are framed in a national context, they succeed in showing how productive this new approach may be. It has not been the ambition of the editors to supply a new unifying narrative, but rather to present a handful of perspectives on the medical past of a particular country. Belgium took shape as a modern nation state from 1830 onwards, when it liberated itself from the Netherlands, its northern neighbour. The bond between them had been an uneasy marriage, arranged at the Congress of Vienna in 1815. The new state was intended to be a middle-sized power, meant to contribute to the post-Napoleonic balance of power in Europe. The marriage had lasted fifteen years, when it ended in a ten-day military campaign. The differences between the north (the former Dutch Republic) and the south (the former Austrian Netherlands, belonging to the Habsburg Empire) had been too big to make for a viable nation state.

In the nineteenth century, the state came to be seen as responsible for the health of the nation. However, before preventive measures for the public benefit could be put in place, health determinants needed to be established first: what factors caused disease, and how could their detrimental effects be prevented or countered? In their quest for answers, the profession and the state relied on each other. While medicine was looking for a way out of its etiological fatalism (e.g. to understand cholera), the state tried to realise its self-imposed goal of catering to the needs of its citizens. Until then, the medical profession had been rather weak and poorly organised, so it needed the support of the state. Building on Hippocratic notions, environmental medicine seemed to provide the answer, and it was considered imperative for the state to act upon advice supplied by the profession. In Chapter 4, Thomas D'haeninck, Jan Vandersmissen, Gita Deneckere and Christophe Verbruggen show how this process slowly materialised over the course of the nineteenth century. At international conferences, physicians and statisticians informed each other about the correlation between health determinants and morbidity patterns in their country. By exchanging and superimposing their observations, they hoped to be able to trace regularities. Ultimately, their deeper understanding of epidemic disease was expected to inform (local) policies at home. In this sense, the profession and the state legitimised each other, one presupposing and reinforcing the other. Their relationship was famously expressed by Rudolf Virchow, when he stated that politics is nothing but medicine on a large scale. This is when the narratives about the beneficial alliance between the profession and the state found their origin, serving an emancipatory goal for the medical profession. Much later, these narratives came to be criticised as being self-serving and celebratory, unduly legitimising a professional monopoly protected by the state. Critics argued that the alliance between the profession and the state had sometimes even done more harm than good. During the interwar years, for example, some states had used medicine to naturalise and support eugenic racial policies, while in the post-war years medicine proved unable of formulating a viable response to chronic disease or to growing inequities in healthcare. In a globalising world there was a growing need to move beyond the profession and the state.

After Belgium had gained independence from the Netherlands in 1830, it faced the challenge to organise the new nation state – and this included setting up a system of medical education. The new state was in need of physicians who could do research on epidemic diseases threatening the nation and who could serve the state by giving advice on health matters. As Renaud Bardez and Pieter Dhondt show in Chapter 5, the new Belgian state was quick in reinventing itself, at least in a formal sense. After drafting its own Constitution, it proceeded by completely reorganising the university system. This also affected the medical faculty and its curriculum. Belgium was the first European state to introduce a single medical degree (it was to take another sixteen years before the Netherlands realised this). In 1849, the patchwork of competences – a legacy of the *Ancien Régime* – was a thing of the past. From then on, physicians were allowed to practise medicine, surgery and obstetrics in all of Belgium. Having said that, we should realise that this was only a legal settlement, accelerated by Belgian independence and the need for the new Belgian state to set up a system of public health and the educational system belonging to it. Bardez and Dhondt show that, more often than not, the educational system and the profession failed to deliver what the state required. First, curriculum reform was paralysed by intense parliamentary discussions between Catholics and liberals on the composition of university boards. Second, medical faculties had to resort to foreign professors – most of them German – due to a lack of Belgian candidates. Third, there was conservative resistance to reform; for example by Liège professors, for whom the transition was moving too fast. Fourth, there was a lack of state funding for the so-called free universities, and the price they had to pay for their freedom of education. And finally, there was the issue of language; it proved to be very difficult to build a nation in a country that is trilingual (French, Dutch and German), especially when the demarcation line is heavily socially charged. Again, by moving beyond the profession and the state, it becomes clear that there is a huge difference between dream and reality and between blueprint and practice. Thus, Bardez and Dhondt's chapter causes us to reconsider the value of professionalisation and medicalisation theories.

Another way to move beyond the older narratives is to resort to other sources, such as material objects. In doing so, more historical actors may be involved in the stories that we tell, like nurses, servants and – last but not least – patients. Although artefacts do not talk, they may contain useful information about the way daily life on the ward was organised, adding layers and nuance to the story. In Chapter 7, Valérie Leclercq and Veronique Deblon argue that the architectural plan of a hospital, for example, may tell us more about the way space was organised. Going to hospital involved a range of segregations, first of all from the outside world. In addition to that, patients were classified and segregated by class, gender, illness and/or behaviour. They were categorised and disciplined by and through medicine, but by religion and morality as well. Thus, the materiality of a hospital reiterated social and moral distinctions in society. The hospital may be considered as a microcosm reflecting cultural values on the outside. In their chapter Leclercq and Deblon are looking at domesticity, religious symbols and social norms as they are expressed through material objects in hospitals. It becomes clear that around 1900, hospitals were still very much involved in charitable care. This started to change at the turn of the century, when the status of medicine improved and the hospital became increasingly accepted as a place for medical treatment. From then on, the artefacts tell a story of physical segregation, the imperative of ventilation and cleanliness and the emergence of the block hospital and new management styles: all of them medical imperatives advocated by medical men. In the process, sanitary goals, medical surveillance and cost effectiveness came to prevail over domesticity, aesthetics and religious symbolism, even though religion continued to be very present until well after the Second World War. Leclercq and Deblon successfully challenge two older teleological narratives – one of medical progress and the other of social control – adding new dimensions of hospital life to their story. Still, its overall trend is one of medicalisation. Over the course of the twentieth century, Belgian hospitals transformed from being charitable institutions for the poor to high-tech, business-oriented centres where patients were redefined as consumers.

This seems to point to an important shift in focus of the alliance between the profession and the state: from preventive measures for the benefit of the nation to curative interventions in the lives of individuals. To fully understand the 'system' of healthcare however, we need to include a third stakeholder complicating the story: the Catholic Church. With poverty and illness being two sides of the same coin, individual care in the nineteenth century was mainly a matter of charity provided by the church. While the young Belgian state did its best to put sanitary measures in place – as much as its liberal ideology would allow – Catholic charity was crucial in supplying the bare minimum of care to individual citizens, either in hospitals or in their homes. In Chapter 6, on the organisation and funding of the healthcare system, Dirk Luyten and David Guilardian introduce funding mechanisms of care and cure as an important dimension. By taking money into account, we are invited to think about the motives for funding and about the entitlements and responsibilities involved. Over the course of the twentieth century the state took over from the church as being the most important funding body of healthcare. In 1853, 75 per cent of all expenditure on care was supplied by the church, with only 18 per cent being supplied by the state. In 2015, this had profoundly changed: 60 per cent of all the expenditure on healthcare was derived from the national compulsory health insurance scheme, 18 per cent from the state, another 18 per cent from out-of-pocket payments by patients and 4 per cent from voluntary insurances. By that time, the church had vanished from the scene. This situation is the result of a complex interaction between many factors. On the one hand, the twentieth century witnessed many scientific and technological breakthroughs, leading to impressive therapeutic results and an increase in the average life expectancy, but to exponentially rising costs as well. On the other hand, secularisation gave rise to new coping strategies with regard to illness, especially after the Second World War. While disease had often been considered as divine fate or as a trial bestowed by God to test a sufferer's belief, it came to be seen as simply bad luck that could and should be remedied at all costs. With the secularisation of society, healthcare increasingly came to be seen as a right to be guaranteed by the state and delivered by the profession; citizens considered themselves to be entitled to all available interventions. In modern neo-liberal society, citizens no longer fatalistically accept their fate. Rather, they expect the state to take care of them from the cradle to the grave and account for its funding priorities in rational and transparent ways.

This brings us to the paradox of our time: although the alliance between the profession and the state has brought a lot to mankind, we are now living in an era of rising costs, diminishing returns and increasing anxiety about the system. In *The Greatest Benefit to Mankind*, Roy Porter took the long view on health, illness and healing in an attempt to contribute to much needed reflection on the system. In his introduction, he observed: 'Medicine is an enormous achievement, but what it will achieve practically for humanity, and what those who hold the power will allow it to do, remain open questions'.[1] Porter concluded his book by formulating a mission for (Western) mankind: 'For centuries medicine was impotent and thus unproblematic ... Today, with "mission accomplished", its triumphs are dissolving in disorientation ... Medicine will have to redefine its limits even as it extends its capacities'.[2] Reflecting and redefining the goals and limits of medicine entails looking beyond the profession and the state. At the same time, we need to rethink the rights and duties of all of us, and the present volume may help us accomplish this. In the past, medical history was written by male, Western physicians. This led to rather unilinear stories of progress through the doings of the profession and the state, referred to as professionalisation and medicalisation. As this volume shows, today's medical history is (also) written by historians, women and non-Westerners, producing multiperspective and multivocal stories. While some may regret this development because of the fragmentation this entails, I would argue that much is to be gained by including *all* historical actors. We should be prepared to take new perspectives, looking at more domains and using more diverse source material. Moving beyond the great doctors, decentring the big picture and provincialising Europe may lead to a diversity of narratives. Yet this is no reason to shy away from it, since it represents the diversity of today's world.

The famous Dutch historian Johan Huizinga once observed that history is the mental form in which a culture takes account of its past. He wrote this in a time when historians were still living under the illusion that the culture of a nation was one and that historians were uniquely equipped to represent its history. We have come to realise that there are many (sub)cultures, both within and between nations, and that each of them is entitled to take account of its past. Of course, there have always been more subcultures than one, but after the emancipation of workers, women, black people, patients and others, they have become vocal – shaping their identities by taking account of their past. Their narratives may be complementary and in line with each other, but more likely they will be in competition with each other, taking their own positions and agendas as their point of departure, showing the sheer richness and diversity of society, both past and present. Like medicine, medical history is not owned by physicians, but by all of us. We should therefore be grateful to our Belgian colleagues, not just for making us realise this, but also for building on that notion by supplying us with wonderful case studies of Belgium, showing the diversity and dynamism of its medical past and inviting all of us to join in the debate.

Notes

1 Roy Porter, *The Greatest Benefit to Mankind: A Medical History of Humanity from Antiquity to the Present* (New York: W. W. Norton, 1997), 12.
2 Ibid., 718.

Timeline of Belgian medical history

Ordering time to make the final outcome of history appear as 'natural' has been for a long time one of the main functions of national histories. Timelines were one of these hermeneutic tools that condensed this willingness to represent a 'neat' and tamed past. Reading them today can be frustrating as they often focus on political and event-driven history, where the historical narrative tries to show the contingency of the past. We asked the contributors of each chapter to propose five dates that were important for their topic. These are assembled here not in a thematic but in a chronological order. At first sight, this timeline appears puzzling. There is no '1796' when the French governance reorganised public health around two institutions: the civil hospitals and the welfare bureaus. Neither does it include '1841', the date of the foundation of the Royal Academy of Medicine of Belgium, or '1944', the voting of the Social Security Act, which laid the basis of Belgium's post-war system of health insurance. Instead, here are forty-five events that, we hope, will lead the reader down sometimes unexpected paths of Belgian medical history.

1803 Foundation of the Sisters of Charity of Jesus and Mary in Ghent, one of the major orders of female religious in Belgian healthcare (p. 68)
1820 Creation of the first institute for deaf girls in Brussels by Jozef Triest (p. 287)
1834 Foundation of the Medical Society of Ghent (p. 139)
1841 Creation of the Catholic Society of St Vincent de Paul (p. 210)
1849 Creation of the single degree of Doctor of Medicine, Surgery and Obstetrics (p. 177)
1849 Establishment of the Superior Health Council, a national commission of non-medical administrators tasked with

	supervising city planning and the construction of public buildings (p. 144)
1850	Adoption of the Mental Treatment Act (p. 286)
1857	Inauguration of the Hospice pour hommes aliénés in Ghent (known as the Guislain asylum) (p. 251)
1868	Miraculé Louise Lateau first displayed the (visible) wounds of Christ, the start of an intense debate among physicians and theologians (p. 79)
1870	First ovariotomy performed in Belgium (p. 43)
1874	Establishment of medical inspection of public schools in Brussels (p. 145)
1876	Law on medical education, introducing laboratory research into the curriculum (p. 185)
1879	A proposition to allow midwives to use forceps is rejected by the majority of members of the Royal Academy of Medicine (p. 34)
1884	Opening of the Stuyvenberg hospital in Antwerp (p. 250)
1884	Isala van Diest is the first female physician allowed to practise in Belgium (p. 37)
1888	The first debate in the Belgian medical press on the occurrence of hysteria among male soldiers (p. 44)
1894	Law on mutual aid societies introducing the regime of 'subsidised liberty' (p. 213)
1895	Health education becomes a compulsory part of the curriculum in both primary and secondary schools (p. 327)
1896	One of the first Lumière screenings in Belgium at the Galerie du Roi in Brussels (p. 334)
1903 –05	Todd/Christy/Dutton Liverpool School of Tropical Medicine sleeping sickness expedition in the Congo Free State (p. 122)
1905	Production of the first clinical research and teaching films by Arthur van Gehuchten at the Catholic University of Leuven (p. 337)
1907	Foundation of the Catholic St Camille School for Nursing in Brussels (p. 71)
1910	Foundation of the School for Tropical Medical Medicine by royal decree (p. 123)
1910	The Dutch physician Pieter Eijkman published *L'internationalisme médical*, an overview of international medical organisations that includes three Belgian initiatives (p. 134)

1911	Creation of the Service d'Assistance Médicale Indigène (SAMI) (p. 107)
1911	Opening of the provincial hygiene museum of Mons (p. 329)
1913	Foundation of the *Bulletin de l'Association belge de Médecine sociale* (p. 151)
1922	Foundation of the Belgian Society of Saint-Luc, a society for Catholic doctors (p. 72)
1927	Informal foundation of the International League for Educational Film (p. 341)
1930	Creation of the Fonds Reine Élisabeth pour l'Assistance aux Indigènes (FOREAMI) (p. 111)
1935	Opening of the new St-Pierre Hospital in Brussels, the first 'block' or 'tower hospital' in Belgium (p. 264)
1937	Premiere of *Un ennemi public*, the first nationally produced public health film by Henri Storck and the Belgian National League Against Tuberculosis (p. 334)
1948	INAMI/RIZIV, the Belgian system of health insurance, registered a deficit for the first time (p. 225)
1949	Ten-year development plan for the Congo (p. 120)
1957	Legal regulation of medical specialisation (p. 193)
1958	The world exhibition takes places in Brussels, with the Atomium as its icon, a breakthrough also for televised science (p. 322)
1961	Foundation of the Institute for Family and Sexuality Studies at the Catholic University of Leuven (p. 84)
1963	Creation of L'Equipe in Anderlecht, the first sector-based mental health service in Belgium (p. 298)
1963	Law 'Leburton', regulating the price setting of medical fees (p. 227)
1968	First professorship in family medicine at the University of Leuven (p. 195)
1985	Inauguration of the university hospitals CHU Sart-Tilman (Liège) and Gasthuisberg (Leuven) (p. 269)
1990	Partial depenalisation of abortion (p. 51)
1990	Adoption of the Act on the Protection of the Mentally Ill (Loi relative à la protection de la personne des malades mentaux) (p. 307)
1994	Foundation of the International Centre for Reproductive Health (ICRH) (p. 157)
1995	First government-led experiments with personal assistance budgets (p. 303)

Index

abortion 17, 32, 41, 47–53, 81, 85, 87, 88, 157, 365, 374
academic degree of Doctor of Medicine, Surgery and Obstetrics (1849) 4, 41, 177, 178, 188, 193, 198, 360, 367, 372
academic hospital (Ghent) 264, 265, 269
academic hospital (Liège) 269, 374
academic hospital St Raphael/Gasthuisberg (Leuven) 65, 231, 269, 374
acquired immune deficiency syndrome (AIDS) 15, 156, 157
Aga Khan Development Network 157
Albania 2
alcoholism 146, 332, 339
Alexians (religious order) 207
Algeria 103, 123
almshouses 207, 208, 286
American Baptist Missionary Society 106
anaesthetics 87
anatomical museum (Liège) 329
anatomy 1, 5, 6, 29, 30, 77, 139, 172, 174, 176, 178, 180, 181, 182, 185, 190, 194, 246, 250, 320–3, 326–30, 332, 333, 363

andrology 41
animal magnetism 180
anti-psychiatry 294
antisepsis 214, 256
Association Internationale du Congo 104
Association internationale pour le Progrès des Sciences sociales 142
Association of Belgian and Immigrant Women 307
asylum 8, 69, 76, 80, 116, 246, 247, 251–3, 256–62, 268, 270–2, 286, 289, 294–7, 303, 304, 309, 362, 373
Austria 80, 270, 340
Austrian Netherlands 366
Auzoux, Louis 329

bacteriology 137, 143, 144, 148, 254, 256, 342
Baeckelmans, Frans 250
Banneux 76, 78
barber surgeons 172
Barella, Hippolyte 146
Baretta, Jules 329
Baudouin (king) 87
Beauraing 76, 78
Beau-Vallon Asylum 69, 76, 257, 259, 262, 268
Becker, Jérôme 148
Beers, Clifford 305

Belgian Federation of University
    Women (Fédération
    Belge des Femmes
    Universitaires) 39, 49
Belgian League for the Rights of
    Women (Ligue belge du droit
    des femmes) 48, 146
Belgian Medical Federation
    (Fédération médicale belge)
    4, 193
Belgian Ministry of Public Health
    4, 143, 218, 231, 232, 304
Belgian Ministry of War 298
Belgian Phreniatric Society
    (Société phréniatrique
    belge), subsequently Society
    for Mental Illness (Société
    de médecine mentale de
    Belgique) 13, 286
Belgian Revolution (1830) 1, 8, 21,
    32, 172, 177, 178, 286, 362,
    364, 365, 367
Belgian Society for Sex Education
    (Belgische vereniging voor
    Seksuele Vorming) 50, 51
Belgian Society of Gynaecology
    and Obstetrics 13, 41
Belhomme, Jacques-Étienne 291
Belval, Théodore 146
Bijloke Hospital (Ghent) 248, 251
birth control 32, 47–51, 80, 82–4,
    150
Black Sisters 207
Blacklock, Thomas 290
Blackwell, Elizabeth 29
blindness 208, 286–8, 290, 293,
    300, 301, 310–12
Blum, Isabelle 50
Boddaert, Richard 186
Boëns, Hubert 79
Bonn 143
Bordet, Jules 192, 222, 264
Bouckaert, Jean-Jacques 171,
    172, 194

Brachet, Albert 192
Brattgard, Sven-Olof 308
British Baptist Missionary
    Society 106
Broeckx, Jean-Corneille 1–2, 21
Brothers of Charity 35, 68–9, 291
Broussais, François 172, 177
Brugmann Hospital (Brussels) 255,
    258, 268, 279, 283
Brunfaut, Gaston 266
Bruyninckx, Edmond 304, 317
Bulckens, Jean 253
*Bulletin de l'Association belge de
    Médecine sociale* 151, 374
*Bulletin de la Société de Médecine
    Mentale de Belgique* 286
Bulletin medical belge 12
*Bulletin of the Belgian Academy of
    Medicine* 13
Bureau International du Travail
    (Geneva) 108
Bureau of Medical
    Verifications 78
Burggraeve, Adolphe 139–42,
    157, 161–2
Burundi 99, 100, 103, 108,
    121, 125

caesarean section 40, 81, 82
Cameroon 108
Canada 264
cancer 15, 25, 59–60, 65, 71,
    222, 229
Cancer Institute Jules Bordet
    (Brussels) 222, 264
Canon, Pierre 124
*Caritas and Caring for the Ill
    (Ziekenverpleging)* 71
Caritas Catholica 72, 74, 75
Carnoy Institute (Leuven) 189
Carton, Charles-Louis 287,
    290, 313–4
Casti Connubii (1930) 51,
    80, 83, 96

Castille, Antoine 337, 341
Catholic Action movement 65, 83
Catholic Hospital Association (1915) 72
Catholic Nursing (De katholieke ziekenverpleging) 71
Catholic Society of St Vincent de Paul 210, 372
Catholic University of Leuven 10, 18, 26, 38, 65, 68, 79, 81, 84–6, 88, 117, 121, 172, 174, 178, 179, 187, 189, 194, 196–8, 287, 329, 337, 364, 373, 374
Centre for Bioethics (Leuven) 85
Centre for Hospital Sciences (Leuven) 231
Centre for Human Genetics (Leuven) 85
Charcot, Jean-Martin 43
Charitable Native Medical Services (Assistance Médicale Indigène Bénévole) (1920) 111, 113, 114
childbirth 32–5, 41, 53, 81, 178, 336
cholera 77, 140, 144, 366
Christian Health/Mutual Funds 75, 225–34
Christomanie 68, 79
Cinémathèque Royale de Belgique 337
Civil hospital (Mons) 250
Claeys, Emilie 48, 49
Claus, Hugo 86
Clinique Héger (Brussels) 222
Congo 6, 9, 13, 15, 17, 40, 73, 83, 99–126, 137, 147, 148, 149, 155, 360, 361, 364, 374
Congo Free State (CFS) (1885–1908) 104–9, 113, 122, 123, 130, 134, 147, 148, 149, 373

contraception 47, 48, 50, 51, 82, 157
Crocq, Jean Joseph 185, 186
Crommelinck, Constant 37–8, 250, 330
CSM network (Centres de santé mentale or mental health centres) 305, 306

Danneels, Godfried 74, 86, 88
de Hoensbroeck, Constantin 288
de Rudder, Pieter 78
de Ruette, Victor 343
De Saeger, Jos 74
De Vaucleroy, Alfred 146
De Vrouw 48, 49
Decroly, Ovide 293, 337, 341
Dehaene, Jean-Luc 231
Dekeukeleire, Charles 339
Delasiauve, Louis 291
Delcour, Albert 39
Demarez, Luc 308
Demeester, Wivina 308, 309
Denys, Joseph 192
Depage, Antoine 190–1, 264
depression 44
Dermine, Jean 84
Deroubaix, Louis 188
Derscheid, Marie 39, 152
Desguin, Victor 145, 157
Desirant, Yvonne 39
Desmyter, Jan 156
Dhont, Julien 301
diabetes 15
Dille-Lobe, Vogelina 50
Dillemans, Roger 85
diphtheria 144
disinfection 257, 264
dissection 77, 180, 183
Doctors of the World (Médecins du Monde/Dokters van de Wereld) 229
Dolle Mina 51
Donum vitae (1987) 85

Doyen, Eugène-Louis 338
Dryepondt, Gustave 148–9
Ducpétiaux, Edouard 286
Dutch Republic 366
Dutton Todd Christy expedition (1903–1905) 122

Ebola 155–6
Eijkman, Pieter 134–7, 158, 373
electrotherapy 256
Élisabeth Hospital (Brussels) 255
Encyclographie des sciences médicales (1833) 12
epidemic 77, 107, 110, 111, 112, 114, 134, 139, 140, 144, 147, 148, 150, 156, 158, 248, 326, 334, 336, 339, 343, 366, 367
Errera Institute (Brussels) 189
Esquirol, Étienne 75, 291
Ethical Perspectives (*Ethische perspectieven*) 88
eugenics 137, 150, 191, 287, 300, 367
euthanasia 86, 87, 365
Everart, Clémence 38
Exhibition *Body Worlds* 328, 332
Exhibition *De Mensch* (The Human Being) 326–9, 331, 333

family planning 48, 51, 84, 157
Fédération des Institutions Hospitalières (FIH, francophone) 75
Finland 2, 195
Fischer, Alfons 153
Flexner, Abraham 189
Fohman, Vincent 181
forensic medicine 178
Foucault, Michel 304, 311, 331, 363
Fourcroy, Antoine 175
France 2, 4, 8, 11, 14, 30, 33, 35–7, 42, 44, 68, 70, 71, 80, 82, 100, 103, 107, 108, 112, 121, 123, 147, 152, 173, 176, 177, 206, 210, 230, 248, 249, 253, 255, 256, 262, 270, 289, 291, 292, 294, 295, 297, 304, 306, 322, 323, 328, 338, 339, 340, 364
Frédéricq, Léon 143, 189
Free University of Brussels (Université Libre de Bruxelles) 10, 18, 38, 81, 108, 118, 149, 153, 174, 178, 179, 182, 184, 185, 194, 221, 264, 305
French Revolution 172, 208, 234, 248, 289
Fund for Indigenous Well-Being (Fonds du bien-être indigene; FBEI) 118, 120

Garrett, Elizabeth 37
Gatti de Gamond, Isabelle 49
Geel colony (model of psychiatric care) 252–3, 271, 294–8, 362
genetics 85, 196, 365
genital mutilation 157
George, Lloyd 217
geriatric psychiatry 304
germ theory 254
Germany 2, 3, 14, 30, 70, 80, 104, 109, 173, 181, 182, 184, 185, 186, 189, 192, 194, 218, 224, 253, 293, 297, 322, 323, 328, 340, 367
Gezelle, Guido 329
Gluge, Gottlieb 181, 182, 184
Goffman, Erving 363
Gottstein, Adolf 153
Great Britain 2, 3, 33, 36, 43, 44, 45, 47, 49 51, 100, 107, 109, 116, 121, 152, 192, 206, 256, 270, 322, 330, 365

Index 379

Gregorian University (Rome) 83
Grotjahn, Alfred 153
Groupe d'Études pour une
 Réforme de la Médecine
 (GERM) 303
Groupe information asiles (GIA)
 303, 304
Grub, Geert 49, 50
Guido, Marie 40
Guinea 103
Guislain, Joseph 76, 249, 253,
 286, 362
gynaecology 6, 17, 40–2, 45, 82,
 156, 157, 255, 338

Haibe, Achille 144
Havelock Ellis, Henry 49
health insurance 4, 11, 73, 154,
 159, 206, 211, 213, 217
 219, 220, 224, 225, 229,
 231, 233, 369, 372, 374
Héger, Paul 143, 188
Heidelberg 143
Herman, Martin 144
Heyman, Jean-Julien 140–1
Hippocrates 366
homeopathy 180, 192
Hôpital Français (Berchem Ste-
 Agathe) 258
Horta, Victor 255
Hospital Brothers of St Vincent 68
Hospital Service of Our Lady of
 the Cross 78
Hubert, Eugène 82
human genome project 196
human immunodeficiency virus
 (HIV) 2, 157, 196
Humanae Vitae (1968) 51, 84, 85
humoral theories 322
Huntington's disease 337
Huysmans, Camille 217
hydropathy, 25 330
hydrotherapy 256, 322
hygiene 2, 3, 13, 100, 134, 139,
 145, 147–53, 158, 178, 247,
 257, 258, 265, 326–31,
 336, 336, 339, 340, 342,
 343, 345
Hygiene museum of Mons 327,
 329, 374
hygienism 17, 322, 326, 331
hypnosis 287
hysterectomy 42
hysteria 30, 31, 43, 44, 78, 80, 373

Illich, Ivan 363
influenza 107
in utero baptism 81
in vitro fertilisation (IVF) 85, 365
Institut des Sciences (Ghent)
 141, 143
Institut national de Géographie
 (Brussels) 147
Institute for Family and Sexuality
 Studies (Leuven) 84, 374
Institute for the Deaf and Blind
 (Bruges) 287, 290
Institute for the Deaf-Mute
 (Ghent) 300
Institute of Biology (Ghent) 189
Institute of Biology (Liège) 189
Institute of Cancer (Leuven) 65
Institute of Physiology (Liège) 189
Institute of Tropical Medicine
 (Antwerp) 155
International AIDS Society 156
International Centre for
 Reproductive Health
 157, 374
International Conferences of Social
 Work 152
International Federation of
 University Women 39
International Labour
 Organisation 152
iron lung 307
Italy 106, 184, 186, 340

Jacobs, Aletta 48
Jamot, Eugène 112

Janssen, Arthur 83–4
Janssens, Eugène 145
Janssens, Louis 85
Japan 253
Jaspar, Henri 108, 134
Jauniaux, Arthur 220
John XXIII (pope) 51, 84
Journal de Neurologie et d'Hypnologie 286
Journal Médical de Bruxelles 39

Kahn Museum 328
Kenya 156, 157
Kenyatta National Hospital (Nairobi) 156
Kerremans, Ilse 40
Keymolen, Denise 38
kidney disease 332
Koch, Robert 254
Kuborn, Hyacinthe 33

L'Equipe 298, 306, 374
La Famille Heureuse 50, 51
La Réforme 38
La technique sanitaire et municipale 135
Laman, Karl 99
Lanval, Marc 49, 50
Laqueur, Thomas 40
Laruelle, Léon 337, 341
Lateau, Louise 79, 80, 373
law on abortion (1990) 53, 87
law on hospitals, 'Custers' law' (1963) 231
law on medical practice (1818) 177
law on medical specialties (1957) 4, 45, 193
law on mutual societies (1851, new law in 1894) 211, 373
law on public assistance (1925) 221, 258
law on sickness and invalidity insurance, 'Leburton law' (1963) 4, 225–6, 374

Le Mouvement hygièniqe 144
Le Scalpel 13, 144, 330
League of Health Care Institutions (Verbond der Verzorgingsinstellingen) 72, 74
Leburton, Edmond 4, 226
Lefèbvre, Ferdinand 79
Lenssens, Jan 227
Leopold II (king) 72, 104, 105, 113, 123, 134, 147, 334, 361
Leopold III (king) 328
leprosy 73, 112, 115, 120, 148
Ley, Auguste 293
Lierneux 297, 315
Ligue nationale belge contre la tuberculose 334, 342, 344, 345
Ligue nationale belge d'hygiène mentale 305
Ligue patriotique contre l'Alcoolisme 146
Lister, Joseph 254
Little Sisters of the Assumption 307
Lovanium, Faculty of Medicine 121, 123
Lovenjoel Psychiatric Hospital 69, 76, 305
Löwy, Ilana 31
Lubumbashi hospital 119
Lumière (brothers) 341

Maertens, Guido 85–6
malaria 108, 148, 336
Malvoz, Ernest 144, 192
Mama Yemo hospital (Kinshasa) 156
Mangion, Carmen 263
Marcq, Léon 181
Mareska, Daniel 140–1
Marie Mineur 51
Marinescu, Gheorghe 337

Martin, Louis 146
Masarykova, Alice 152
Mascart, Louis 33
Mascaux, Fernand 47
M-Decree 302–3
Medical and Scientific Centre of the Free University of Brussels (Centre scientifique et médical de l'Université Libre de Bruxelles; CEMUBAC) 118
Medical Foundation of the University of Leuven (Fondation médicale de l'Université de Louvain; FOMULAC) 113, 118, 124
Medical Missionary Aid Society (1925) 83
Medical Society of Antwerp (Société de médecine d'Anvers) 139, 145
Medical Society of Ghent (Société de médecine de Gand) 139, 141
Medical Treatment Act (1850) 4, 14, 288
Medical Women's International Association (1919) 39
melancholy 44, 80
mental illness 13, 19, 43, 44, 68, 75, 76, 179, 183, 186, 252, 283–8, 291–5, 302, 309, 310, 312
Mercier, Joseph-Désiré 82, 83
miasma 248, 254
microbiology 110, 155
midwifery 32–7, 40, 48, 49, 109, 172, 360
migraine 15
Mont Thabor (Berg Thabor) 72
Montefiore Institute (Liège) 189
moral therapy 67, 75, 76, 252–3, 292
Mozambique 157
Müller, Johannes 182

Musée Consael 332
Museum Dupuytren (Paris) 329

Namèche, Alexandre 186–7
National Committee on Bioethics 86
National Institute for Health and Disability Insurance (INAMI/RIZIV) 224, 228, 230, 232, 374
National Joint Commission 230
National League Against Depopulation (Ligue nationale contre l'infécondité intentionnelle) 82
National Relief and Food Committee 218
Native Medical Services (Service d'Assistance Médicale Indigène; SAMI) 105, 107, 111, 112, 113, 122, 374
Ndgongala, Gaston Diomi 124
Neefs, Hans 156
neo-malthusianism 47, 48
Netherlands, the 35, 36, 51, 123, 152, 177, 184, 192, 206, 233, 288, 297, 329, 347, 365, 367
neurology 337, 341
Nolf, Pierre 192
nursing 34, 35, 37, 40, 49, 66, 70, 72, 109, 116, 191, 207, 210, 221, 227, 246, 248, 250, 262–7, 283, 292, 304, 308, 360, 373

obstetrics 4, 13, 33, 41, 45, 82, 157, 175, 177, 178, 188, 193, 198, 367, 372
Océan (l') (military hospital) 190, 264, 277
Office international d'hygiène publique 153
oncology 196

Onze-Lieve-Vrouw Hospital
    (Oudenaarde) 261
ophthalmology 179, 180, 183,
    187, 255
Order of Physicians (Orde der
    Geneesheren) 4
otorhinolaryngology 255
ovariotomy 41, 43, 373

Parent, Marie 146
Parkinson's disease 337
Partoes, Henri-François 249
Pasteur Institute (Brussels) 192
Pasteur Institute(s) (France) 123
Pasteur, Louis 123, 192, 254, 316
Pasteurian (bacteriological)
    revolution 143, 144, 256
Paul VI (pope) 51, 84
Pauli, Adolphe 251
Peers, Willy 51
Peeters, Ferdinand 51
People's Clinic (Ghent) 219
People's Movement for Families
    (Mouvement Populaire des
    Familles) 84
personal assistance budget 303,
    307, 308, 310, 374
pharmaceutical industries 196–7
pharmacy 15, 177, 207
physicians' strike (1964) 230
physiology 43, 178, 180,
    181, 189
Pinel, Philippe 75
Piot, Peter 155–7
Pirmez, Eudore 29, 30
Pius X (pope) 83
Pius XI (pope) 83
Pius XII (pope) 84
plague ('pesthuyskens') 207
Platform for Christian Ethics
    (Overlegplatform
    Christelijke Ethiek) 88
pneumonia 78
polio 15, 307

Popelin, Marie 47–8
Porter, Roy 5, 20, 370
Portugal 2
Prauscher Museum 328
pre-implantation genetic diagnosis
    (PGD) 88
pre-marital check-ups 150
Project SIDA 156
Prussia 177, 184
Psychiatric Institute of the Brothers
    of Charity (Ghent) 291
psychology 150, 171, 187, 285,
    306, 337
psychotherapy 306
public health film 14, 20, 323,
    335–45, 364, 374

Queen Elizabeth Funds for
    Native Medical Assistance
    (Fonds Reine Elisabeth
    pour l'assistance médicale
    indigene; FOREAMI) 111–4,
    118, 120, 124, 374

rabies 144
radiotherapy 71
Ratzka, Adolf 308
Red Cross 72, 152, 191, 326,
    328
Renaer, Marcel 85
Revue d'eugénique 151
Richmond, Mary 152
Roberts, Edward 307–8
Rockefeller Foundation 153,
    221, 264
Rodhain, Jérôme 110, 150
Rommelaere, Guillaume 188
Rops, Félicien 325–6, 333
Royal Academy of Medicine of
    Belgium (Académie royale
    de Médecine de Belgique) 4,
    10, 30, 33, 67, 81, 139, 173,
    179, 185, 191, 193, 194,
    360, 372

Royal Academy of Sciences, Letters and Fine Arts of Belgium (Académie royale des Sciences, des Lettres et des Beaux-Arts de Belgique) 79, 139
Royal Institute for the Belgian War-Blinded 301
Royal Society of Public Health (Société royale de Médecine publique) 144
Ruanda-Urundi 13, 17, 40, 99, 101, 103, 104, 106, 112, 121, 123, 124
Russia 30, 184
Ryspeert, Louise 290–1

Sabbe, Jan-Jan 308
Saint-Luc Médical 83
Sand, René 151–3, 158, 334, 340, 341
Sasz, Thomas 363
Saunier, Pierre-Yves 137, 142, 153
Sauveur, Maurice 286, 287
Schiebinger, Londa 31
Schockaert, Rufin 46, 47, 50, 82
School of Tropical Medicine (École de Médecine Tropicale) (Brussels) 73, 114, 148, 149
School of Tropical Medicine (Liverpool) 122, 134, 147
School of Tropical Medicine (London) 147
Schotsmans, Paul 85
Schulten, Hans 194–5
Schuster, August 134, 136
Schwann, Theodor 181, 182
Superior Health Council (Conseil supérieur de la Santé) 144, 249–50, 254, 256, 263–4, 266, 271
Séguin, Edouard 291
Seutin, Joseph 175
sexually transmitted diseases 157

shell shock 44
Sisters of Charity of Jesus and Mary 65–9, 372, 72, 262
Sisters of St Marie of Namur 106
Sisters of St Vincent de Paul (1818) 68, 72
sleeping sickness (human trypanosomiasis) 15, 105, 107, 109–12, 114, 115, 117, 122, 125, 134, 148, 150, 373
smallpox 125, 148
social security 4, 11, 18, 154, 206, 224, 226, 227, 228, 231, 233, 234, 267, 372
social work/service 152, 264, 285, 304, 306, 307
Socialist's Women Federation 50
Société (royale) belge d'Etudes coloniales 147, 149
Société Belge d'histoire des hôpitaux/Belgische vereniging voor de Geschiedenis van de Hospitalen 246
Société Huet 139
Société royale d'Histoire naturelle de Gand 139
Society of Medical and Natural Sciences of Brussels (Société des Sciences médicales et naturelles de Bruxelles) 139
Society of Saint-Luc (Belgian) 50, 67, 72, 83, 84, 374
Society of St Luc, St Cosmas and St Damian (French) 83
Solvay Institute in Brussels 189
South Africa 116
Southern Netherlands, the 32, 33, 68, 171, 172, 175, 248
Specola Museum (Florence) 333
Spillemaekers, Ghislena 300
Spitzner Museum 44, 328, 329, 330, 332, 347

Spring, Antoine Frédéric 181, 187
St Camille School (Brussels) 71, 373
St Dymphna 294
St Elizabeth Institute (Leuven) 66, 71
St-Elisabeth hospital (Antwerp) 221, 229
St-Jean Hospital (Brussels) 222, 244, 249, 250, 251, 252, 262
St-Pierre Hospital (Brussels) 181, 209, 221, 222, 260–2, 264, 267, 374
Stampar, Andrija 153
Stanley, Henry Morton 106
sterilisation 70, 84, 85, 150
Stopes, Mary 49
Storck, Henri 334, 340, 341, 342, 344, 374
Stuyvenberg Hospital (Antwerp) 221, 250, 267, 268, 373
Suenens, Leo Jozef 51, 74, 84
surgery 40, 41, 42, 45, 71, 115, 139, 174, 175, 177, 180, 186, 188, 190, 193, 195, 198, 207, 214, 220, 222, 255, 259, 264, 334, 337, 338, 367, 372
Sweden 116, 307, 308
Swedish Mission Society 106
Switzerland 37
syphilis 30, 139, 183, 260, 326, 336

Teleky, Ludwig 153
Temmerman, Marleen 155, 156, 157
Terwagne, Modeste 71
Tihon, André 69
Timmerman, Anna 287
Triest, Petrus-Joseph 69, 372
Trisca, Peter 150

tropical medicine 17, 73, 100, 107, 114, 116, 118, 122, 134, 147–50, 155
tuberculosis 15, 115, 118, 120, 144, 218, 334–6, 339, 342, 344, 345

Uganda 110, 134
Un ennemi public (film, 1937) 20, 334, 335, 340, 344, 345
Union of Belgian Colonial Women (L'Union Des Femmes Coloniales) 40
Union of the Associations of Freethinkers 74
Union of Women of the Belgian Congo and Ruanda-Urundi 40
United Kingdom 11, 14, 32, 147, 177, 184, 263, 264, 340, 365
United Kingdom of the Netherlands 1, 172, 289
United Nations 120, 156
United States 2, 29, 30, 32, 33, 36, 43, 66, 72, 83, 85, 116, 152, 192, 263, 264, 270, 294, 305, 307, 328, 336, 339, 340, 346
University of Ghent 39, 118, 139, 152, 156, 171, 178, 182, 184
University of Liège 118, 152, 178
urology 40, 255
Uytterhoeven, André 249

van Bogaert, Ludo 337
van Campenhout, Jean E. 150
van der Bracht, Irène 39
van Diest, Isala 37, 38, 39, 373
van Gehuchten, Arthur 337, 373
van Gehuchten, Paul 337
van Helmont, Jan Baptist 1

van Humbeeck, Pierre 143
van Meerbeeck, Pierre 182
van Rotterdam, Jean-Charles 177
van Vlasselaer, Isidore 301
van Wing 99
Vandenbroucke, Jozuë 194, 195
Vandevelde, Henry 266
Vatican 68, 80, 84, 86, 88, 113, 364
Vatican Council, Second 51, 74, 84, 87
venereal diseases 44, 140, 150, 260, 326, 329, 332, 333, 336, 339
Vermeersch, Arthur 83
Vermeylen, Jean 298
Virchow, Rudolf 366
virology 196
Vives, Juan Luis 288
Voisin, Félix 291
von Hagens, Gunther 326

Wauters, Joseph 219
White Fury (Witte Woede) 227

Windischmann, Karl 181
Work of the Calvary 71
World Health Organization (WHO) 138, 154, 156, 157, 193
World War I 12, 14, 38, 42, 44, 72, 105, 107, 113, 150, 152, 184, 190–2, 217, 221, 233–4, 264–6, 294, 297–301, 336, 338, 341
World War II 14, 36, 73, 84, 103, 104, 112, 116, 118, 120, 121, 123, 124, 126, 131, 154, 194, 197, 218, 224, 230, 231, 233, 234, 296, 297, 306, 364, 368, 369

x-ray 256, 264, 337, 341, 344

Yambuku 155
Yperman, Jan 1

Ziekenhuis Netwerk Antwerpen 232

EU authorised representative for GPSR:
Easy Access System Europe, Mustamäe tee 50,
10621 Tallinn, Estonia
gpsr.requests@easproject.com